OTHER BOOKS BY LEONARD STEVENS

The Elizabeth: Passage of a Queen (*1968*)

The Ill-Spoken Word (*1966*)

On Growing Older (*1964*)

Are You Listening? *with Dr. Ralph Nichols* (*1957*)

EXPLORERS
OF THE
BRAIN

EXPLORERS

OF THE

BRAIN

LEONARD A. STEVENS

ALFRED A. KNOPF, NEW YORK, 1971

TO APRIL, BROOKE, CARLA, SARA, AND TIM

ACKNOWLEDGMENTS

As I turned to the research for this book, the forbidding nature of the subject was soon evident in its breadth and complexity—and I needed help. The person who first drew my interest to the topic also kept me afloat for several months thereafter with encouragement and guidance. She is Mrs. Ruth Dudley, Information Officer of the National Institute of Neurological Diseases and Stroke (NINDS), Bethesda, Maryland. As I visited Bethesda on several occasions, Mrs. Dudley and the Institute's Director, Richard L. Masland (now at Columbia University), generously offered their counsel and arranged for meetings with scientists who would further my research. To Mrs. Dudley and Dr. Masland I am most appreciative for their interest, patience, encouragement, and faith in my efforts.

From Bethesda I went on to visit the offices and laboratories of some of the world's leading neuroscientists, from Paris to Los Angeles. Many others responded to my letters and provided reprints of their papers. To all of these people I extend my thanks for giving their time and assistance with the grace and patience I needed.

Those who personally spent time with me are as follows:

W. R. Adey, University of California at Los Angeles (UCLA); Maitland Baldwin, NINDS; Nicole Baumann,

Hospital of the Salpêtrière, Paris; Mary A. B. Brazier, UCLA; Kao Liang Chow, Stanford Medical Center; C. D. Clemente, UCLA; Kenneth S. Cole, NINDS and Marine Biological Laboratory, Woods Hole.

Also, Alfred Coulombre, NINDS; Paul H. Crandall, UCLA; José M. R. Delgado, Yale University; Raymond Escourolle, Hospital of the Salpêtrière, Paris; Derek Fender, California Institute of Technology; Karl Frank, NINDS; John D. French, UCLA.

Also, Edward Geller, UCLA; Ward C. Halstead, University of Chicago; A. van Harreveld, California Institute of Technology; John Hubbard, Northwestern University; David Krech, University of California at Berkeley; Lewis Lipkin, NINDS; Robert B. Livingston, University of California at San Diego.

Also, H. W. Magoun, UCLA; Frank Morrell, Stanford Medical Center; N. C. Myrianthopoulis, NINDS; Walter D. Obrist, Duke University; Karl H. Pribram, Stanford Medical Center; Antoine Rémond, Hospital of the Salpêtrière, Paris; J. P. Segundo, UCLA.

Also, Eric M. Shooter, Stanford Medical Center; Roger W. Sperry, California Institute of Technology; Arnold Starr, Stanford Medical Center; Sylvius Varon, Stanford Medical Center; Richard D. Walter, UCLA; C. A. G. Wiersma, California Institute of Technology; J. Z. Young, University College, London.

And Spyros Andreopoulos, Stanford Medical Center, and Al Hicks, UCLA, two information officers who spent many hours assisting me.

While visits to the above required considerable travel, the distance falls short of the total miles traveled between my home and New Haven, Connecticut, where I spent countless hours at the Yale Medical Library. Whenever possible I consulted the original scientific papers for the work discussed in this book. Yale's library stacks provided the opportunity and the Library's staff members kindly helped me use the voluminous material to the best advantage. I am grateful to the Yale Medical Library and all the people who make it such an excellent and efficient place for research.

Because this book covers many fields of neurology and much of the history of the science, few persons could be expected to verify all that is covered; therefore, I assume full responsibility for any errors herein. However, the manuscript was read by five well-qualified individuals who helped ensure the book's accuracy. They are: Alan K. Percy, Department of Neurology, The Johns Hopkins Hospital; Sue Friedman and Paul Scott, Department of Pharmacology, Yale University; and Philip Skehan and Paul Weatherly, Department of Biology, Yale University. I wish to thank all of them for their special efforts in behalf of this book.

Finally, my appreciation for many hours of careful and considerate work goes to Miss Ellen Moore, New Milford, Connecticut, who typed the manuscript.

Leonard A. Stevens

CONTENTS

ILLUSTRATIONS

HEMISPHERES

(RIGHT)   (LEFT)

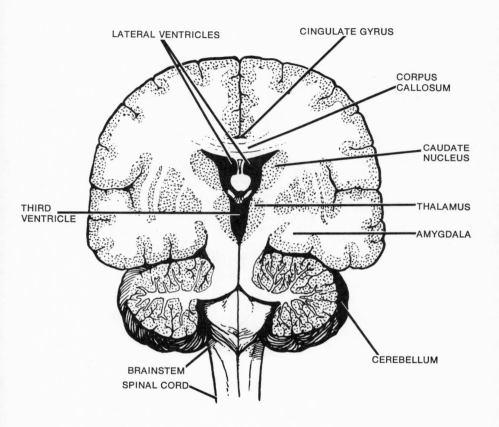

LATERAL VENTRICLES

CINGULATE GYRUS

CORPUS
CALLOSUM

CAUDATE
NUCLEUS

THIRD
VENTRICLE

THALAMUS

AMYGDALA

CEREBELLUM

BRAINSTEM
SPINAL CORD

*Both hemispheres of human brain shown by vertical section cutting
down across organ to the spinal cord.*

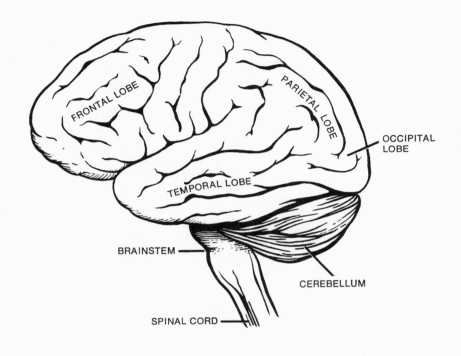

Left hemisphere of human brain showing cortex as viewed from the side.

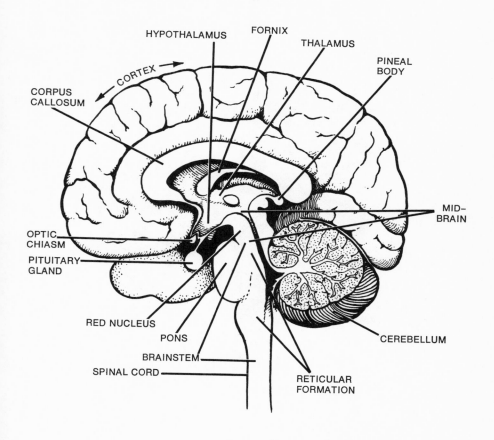

Vertical section of human brain cutting down between the two hemispheres and through brainstem and cerebellum.

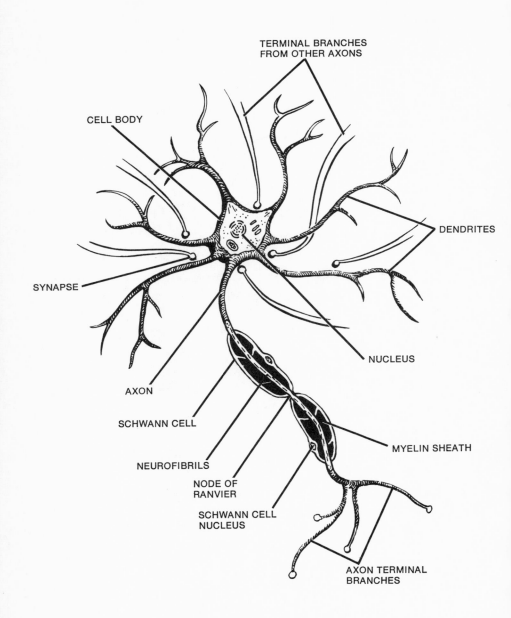

TERMINAL BRANCHES
FROM OTHER AXONS

CELL BODY

DENDRITES

SYNAPSE

NUCLEUS

AXON

SCHWANN CELL

NEUROFIBRILS

NODE OF
RANVIER

SCHWANN CELL
NUCLEUS

MYELIN SHEATH

AXON TERMINAL
BRANCHES

Highly schematic drawing of a nerve cell, with part of the body and axon cut away to reveal internal structures.

EXPLORERS
OF THE
BRAIN

1

THE MOST DIFFICULT LESSON

Soon after completing the world's first heart transplant, Christian Barnard declared that a brain transplant was unlikely in the near future, for the nature of tissue in the central nervous system (which includes the brain) made the operation virtually impossible. The renowned surgeon then added that one cannot really talk of transplanting a human brain, even if techniques were available, because the transfer of the organ could only be looked upon as providing it with a new body. The operation would therefore be a body transplant, not a brain transplant.

This semantic distinction pointed up the unique place of the nervous system among all other human parts. It represents the "thou" of the individual, while all else represents only biological functions. A surgeon might replace a person's heart, liver, bone, lung, and skin without altering his essential nature, but this would not hold for a change in brains. The recipient would be certain to see himself as the donor fitted out with a new body.

Christian Barnard's comment emphasized something few of us can easily accept, that the wet, gray, gelatinous mass of material called the brain is one and the same with our conscious selves. It is both mind and body, the most important organ in the living system. Its cells keep secrets that men have wanted to understand for thousands of years.

The physical exploration of the brain, which seeks to compromise these secrets by learning how the organ functions, may be history's ultimate scientific quest, for it concerns the most fundamental subject that man can take up, the physiological basis of the controls determining his life and thought. The search was well characterized more than three hundred years ago by Cervantes when he wrote, "Make it thy business to know thyself, which is the most difficult lesson in the world." To know the nervous system is the most difficult of all sciences. Its fantastic intricacy has always been an impenetrable bastion against the efforts of man's brain to fully understand man's brain, which is undoubtedly composed of the most complicated material in the universe.

For ages the organ was so little understood that it could only be regarded as a magic black box by most men. Analogies for the brain were always drawn from the most complicated things of the period. In ancient Greece and Rome, the system of brain and nerves was compared to the reservoirs, aqueducts, fountains, baths, and sewers of that age. When machines began to serve man, the brain was said to resemble the most complicated one at the time: the clock was once used as the analogy. Later, telephone systems, with their nerve-like lines feeding through brain-like switchboards, provided another model of the brain. In recent years, of course, the computer seemed like the perfect analogue of the brain; it's closer, but far from perfect. At the New York World's Fair in the mid-1960's thousands of visitors stopped at a display described by its sponsors as "a giant electrified model of the brain." It had thirty-eight miles of electrical wiring, and an "assemblage of humming motors, flashing electric lights [38,000 in all], huge aluminum discs, and tortuous metal tubes . . . ," according to a press release. Yet, the publicity writer admitted, "it only faintly resembles" the actual physical structure of the real brain—a statement that scarcely indicates how little the complexity of the model resembled that of the brain.

The difficult science of brain and nerve is by no means a new study, as people often assume. Some of the more important and exciting discoveries were made over a century ago with primitive instruments applied with unprecedented skill and patience. In recent years, entire institutes of experimenters with highly sophisticated instruments have found that mining knowledge of the nervous system grows harder and harder because the most difficult and revealing lessons are still to be learned.

The story of this exploration is among the more fascinating tales that science can offer. Many of the accomplishments have been remarkable in that they happened at all. The odds were always unusually high against investigators making headway in this incredibly complex field. Furthermore, their searches often seemed to trespass upon forbidden territory, where physical explanations were not welcomed for fear that they might undermine some of the most dearly held "truths" of mind and soul—so the explorers frequently found themselves accused of heresy and materialism of the worst kind. But when discoveries were made, their fundamentally important nature often brought great honors to the scientists, as shown by the fact that eighteen of them have won Nobel Prizes since the awards were first established in 1901.

The explorers seeking to explain the functions of brain and nerve have also learned much about the dysfunctions, but again the most difficult, trying problems remain. Above all, the tissue of the brain and spinal cord, the central nervous system, is unrepairable and irreplaceable. It can be punctured, cut, and mutilated without pain to the owner, but such physical damage does not heal, for the nerve cells, unlike other cells, do not reproduce. Therefore harm to the nervous system is irreversible unless undamaged areas of tissue take over the lost functions of the damaged parts. If, however, the failure is unrelieved, the victim may suffer in ways that strike at his very core, the "thou" of human life. Diseases and injuries affecting the nerves and brain can cripple and immobilize people. They can erase memories and destroy the ability to learn anew. Malfunctions of the nervous system can transform an individual of purpose and direction into one who has lost his will and way. They can steal his sight, block his hearing, or seal him within himself by shutting off the precious gift of speech. Such failings represent the worst of human calamities and by themselves provide more than enough reason to explore the nervous system. The problems include stroke, Parkinsonism, epilepsy, multiple sclerosis, mental retardation, head injury, and others.

Scientists have slowly undone many of the mysteries of the nervous system. The ethereal mind and soul have less and less room to hide within the brain, which previously could not be subjected to physical examination. It is no longer unreasonable to think of a surgeon's tools removing the "thou" of a man to fit it into a new body. And one can also imagine changing the "thou" of a body by altering the brain—perhaps with an injection that expands the mind and cleanses the soul. As men learn about the functioning of the nervous system it often forces them to change or question ancient dogma. Consider two examples:

For thousands of years people felt that the heartbeat and breath indicated the difference between life and death. Now, however, there are machines (resuscitators) that can restore the breath and reinstate the beat of a heart that has failed. In some instances, however, the patient may remain in a deep, irreversible coma, the result of brain damage. The person's conscious life, all that he knows and feels, is gone forever, although his heart may continue beating for years (twelve years in the case of a young man in Minnesota, the victim of an automobile accident). Such a fate is now called "brain death," and it can be ascertained electrically. It's the definition of the death suffered by the donor of a beating heart that is lifted from the person's breast and transplanted, still beating, into another individual. After the first heart transplants in the 1960's, many eminent doctors pressed for a change in the rules of death; among them was the Ad Hoc Committee of the Harvard Medical School to Examine the Definition of Brain Death. The recommendation to turn from the heart to the brain had an immediate impact in law, religion, philosophy, and on the minds of everyone who ever thought about the nature of death. It added emphasis to the growing realization that the brain, of all organs, plays the key role in matters most central to life.

For a second example, consider how men have assumed for centuries that one could be certain of his knowledge as long as he could make objective observations and judgments of the world. Assurance of this came from the seventeenth-century French philosopher, mathematician, and scientist René Descartes, whose ideas still exert a strong influence on our thinking. He believed that a man could see the world as it really is if he was able to divest himself of his passions. But modern neurological scientists (neuroscientists) are finding physical evidence of nervous action that weakens this axiom, and this evidence leads to serious questions about the validity of the view that has influenced civilization for three centuries. They are becoming aware of built-in distortions among electrochemical paths forming the neural circuits of our senses. Until these distortions can be more clearly defined and taken into account, how can the most dispassionate man know he is really objective?

The scientist who looks for the answers to such questions searches among the "neurons," the given name of nerve cells. The neuron, the basic building block of the nervous system, is probably the most interesting of all living cells. It is, on the one hand, an electrical unit that (in most cases) is either on or off, no in betweens, one that supplies its own current from a constantly available power potential. When it acts, the neuron conducts an electrical impulse, the "nerve impulse," outward along a fiber called an "axon." On the other hand, the neuron is a chemical unit, and when a nerve impulse is transmitted from one cell to another (or to a muscle or gland) the momentary transfer usually becomes a chemical rather than an electrical event. The chemical activity takes place at a complex junction, the "synapse," between the axon of the transmitting cell and the body or a "dendrite" of the receiving cell. A dendrite is one of several branches (besides the single axon) projecting from a cell body. What happens at the synapse determines the all-important communication between neurons.

With few exceptions, nerve cells, which come in many varieties, are microscopic, even though their ultra-slender axons may in some cases extend several feet. The minute dimensions are emphasized by the fact that the human brain contains ten to twelve billion neurons—all of which are packed in with and are far outnumbered by another type of cell, the "glia." Even a nerve running through the body consists of a bundle of nerve cell fibers, axons, and in a single nerve, which might be pictured as a trunkline, there may be 100,000 fibers, each the extension of a neuron.

All these cells, three or four times the number of persons on earth, somehow work in harmony to conduct the electrical-chemical business of an infinitely complex information and control system that decides what each human being is all about. Its most mysterious and remarkable capability is one blithely accepted by most of us: it can store an astonishing amount of information and recall it at will. The marvelous process of memory is seen in the man of eighty or ninety who relates the details of an experience from the age of six. One is awed by the reported case of a bricklayer who was able, under hypnosis, to describe every bump and grain in a brick that he had placed in a wall twenty years earlier. Scientists estimated several decades ago that in seventy years of life the human brain, only when awake, receives and possibly stores some fifteen trillion "bits" of information (a bit is the smallest single unit of information for a storage device, like a computer). But this is a meaningless statistic that can hardly describe the magical quality of memory, the functions of which we have barely started to comprehend, even though it is central to all human abilities.

In 1906 one of the most famous neurological scientists of all time, Charles S. Sherrington, an English physiologist, proposed that regardless of the nervous system's complexity, its functional foundations rest on two basic factors—and his theory has yet to be discounted.

First, he said, there are nerve cells whose fibrous projections transmit information.

Second, connections between nerve cells are the sites of decisions behind the transmittal of information.

This fundamental understanding of the nervous system came from momentous discoveries by the earliest pioneers of the neurological sciences, giants of their times, and their contributions guided other great explorers to discoveries that are still being made.

This is the story of explorers in search of a physiological reply to one of man's oldest puzzles: Who am I? How do I relate to the world around me? Or as Shakespeare wrote in *The Merchant of Venice*:

> *Tell me, where is fancy bred,*
> *Or in the heart, or in the head?*
> *How begot, how nourished?*
> *Reply, reply.*

2

FROM SPIRITS TO ELECTRICITY

One day in 1784 a Naples professor of anatomy, Domenico Cotugno, was dissecting a live mouse for a demonstration. As he carefully cut across the animal's stomach, the professor held the wiggling specimen upside down by grasping the skin of its back between a thumb and two fingers and clasping the tail between the last two fingers of the same hand.

"I had hardly cut through part of the skin of that region," said Cotugno in a letter dated October 2, 1784, "when the mouse vibrated his tail between the fingers, and was so violently agitated against the third finger, that to my great astonishment, I felt a shock through my left arm as far as the neck, attended with an internal tremor, a painful sensation in the muscles of the arm, and with such giddiness of the head, that being affrighted, I dropped the mouse. The stupor of the arm lasted upwards of a quarter of an hour, nor could I afterwards think of the accident without emotion. I had no idea that such an animal was electrical; but in this I had the positive proof of experience."

Whatever the origin, Cotugno's shock never proved mice are electrical, like certain fish that deliver shocks, but his experience caught the attention of leading scientists in the late eighteenth century, including Alessandro Volta. The phenomenon of "animal electricity" was in Europe's scientific air, and scientists were hoping to prove whether or not such electricity existed and, if so, what caused it. However, few accepted the report from Naples. It was concluded that Cotugno's shock came, not from the mouse, but from his own mind, which in those anticipatory times was ready and willing to perceive electricity in most any animal.

For the first time in more than fifteen hundred years, scientists of the eighteenth century were seriously questioning a theory of nerves and nervous systems that had been firmly fixed in medical minds by Galen, the physician of Greek parentage who lived from A.D. 130 to about 200. From his anatomical observations, Galen developed a surprisingly accurate understanding of underlying functions, enough so that he became known as the father of experimental physiology. His work, which included some basic descriptions of nervous system functions, was unrivaled in antiquity, and his teachings virtually stood as law in medicine for hundreds of years.

Before Galen's time the brain and nerves had been recognized, but as something of little consequence to a living organism. The Greek historian Herodotus (c. 484–425 B.C.) described how the early Egyptians, who thought of the brain as an inconsequential mass, removed the organ from the dead by scooping it out through the nostrils with a bent metal tool. They believed the heart and the liver were the seats of human emotions.

By 450 B.C. the significance of the brain had become more obvious. Plato claimed that its spherical shape made it the ideal residence for reason, which, along with desire and passion, formed the human soul. Some three decades later Hippocrates, in his observations of epileptic patients, came close to a modern description of the brain's function. The father of medicine said: "Man should be fully aware of the fact that it is from the brain and from the brain only that our feelings of joy, of pleasure, of laughing arise as well as our sorrow, our pain, our grief and our tears. We are thinking with the brain and we can see and hear and we are able to draw a distinction between ugliness and beauty, bad and good and what is pleasant and unpleasant."

In another hundred years particular parts of the nervous system were being recognized and studied. The Greek anatomist Herophilus accurately described the brain's four small chambers, the cerebral ventricles, and he believed that all bodily powers originated in these small spaces.

When Galen analyzed the nervous system, he concerned himself with its functions and correctly concluded that all nerves are divided into two pathways, one for the senses and one for physical actions (the two eventually became known as the sensory and motor pathways). Galen found evidence of these double functions in a patient, Pausania, who had injured his spine in a fall from a chariot. The sense of feeling was missing from Pausania's fingers, yet he could move them normally, which proved to the Greek physician that one pathway (motor) remained intact while the other (sensory) had been damaged. Galen experimentally supported the double-pathway theory by selectively cutting the longitudinal sections of an animal's spinal cords so as to interrupt one path or the other and to note the resulting sensory and motor disturbances.

But if nerves could be grouped into a double-track system, what traveled along the two pathways? In answer Galen offered a theory that was to survive some fifteen hundred years. He decided that the nervous system was a pneumatic network of hollow tubes conducting "animal spirits" from their point of origin, the cerebral ventricles, through the body's sensory and motor pathways. To explain how animal spirits were created and replenished, the Greek physician said that digested food was transferred from the human gut to the liver, where it was used to make "natural spirits." The liver passed the natural spirits to the right side of the heart for conversion to "vital spirits," which were pumped with arterial blood to the brain's ventricles and made into animal spirits.

For centuries Galen's was an amazingly durable theory, widely accepted and used by scientists and doctors. In the seventeenth century Thomas Willis, a London physician, noted that if blood was blocked from the brain, nerve functions ceased because vital spirits could not reach the ventricles for conversion into the essential animal spirits. Willis demonstrated how parts of the body could be paralyzed by ligating connecting nerves and interrupting the flow of animal spirits. In a paper written in 1671 he gave an involved but colorful summary of how animal spirits carried out their work.

"Therefore as to the Musculary Motion in general," he wrote, "we shall conclude after this manner, with a sufficiently probable conjecture, that the animal Spirits being brought from the Head by the passage of the Nerves to every Muscle (and as it is very likely), received from the membranaceous fibrils, are carried by their passage into the tendinous fibres, and there they are plentifully laid up as in fit Storehouses; which Spirits, as they are naturally nimble and elastick, where ever they may, and are permitted, expanding themselves, leap into the fleshy fibres; then the force being finished, presently sinking down, they slide back into the Tendons, and so vicissively . . ."

But as these words were set down in London, questions were arising about Galen's animal spirits. For one thing, men were having a new look at nerves with the compound microscope employed by Robert Hooke in 1665. While the magnification was limited by chromatic aberrations, it was still much more powerful than the simple glasses of the past, and it gave microscopists a fair view of the coarse nerves in animal and human limbs. But the new look only emphasized the complexity of the subject matter, and added little agreement as to what nerves were like. Certainly their apparent design did not always support the idea that they conducted ethereal animal spirits. A German, Martin Ledermüller, said that nearly three dozen empty tubes were packed in parallel to form a nerve fiber. Others agreed, but claimed the tubes were filled with something. One microscopist reported that it was a gelatinous fluid. Another saw globules lined up like the beads of a necklace strung within the tubes. A French scientist said the beads were stuck to the outside of tubes filled with a transparent fluid. Obviously the new microscope was misleading, and truer images of nerves would have to wait for the improved magnification of the achromatic microscope developed in the nineteenth century.

Actually the undermining of Galen's theory was most evident in the attacks by experimentalists who began questioning its veracity toward the end of the seventeenth century. The man credited with first denying the ancient theory was Francis Glisson, Regius Professor of Physic at Cambridge from 1636 until his death in 1677. In a paper published the year he died Glisson recommended an experiment which, he said, disproved the notion that animal spirits caused muscular contractions. It called for a glass tube, closed at one end and large enough for a "strong brawny man" to insert his full arm, which was then fixed in place with a watertight seal around the skin of the shoulder. An attached, upright funnel allowed the investigator to fill the sealed tube with water.

". . . pour through the funnel as much water as the glass can hold and allow some water to overflow into the funnel," Glisson instructed. "When this has been done, order the man now alternately to contract strongly, and now to relax, all his arm muscles. During contraction the water in the tube sinks, but during relaxation rises. Hence it is clear that muscles when taut or contracted, are not at that time inflated or swollen, but are on the contrary unswollen and actually diminished. For if they were swollen, the water would ascend higher in the glass and would not descend. Therefore one must conclude that the fibres are shortened by their own vital motion, and have no need of plentiful afflux of animal or vital spirits by which they might be inflated in order to be shortened and in order that their movements might obey the commands of the brain."

While Glisson's experiment appeared to disprove Galen's ideas on muscular movement, the Englishman replaced the ancient theory with a vague counter-proposal attributing the action to an intrinsic "irritability" of the involved tissue, although its connection with the brain was never clear to the Cambridge professor. Largely meaningless, the word "irritability" remained in use by a number of authorities for a century or so.

In Italy one of Glisson's contemporaries also had doubts about animal spirits. Giovanni Alfonso Borelli of Naples was an experimenter with wide interests. On the one hand he designed a submarine to be rowed around the bottom of the sea; on the other, he was interested in the way nerves and muscles related to the mechanics of man. He questioned the theory that ethereal animal spirits actuated muscle, and he devised an experiment to check his doubts. Borelli submerged the limb of a laboratory animal and cut into a muscle to see if bubbles would rise from the wound. There being none, the Italian experimenter decided that the nerves did not carry gaseous spirits. He then adopted the comparatively new "fermentation" theory that had already been set forth by William Croone, the English physiologist. It still involved spirits, but replaced much of their magical qualities with a somewhat scientifically explained process.

Croone proposed that "if faith may be placed in the eyes," nerves carried, not a gas, but a liquid, a "very rich and spiritous juice which is drawn all through the nerves in a constant circuit. . . ." Upon a command from the brain, "some impulses" sent droplets of these into the muscles, and when they mixed with spirits of the blood, there occurred "continuously a great agitation of all the spiritous particles which are present in the vital juices of the whole muscle, as when spirit of wine is mixed with the spirit of human blood." The agitation, confined within the muscle, caused it to swell, and "no sooner does [it] begin to swell at its boundaries than are fibres also contracted, and so everything occurs at one and the same time in the twinkling of an eye."

Around 1713 a third theory joined the fermentation and irritability theories. Sir Isaac Newton, a man of many scientific ideas, proposed that Galen's animal spirits were really ethereal vibrations conducted from the brain via the nerves to muscles, where they motivated mechanical action. For a time Newton's idea was widely accepted by English physiologists.

As the eighteenth century began, however, increasing numbers of scientists and physicians were attracted by still another theory, which developed from a general interest in "animal electricity." The theory proposed that an electric fluid conducted animal spirits over the nerves from the brain to muscles. The will of the mind, said the theory, controlled the flow of the electric fluid. The idea gained support from some of the century's most fascinating inventions and experiments.

An "electric influence machine" that generated static electricity with friction had been available to scientists from the late 1600's, and in 1745 they acquired the Leyden jar, which could store static electricity. With these inventions it was discovered that a static charge applied to living organisms caused violent contractions of skeletal muscles. In humans, a shock quickened the pulse and increased glandular activity. Indeed, physicians began using electricity as a stimulant. They assumed it benefited the human system because it stirred up and released animal spirits.

The effect of electrical phenomena upon living organisms led eighteenth-century scientists to a number of electrical experiments with animals and humans. The Englishman Stephen Gray, who discovered that a static charge could be transferred from one body to another, described an unusual experiment he did in 1730. His subject was a forty-seven-pound-ten-ounce boy suspended horizontally above the ground by two "hairlines such as cloaths are dried on." A flint-glass tube was held near the subject's feet while a leaf-brass electroscope (a device for detecting a static charge) was placed near the boy's nose. As the tube was charged by rubbing with a cloth, the electroscope was deflected with "much vigour" by the youngster's nose. The Frenchman Jean Antoine Nollet performed the experiment before members of the court of Louis XV and amused the audience as he ended the demonstration by drawing a crackling blue spark from the poor boy's nose.

Though provocative, such electrical experiments added little to an understanding of the nervous system. If the system were electrical, a living organism obviously had to have an intrinsic electricity, of which no evidence existed, except for some possible indications in certain kinds of fish, notably the torpedo.

From antiquity it had been recognized that a torpedo could deliver an unpleasant sensation to the person who touched it. This was described by Galen, Aristotle, and Pliny. Roman physicians treating gout prescribed that the patient stand on the fish until its mysterious power subsided. In an Abyssinian treatment for fever, the patient was bound to a table while a torpedo was repeatedly touched to his body until the temperature dropped. But no one could explain the sensation peculiar to the fish. In 1678 an experimenter in Florence inspected a dissected torpedo and suggested that it had an abundance of corpuscles which "enter into his hand who toucheth it." "These Corpuscles or *Effluviums*," he continued, "do not come thence from themselves, but they are driven, and as it were darted forth. . . ." A French scientist postulated that when a torpedo was touched, its muscles were rapidly contracted and abruptly released to deliver a sharp, mechanical blow to the victim. One writer decided that the torpedo's power was comparable to lightning. He was on the right track, but could hardly know for sure, since his observation came nearly a half century before Benjamin Franklin proved that lightning was electricity.

For some time Europeans puzzling over the torpedo failed to notice that a similar fish had been reported from South America in 1671 and again in 1745. Finally in 1755 the second report was seen by a Dutch physicist, who wrote for details from his friend Willem Gravesande, governor of Essequibo, a Dutch colony in South America. The governor replied that the fish was the *sidder-vis*, which in Dutch meant "tremble fish." Gravesande, who was knowledgeable about electricity and the new Leyden jar, remarked that the effect of the fish appeared to be electric.

The governor had touched upon the truth, but it took several years to prove. Subsequently some experimental attempts to understand the tremble fish (eventually known as the electric eel) were reported in two natural histories of South America. One told of how the writer and fourteen servants joined hands to make an open loop, and the two end people simultaneously touched a tremble fish. A sensation was transmitted from person to person like an electric shock, the author reported. In "An Essay on the Natural History of Guiana," an English doctor named Bancroft pointed out that "when it [the fish] is touched either by the naked hand, or by a rod of iron, gold, silver, copper, etc., held in the hand, or by a stick of some particular kinds of heavy American wood, it communicates a shock so perfectly resembling that of electricity, which is commonly so violent that but few are willing to suffer a second time."

Bancroft's essay was read in England by a member of Parliament, John Walsh, who decided to try a similar experiment with the torpedo on the Île de Ré near La Rochelle, France, where the fish were plentiful. In the summer of 1772 Walsh conducted his investigations, which he reported in letters to Benjamin Franklin. In one test a torpedo was placed on its side upon a damp cloth spread over a table. The underside of the fish was connected to a thirteen-foot brass wire suspended from the ceiling by silk cords; the wire led to the first of five water-filled basins on a second table. From the last of the five vessels another suspended wire led back around the room to a point just above the fish. Four people stood beside the basins, each with his hands immersed in two of the dishes so as to form a human link between them. Walsh then touched the torpedo's top side with the wire from the fifth basin, and all the participants "felt a commotion which differed in nothing from that of the Leyden experiment, except in the degree of force." A similar test was made with two people placing their hands in three basins while a third subject made a separate and independent contact with both sides of the fish. In this case Walsh reported that all three persons felt the shock simultaneously. It was evidently electricity generated by the fish. Walsh and his subjects noted that the torpedo's eyes were momentarily depressed as the electricity was delivered. The experimenter decided that this proved the shock was released through the exertion of the fish's will.

Walsh's work with the torpedo brought him the coveted Copley Medal from the Royal Society of London for Improving Natural Knowledge. However, his continuing investigations were soon questioned by members of the Royal Society, who decided he really couldn't prove that the torpedo produced electricity. They cited a second experiment in which Walsh tried to make the torpedo's electricity jump a small spark gap. He made a series circuit of the fish, wire, people, and a strip of tinfoil pasted to sealing wax. The human subjects experienced the shock as usual, but when Walsh separated the tinfoil with a fine slit cut by a penknife, the sensation ceased, for the electricity failed to jump the tiny gap, as it would when delivered by a Leyden jar. The critics thus decided that the fish was not producing electricity. Walsh adhered to his theory, and the debate continued for months while a number of experiments appeared both to prove and to disprove his conclusions.

The greatest support for the electrical theory came in 1776, when the renowned scientist Henry Cavendish published a paper entitled "An Account of Some Attempts to Imitate the Effects of the Torpedo by Electricity." Supporting Walsh's contention, Cavendish described how he had constructed a model torpedo of wood, sheepskin, glass, and metal, and electrically excited it with forty-nine Leyden jars. It acted much like the real torpedo, he reported. It could even perform in the fish's natural habitat (torpedoes bury themselves in wet sand along a beach—woe to the barefoot walker). Cavendish planted his charged model on a beach and tested it with his hand, receiving the electrical shock through wet leather. He also revealed that the model's charge, like that of the real fish, appeared incapable of jumping a tinfoil gap. Cavendish concluded that "there seems nothing in the phenomenon of the torpedo at all incompatible with electricity."

Walsh, however, finally and conclusively proved that the real fish was electrical, and he did so with a tinfoil gap. He carefully made an extremely narrow opening in the foil and then conducted his old experiment in a dark room. When a human subject in the same circuit with the fish and foil felt the usual sensation, Walsh could see a tiny spark jump the gap.

The Englishman asked a fellow scientist, John Hunter, to make an anatomical investigation of the male and female torpedo. Hunter's dissections revealed that the parts which issued the electric shock were related to the fish's nervous system. No other organs, including those for seeing, hearing, smelling, and tasting, were so heavily supplied with nerves as were those producing the shock. Hunter surmised that the torpedo's nervous system was ". . . subservient to the formation, collection or management of the electric fluid: especially as it appears evident, from Mr. Walsh's experiments, that the will of the animal does absolutely control the electric power of its body; which must depend on the energy of the nerves." Hunter concluded: "How far this may be connected with the power of the nerves in general, or how far it may lead to an explanation of their operations, time and future discoveries alone can fully determine."

The time and the discoveries were at hand. Toward the final quarter of the eighteenth century, the possible connection of animal electricity with nerves was a leading subject in science. It was at this time that Professor Cotugno of Naples thought he had been shocked by a laboratory mouse. But far more important, the subject had caught the interest of another Italian professor in Bologna, Luigi Galvani, whose work with animal electricity was to make one of history's most significant contributions toward the understanding of how a nerve functions.

Galvani first used an electric influence machine to experiment with frog muscles. As the machine was cranked and sparks flew from its parts, the Italian found that a frog's muscles, not connected with the machine and even located across his laboratory, would contract if simply touched with a metal scalpel held by an assistant. Wiring a frog directly to the machine, Galvani found the muscles would contract in unison with the intermittent production of electricity. He put the machine and frog in separate rooms and connected them with a long wire. The results were the same, but he noted that the longer the connecting wire the weaker the muscular response.

The Bologna experiments took an interesting but dangerous turn when Galvani used the atmospheric effects of natural lightning as his electrical source. He had heard of Benjamin Franklin's famous kite experiments in America, and of Thomas Dalibard, a Paris botanist who had collected atmospheric electricity with a forty-foot iron rod. Galvani had not read, or had ignored, later reports of how lightning had killed other investigators in similar experiments. He strung a wire (like today's radio antenna) across the roof of his father-in-law's Bologna home and led it to a downstairs laboratory. When lightning flashed over the city and generally charged the air, the muscles of Galvani's frogs responded to the small amount of electricity arriving over the wire. Indeed, the experiment worked even when only a dark cloud passed overhead. Good luck prevented a direct enough strike of the lightning from incinerating the frogs, Galvani, and his father-in-law's house. It could have drastically changed the history of nerves, electricity, and science in general.

Galvani is best remembered for a discovery he made in 1786, one that had apparently been made over 100 years earlier. A Dutch naturalist, Jan Swammerdam, had shown the grand duke of Tuscany an experiment that was possibly the first ever conducted in electrophysiology. Swammerdam had wrapped a frog's leg in silver wire and mounted it on a copper support. When the loose end of the wire was touched back upon the copper, the frog's muscles contracted. Swammerdam hardly could have attributed his results to electrical phenomena because electricity was a mystery at the time. It was a different matter at the time Galvani accidentally encountered similar results when he went out onto his parapet one evening while conducting an experiment that required hanging frogs on an iron railing.

"So on an evening at the beginning of September," wrote Galvani, "we set up frogs prepared in the usual way, piercing each spinal medulla with an iron hook and hanging them in a horizontal line above the parapet. If the hook touched the iron railing, behold, there were spontaneous single contractions in the frogs, quite frequently. If one used a finger to push the hook against the surface of the iron, the quiescent muscles were excited, as often as the push was given."

Here Galvani had made one of the greatest accidental discoveries in the history of science, but only after many years and a famous debate was the relationship between the contractions, the hooks, and the railing understood. For the next five years Galvani conducted many such experiments to produce contractions in frogs' muscles. Most were done in his laboratory, where an iron plate took the place of the railing. Originally his hooks and the railing had been iron and the contractions had been very small. Later he discovered that the results could be more "vehement" when the metal of the hooks differed from that of the railing. He then designed "arcs," bent rods made by joining two different metals, and they served in place of both the hooks and railing. Galvani found that silver and iron produced a relatively strong reaction in the frog. And he demonstrated that non-conductors of electricity—glass, stone, or wood—did not work in place of the metal for either the hooks or the railing.

Galvani's many experiments were published in 1791 in his famous book, *De Viribus Electricitatis in Motu Musculari Commentarius*. In it he proposed that an inherent electricity existed in the frog itself—and supposedly in all other living organisms. In reference to the frog's muscular contractions, Galvani wrote: "Naturally such a result evoked no little wonderment within us and began to give rise to a suspicion that electricity was inherent in the animal itself. Both of these were increased by the flow, so to speak, of a very fine nerve fluid from the nerves to the muscles, which we noticed took place during the phenomenon, in the same way as the electric fluid is set free in a Leyden jar."

Galvani apparently assumed that the brain was the source of an animal's inherent electricity and that it was distributed by the nervous system. At the nerves' extremities, he decided, the electricity was transferred to muscle fibers, each of which acted as a tiny Leyden jar, condensing and storing the electricity. The fibers, as would a Leyden jar, discharged through the metal hooks as they contacted another metal (the railing).

The most important reaction to Galvani's "Commentary" came from Alessandro Volta, the Italian physicist, who at first greeted the findings with great acclaim but then turned upon them as false. In the first instance, he wrote:

"The treatise which appeared a few months ago concerning the action of electricity on the movement of muscles, written by Signor A. Galvani, member of the Institute of Bologna and Professor of the University of that place, who has already distinguished himself by other anatomical and physiological discoveries, contains one of those great and brilliant discoveries which deserves to mark a new era in the annals of physics and medicine.

"The existence of a real and inherent animal electricity which arises of itself in the living organs without extraneous assistance . . . which is associated with all animals with either cold or warm blood, which has its origin in the organism itself, which is preserved and continues in the dissected limbs so long as some vitality is there, the play and movement of which takes place primarily between nerves and muscles; it is that which is proved and described at length in the third part of the work of Signor Galvani to the extent of certainty through many well ordered and accurately described experiments."

Volta must have regretted these words, for he soon changed his mind. He decided that the current did not come from the frog, but was generated by the contact of the two metals in the hook and the railing. Galvani stood by his theory of self-contained animal electricity. The difference in opinion led to a famous debate, with many scientists choosing sides in support of either Galvani or Volta. Oddly enough, both men were both right and wrong at the same time.

In questioning Galvani's work, Volta recalled a 1761 report made by Johann Georg Sulzer to the Berlin Academy of Science describing a sensation experienced when two metal strips (one lead, one silver) were touched to the tongue. The strips, said Sulzer, had been held to form a "V." The two open ends of the "V" had been in contact with the tongue while the pointed end had been joined outside the mouth. As the strips had come together, Sulzer had tasted something like ferric sulphate. When the contact was broken, the taste had disappeared. Volta successfully repeated the experiment using the same two types of metals found in Galvani's bimetallic arcs. It not only produced the taste in Volta's mouth, but also made him see flashing lights. He decided that the joining of disparate metals generated electricity which produced the taste and the lights. This was when he changed his mind and turned his praise of Galvani's findings to severe criticism. He even dropped the term "animal electricity" from his writings. Torpedoes might be electric, said Volta, but Galvani's frogs were not. They were simply acting as sensitive electrometers that detected the tiny currents generated by the contact of disparate metals. From 1793 to 1880 Volta published many papers supporting his theory of "bimetallic electricity" and often attacking his fellow countryman.

Galvani refused to debate Volta publicly. Not only was he shy, but also all of his life he had intensely disliked public controversy. Volta's charges, however, were answered. The silent man in Bologna had several avid defenders. The most vigorous and persistent was Galvani's nephew, Giovanni Aldini, who was probably guided, at least in the beginning, by his uncle. Actually, Aldini practically made a lifelong career of defending Galvani. He became so emotionally involved with the mission that his judgment and reliability were questioned.

The most important support for Galvani's claim of having discovered intrinsic animal electricity was anonymously written and published as a scientific paper followed by a supplement. It was thought to have come from Galvani's pen, or from a joint effort between him and Aldini. The mysterious paper reported an experiment that seemed definitely to prove the case for animal electricity. The experimenter told of baring the muscle of a frog, touching the open area with the loose end of the animal's spinal cord, and observing a contraction of the muscle. A contraction was also obtained, the paper stated, when an exposed muscle was drawn up so as to touch an exposed nerve. Here the experimenter was apparently dealing with what became known as the "current of injury," and it was good evidence of an intrinsic animal electricity.

Meanwhile Galvani apparently did not abandon his original idea that his hooks released animal electricity. He died in 1798, before his theory was conclusively proven wrong by Volta. In 1800 the physicist invented the Voltaic pile, the first battery, with discs of different metals separated by pads moistened in acid. The invention proved that the disparate metals in Galvani's experiments had been the electrical source for the frogs' muscular contractions. Thus Galvani had accidentally opened the way for one of the greatest discoveries of all time, but not the one he had in mind as he went to his grave.

Discussions assessing the Volta–Galvani contributions have been carried into modern times. Many agree that Volta was the greater scientist of the two. While Galvani's accidental discovery of muscular stimulation led him to a hasty, false conclusion, Volta eventually arrived closer to the truth through experimentation, and in the process he provided one of the greatest of all inventions, the electric battery. Galvani did not stand on such firm scientific ground. He revealed that in addition to certain fish all animals exhibit an intrinsic electricity, but he neither described nor measured the electricity—which left him unable to say conclusively that it was electricity he had uncovered. However, the professor of Bologna unquestionably made a major contribution, one that led others to open up the new science of electrophysiology.

At the turn of the nineteenth century, then, Galen's theory of the nervous system was fading, although his animal spirits were not easily unseated, having been firmly in charge of the neurological sciences for many centuries.

3

THE DETECTION OF
IMPULSES AND WAVES

Although Galvani claimed that electricity was the nerve power, prompt and firm scientific proof was impossible for lack of instruments capable of detecting or measuring extremely small currents. The first break came in 1820 with another accidental discovery, this time at the University of Copenhagen, where Hans Christian Oersted, conducting a classroom experiment, found that a compass needle was affected by a current-carrying wire. He noted that when the compass was near the wire, the needle turned and stopped at a right angle to the flow of electricity. His report of the discovery soon led Johann Schweigger, a professor of physics and chemistry at Halle, Germany, to develop what became known as a galvanometer, galvanoscope, or multiplier. It consisted of a wire and coil on a frame around a suspended compass needle. While it could detect electrical currents, it was extremely insensitive, since the earth's magnetism was a drag upon the needle's action. The instrument was far from good enough to detect the tiny amounts of electricity in nerves.

Five years later the device was improved by Leopoldo Nobili, professor of physics at Florence. Nobili countered the earth's effect by suspending two needles on a common thread so their polarities canceled the pull of natural magnetism. It was a major improvement; even so, it required the large part of a minute to react fully—still far too sluggish for nerve currents.

The handicap, however, did not deter investigators from detecting animal electricity—or so they thought. One even believed he was picking up electricity from apples, pears, peaches, plums, and apricots. In some instances Nobili's galvanometer responded to "frog currents" that appeared to flow from the frog's leg muscles toward its spinal cord. In 1830 an experimenter, identified only as David, reported on galvanometer readings he claimed to have obtained from fine brass wires inserted in the nerves of rabbits and hens. He tapped a rabbit's sciatic nerve that had been withdrawn from the animal and spread on a glass surface. Whenever the creature struggled, David's instrument deflected. In addition, a French investigator, Alfred Donne, reported that one galvanometer electrode placed on his tongue and the other somewhere on his skin caused a violent deflection of the needle. Donne is the man who thought he had discovered electricity in fruit. As the results might indicate, these experiments were not dealing with the true electrical activity of the nervous system. They were more likely detecting currents generated by clinical differences between the galvanometer probes and whatever they touched—as some scientists of the time recognized.

Toward the middle of the nineteenth century no one could say with assurance that nerves were electrical. For example, the English scientist Michael Faraday felt that nerve force might be electricity, but he would not firmly commit himself. Instruments were still too insensitive to verify the truth of the matter.

At this time, a well-known Italian physicist, Carlo Matteucci, was struggling under the technical handicaps to define and measure what Galvani had inconclusively decided was electricity. In the 1840's Matteucci made a "galvanoscopic frog," consisting of a glass container enclosing a special preparation of a frog's muscle and nerve. When the device was contacted by the exposed nerve of a live frog or other animal, the galvanoscopic frog muscle contracted. Matteucci also developed a "frog battery," designed like a Voltaic pile, but with the thighs of several frogs substituting for metal plates. When galvanometer leads were connected to the frog-thigh pile, the instrument detected electricity, and when the thighs were wet with sulphuric acid, the reading increased. The intrepid Matteucci obtained like results from similar piles of muscles from eels and pigeons. But such efforts proved little about the true electrical nature of nerves.

Matteucci and another scientist, François Longet, obtained one of the most sensitive galvanometers of the time, constructed by a renowned Paris instrument maker, Heinrich Ruhmkorff, and they attempted to measure electricity in the sciatic nerve of a horse, where they assumed the current would be greater because of the animal's size. It didn't work. Matteucci also tried unsuccessfully to measure the electricity in a torpedo, which he clamped between two metal plates, each connected to one side of a narrow spark gap made from two metal balls. When the plates were pressed in upon the torpedo, Matteucci observed (in a dark room) that a spark jumped the gap, but his galvanometer failed to respond when connected to the same circuit.

While he never quite succeeded in explaining the nerve force scientifically, young scientists who would succeed were emerging. The most important were students of a single teacher, Johannes Peter Müller, the founder of scientific medicine in Germany and a giant in the history of physiology. In the first half of the nineteenth century Müller made many contributions to different fields of biological thought, particularly with regard to the nervous system. In a famous textbook published in 1826 he revealed the depth of his insight when he pointed out that sensory nerves, while all appearing to work exactly alike, are actually different, depending on the senses to which they connect.

". . . in one," he said, "the sensation of light is produced; in another, that of sound; in another, taste; while in a fourth, pain and the sensation of a shock are felt. Mechanical irritation excites in one nerve a luminous spectrum; in another a humming sound; in a third, pain. . . . A consideration of such facts could not but lead to the inference . . . that the nerves of the senses are not mere passive conductors, but that each peculiar nerve of sense has special powers or qualities which the exciting causes merely manifest."

Two of Müller's students dramatically advanced the neurological sciences from the point arrived at by Galvani. They were Emil du Bois-Reymond and Hermann von Helmholtz.

Du Bois-Reymond, a young German scientist of Huguenot stock, was so incensed by Matteucci's perplexing, contradictory efforts that he openly attacked them and was consequently motivated to attempt the detection of electrical nerve force himself. He recognized that the Italian was often led astray by the extraneous currents arising from chemical dissimilarities involved when metallic electrodes touched the subject material. To overcome this effect du Bois-Reymond developed a set of "non-polarizable electrodes" to eliminate the extraneous currents. Then he made a special "multiplicator for nerve currents," or "nerve galvanometer." It was conventional except that the moving parts were exceptionally light, and the wire windings were drawn much finer (0.15 millimeter diameter) than was ordinary. The fineness allowed the scientist to use a single strand of wire a mile and a quarter long, double the length found in previous models. This instrument, with non-polarizable electrodes, was fully capable of confining itself to and measuring the minute electrical forces within a nerve. At long last du Bois-Reymond finally settled the basic question of the nature of the nerve force.

In his memorable experiments, conducted around 1850, the German physiologist attached his galvanometer electrodes to the peripheral nerve of a laboratory animal, one lead to an intact section and the other a short distance away on the cut end of the nerve. The sensitive device then showed him that electricity was flowing from the intact part of the nerve through the instrument to the injured end. But, most remarkable, du Bois-Reymond found that when the nerve was stimulated somewhere along its length (by a small electric shock or a light physical tap), waves of electrical change moved along the nerve away from the stimulus in both directions. It was evident as a wave passed the electrode on the intact section of nerve, for the current abruptly reversed directions through the galvanometer. For a moment it flowed from the injury to the intact part of the nerve. This indicated that during that moment the electrical potential at the electrode shifted from positive to negative back to positive. Du Bois-Reymond called the phenomenon "negative variation." Actually he had discovered the nerve impulse, a basic characteristic of the electrical activity of the nervous system.

Du Bois-Reymond recognized that his accomplishments were considerable, and he wrote: "If I do not greatly deceive myself, I have succeeded in realizing in full actuality (albeit under a slightly different aspect) the hundred years' dream of physicists and physiologists, to wit, the identification of the nervous principle with electricity."

As more sensitive galvanometers were developed, du Bois-Reymond's basic work was confirmed. Galen's animal spirits were finally and unquestionably revealed to be electricity.

Hermann von Helmholtz, the other Müller student, was a close friend of du Bois-Reymond. He is most noted for his part in developing the concept of the conservation of energy, but he was also a major contributor to the science of the nervous system. As du Bois-Reymond reported his famous work, Helmholtz attempted to measure the speed of a nerve impulse through animal and man.

At the time it was easy to conclude that nerves were like

the wires of the recently invented telegraph, and that messages to various sensory and motor functions coursed through the body at a speed comparable to that of wire-borne electricity, which was not definitely known but was apparently as fast as lightning. Before Helmholtz the rate of nervous action had been estimated at various velocities, all very high. The Swiss scientist Albrecht von Haller had

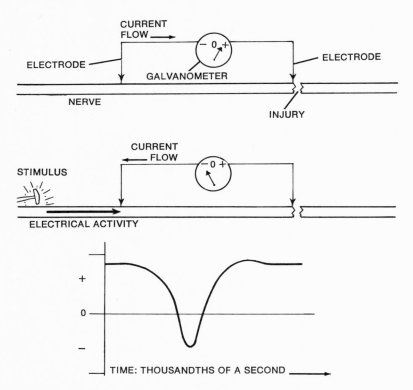

Negative variation seen by du Bois-Reymond. Top: With electrodes placed on both intact and injured sections of nerve, current flows through wire and galvanometer from left to right. Middle: Stimulation of nerve causes wave of electrical activity which momentarily reverses flow between electrodes. Bottom: Curve of electrical values (positive + and negative —) plotted against time indicates negative variation immediately following stimulation.

said in the eighteenth century that nerve messages move 9,000 feet a minute. Another estimate set the velocity at 57,600,000,000 feet per second. In 1833 Müller claimed that the whole question was academic, for in truth (he assumed) the high speed of nervous activity would be impossible to measure over the short distances in a living organism.

The high estimates, along with Müller's assumption, were all proven wrong in 1850 when Helmholtz succeeded in measuring the speed of the nerve impulse with a comparatively simple technique. He found that by stimulating a frog's nerve at successive points away from the related muscle he could discern differences in the time it took for the muscle to contract. Moreover, he recognized that the time differences were great enough to measure, which allowed him to figure out the velocity of the nerve impulse. As compared to earlier estimates, Helmholtz established, the speed was surprisingly slow, only twenty-five to forty meters per second. Helmholtz then tested a human subject with a primitive instrument that recorded the contraction and relaxation of muscles, and he discovered the nerve impulse moved at some thirty-five meters per second. Helmholtz's experiments, though simple, were sound, and when repeated by others, they produced the same results.

The findings of Müller's two students were major contributions to nerve physiology, but in combination they created a vexing new puzzle for scientists. Du Bois-Reymond's proof that nerves were electrical seemed to establish that the nervous system was comparable to the high-speed, message-flashing telegraph. But Helmholtz quickly upset the comparison in proving that nerve messages move at a minor fraction of the speed of telegraphic messages. How did this electrical system work?

Again the answer was dependent on technological advance. And the question was so basic that it had a very long wait for a full answer, since it required an understanding of the minute electrical and chemical activities of the nervous system. It had to wait until twentieth-century technical apparatus was available.

While Matteucci, du Bois-Reymond, and Helmholtz were unveiling the secret of the nerve force, the brain remained a deep mystery. To most physicians and physiologists it was a complex, unfathomable organ, a "black box" that magically controlled the senses and physical actions of animals and men. The brain's complexity was so impossible to compre-hend that it was accepted as a sacred unit, not to be tampered with for fear of disturbing its magical forces. This attitude is reflected in a strange tale that came from Cavendish, Vermont, in 1848.

On September 13 of that year a twenty-five-year-old construction foreman, Phineas Gage, employed by the Rutland and Burlington Railroad, was preparing a blast hole when the powder accidentally exploded and propelled an iron tamping rod skyward so that it passed completely through the man's head. The rod—13¼ pounds, 3½ feet long, and 1¼ inches in diameter—entered Gage's left cheek and emerged from the front right side of his skull. The foreman fell to the ground as the rod landed on the rocks several yards away. The holes in Gage's head indicated that death was at hand, but then the foreman sat up, touched the wounds and asked his astonished workmen: "Where's my rod?" Gage was taken by oxcart to the Cavendish Hotel, where an equally astonished local physician, John M. Harlow, discovered he could insert his fingers into the hole in Gage's brain without the victim feeling it. The doctor advised that the poor man be carried to bed, but refusing assistance, Gage rose and walked upstairs to his room. That night a Cavendish cabinet maker, Thomas Winslow, measured Gage and built a coffin that the prospective customer never used. He was soon active again, but it was evident that he was not the same man who had been one of the railroad's outstanding foremen. His soft-spoken nature had given way to a bombastic personality marked by continual cursing. His purposefulness had been displaced by the whims of wanderlust. They eventually led him, via South America, to San Francisco, where he died in 1860. Dr. Harlow answered untold inquiries about the man with the hole in his head, but could offer no explanation of the strange case he had doctored.

A Vermont country doctor could hardly have explained why Gage's mutilated brain had allowed its owner to wander the earth for twelve years. Even the foremost physiologists, with a few exceptions, would have been at a loss to offer a reason. The human brain had not been mapped out as an organ that contained fairly distinct regions having functional assignments in the control of life and thought. Gage's tamping rod obviously tore away parts of his brain dealing with thought rather than the physical control of life.

Prior to the event a few European scientists had considered that the brain might be made up of components with different functions. This idea had occurred to a Paris surgeon, Julien Legallois, in 1811, when he found that an injury to a part of the brainstem, the "medulla oblongata," interfered with breathing. At the same time a Viennese physician, Franz Joseph Gall, tried to develop a functional map of the brain's surface, for he believed that different areas had different responsibilities. Gall speculated that outstanding character traits might be revealed by enlarged areas of a person's brain. This conjecture started the pseudoscience of phrenology, which looked to the shapes and bumps of the human skull as indicators of intelligence and character.

One of the most comprehensive portrayals of the brain as an organ of different functional parts was offered in 1811 by an English anatomist, Sir Charles Bell. He outlined his thoughts in a private paper of which only a few copies were printed and submitted only to his friends. In an early paragraph he expressed fear that his readers might consider he was in search of the seat of the soul, but he explained:

"I wish only to investigate the structure of the brain, as we examine the structure of the eye and ear.

"The prevailing doctrine of the anatomical schools," added Sir Charles, "is that the whole brain is a common sensorium. . . .

"It is imagined that impressions . . . are carried along the nerves to the sensorium, and presented to the mind; and that the mind, by the same nerves which receive sensation, sends out the mandate of the will to the moving parts of the body.

"This appears sufficiently simple and consistent, until we begin to examine anatomically the structure of the brain, and the course of the nerves—then all is confusion: the divisions and subdivisions of the brain, the circuitous course of nerves, their intricate connections, their separation and re-union, are puzzling in the last degree, and are indeed considered as things inscrutable. Thus it is, that he who knows the parts the best, is most in a maze, and he who knows least of anatomy, sees least inconsistency in the commonly received opinion."

Sir Charles continued through several well reasoned pages to "shew why there are divisions, and many distinct parts in the brain. . . ."

In this vein a French physiologist, François Magendie, conducted some interesting experiments in 1822 on the nerves of dogs. He surgically severed various nerve roots connecting the brain and spinal column, and observed the effect on the dog's actions. As a result, Magendie is generally credited with discovering that the nerves connecting the brain to the body are morphologically divided into separate incoming and outgoing pathways. This same discovery was written up by Sir Charles Bell in a paper dated 1821, but it is now thought that he dishonestly tried to take credit for the discovery by dating the paper considerably in advance of its true time of preparation.

In 1824 a French anatomist, Pierre Jean Marie Flourens, conducted experiments on dogs at the University of Paris and produced evidence indicating that the brain is an organ of separate functional parts. He experimented surgically with the cerebellum, a brain center related to the general supervision of muscular movements, particularly balance. "I made a lesion in the cerebellum of a young and healthy dog by means of incisions which extended deeper and deeper," wrote Flourens. "The animal gradually lost the power of ordered and regular movement, and when the mid-region of the cerebellum was reached he could only totter along with a zigzag motion. When he tried to go forward he would go back and when he wished to turn . . . left he would turn right. He made great efforts to move, but being unable to control them he would bound forward suddenly and fall all over himself. . . ."

For the next quarter of the nineteenth century few scientists appear to have studied the brain as a box of separate functional units. However, clinical evidence produced by nervous-system diseases and accidents, such as the Gage case, frequently indicated that the brain was more than a "common sensorium." A young English physician, John Hughlings Jackson, at the National Hospital for Epileptics at Queen Square, London, recognized that specific brain impairments from disease and physical injury clearly affected the use of limbs and other parts of the body. In 1864 and 1870 Jackson wrote that the brain, among its functional areas, contained a motor region that governed a person's individual movements.

Meanwhile a French surgeon, Paul Broca, conducted some revealing post-mortem studies of the brains of people who had suffered from aphasia, the inability to speak or understand speech. In these cases, studied in the 1860's, he found damage to certain areas of the cortex, predominantly on the left side of the brain, and his observations allowed him to outline the regions of the brain related to human speech. In the following decade a twenty-six-year-old professor at the University of Breslau, Carl Wernicke, published a classic paper, "The Symptom Complex of Aphasia," which pointed out important differences between the two major speech-related areas of the brain and initiated the modern study of the subject. The two cerebral regions have long been identified as "Broca's area" and "Wernicke's area."

A valuable method for mapping the functions of brain areas was developed around 1870 by two Berlin physicians, Gustav Fritsch and Eduard Hitzig. A few years earlier Hitzig had been the head physician in a military hospital where he conducted what have been described as "brilliant but ghoulish" experiments. His subjects were patients with parts of their skulls blown away in battle so the surfaces of their brains were exposed. Hitzig stimulated these open patches of brain with wires from a galvanic battery that could deliver a tiny shock. He observed that applying stimulation near the back of the brain caused a patient's eyes to move in response to the shocks. Later Fritsch and Hitzig wrote a classic paper in which they claimed that the latter's experiments produced "the first movements of voluntary muscles . . . brought about by direct stimulation of the cerebral organs and observed on man." The two physicians reported upon similar experiments on animals. Lacking a laboratory, they had worked at Hitzig's home on Frau Hitzig's dressing table and had electrically stimulated the brains of live dogs after surgically opening the animal's skulls. As they continued these experiments, Fritsch and Hitzig recognized that stimulation of specific cortical areas made certain muscles react in the body. Other areas did not prompt muscular movement. Those that did were recognized by the Germans as motor regions. This investigation put electrical stimulation of the brain (ESB) on firm ground, and it became an important tool for mapping out many brain functions. It remains valuable today as scientists continue to unravel the vastly complicated structure that controls life and thought.

In the United States an account of electrical stimulation of the human brain appeared in the *American Journal of the*

Medical Sciences for April 1874. Roberts Bartholow, Professor of Materia Medica and Therapeutics and of Clinical Medicine in the Medical College of Ohio, reported that a patient, Mary Rafferty, a thirty-year-old Irish housekeeper, had arrived at the Good Samaritan Hospital of Cincinnati with a cancerous ulcer on her scalp that had eroded a large hole in the skull, exposing the dura mater, a membrane that envelops the brain. In the few days before the patient's death, Bartholow, who attended her, electrically stimulated the woman's brain, using needle electrodes connected to a battery. Bartholow described one of his first observations as follows: "Two needles insulated were introduced into left side until their points were well engaged in the dura mater. When the circuit was closed, distinct muscular contractions occurred in the right arm and leg. The arm was thrown out, the fingers extended, and the leg was projected forward. The muscles of the neck were thrown into action, and the head was strongly deflected to the right." Other tests with needles placed at different points in the exposed dura mater prompted different reactions in the subject. When Miss Rafferty died, Bartholow removed her brain, sectioned it, and noted the precise location at which his needles had entered the cortex. The doctor's report doesn't mention public reaction to his experiments, which was adverse enough to force him to leave the Ohio community.

Despite such beginnings, ESB was soon put to work to explore the functions of the brain in a systematic way. The subjects, with a few exceptions, were animals. One of the leading pioneers was an English neurologist, Sir David Ferrier, whose work began about 1873. Sir David, employing electrical stimulation with other experimental and clinical methods, was amazingly precise in defining areas responsible for brain functions. His place in neurology was summarized at his death in 1928, when another great English neurologist, Sir Charles S. Sherrington, wrote Ferrier's obituary for the Royal Society. "He established the localization of the motor cortex very much as we know it," said Sherrington (the cortex is the convoluted outer tissue layer of the brain). " . . . He pointed out that its extent was greater and its character more detailed in the ape than in any of the types less near to man. He showed that its focal movements were obtainable with such definition and precision that 'the experimenter can predict with certainty the results of [electrical] stimulation of a given region.' He went on to determine the effects of destruction of limited portions of the cerebral cortex. He allocated regions specially concerned with vision and with hearing respectively. He showed that the hemiplegias [paralysis of one side of the body] and monoplegias [paralysis of a single limb], ensuing on injuries within the motor region of the ape, were characteristically greater than those produced by similar cerebral lesions in the dog. The symptoms in the ape he stressed as being strikingly akin to those familiar in the clinic. . . ."

The best-known pioneers with ESB also include two other Englishmen, Charles Beevor and Victor Horsley. They first experimented on the brain of the Bonnet monkey, but then turned to the anthropoid ape, "in order that we might form a more correct estimate of the mode of localisation in Man." Their subject was an orangutan whose brain was surgically exposed. Aided by fine pairs of compasses, they copied the configuration of the animal's cortex onto paper lined off in numbered squares of two millimeters on each side. An electric current for stimulation was fed to platinum electrodes through an induction coil from a battery. "This current," said the English scientists, "was such as to cause discomfort bordering on pain when applied to the tip of the tongue of the experimenter." As they systematically stimulated point after point on the animal cortex and observed the results, the findings were recorded with reference to the numbered squares on the paper configuration of the creature's brain. Thus they built up a comprehensive functional map of each tiny segment of the brain. For instance, in areas corresponding to squares on the left side of the cortex, numbered 95, 96, 121, and 127, electrical stimulation caused elevation of the animal's upper lip on the right side of the mouth. Stimulation of squares 24 through 27 and 111 through 119 produced the combined movements of the brisk opening of the animal's eyelids and the turning of its eyeballs and head to the right.

Electrical stimulation was an excellent tool for the early cerebral explorer, but it was necessarily limited to a one-way view of the nervous system. An experimenter could define brain areas with nerve circuitry leading outward to the body's various organs and muscles, but the technique offered no information about areas related to pathways inbound from the senses to the brain. Exploration of these sensory regions had to wait for more sensitive measuring equipment than was then available, since currents drawn from specific points on the brain were much less than those detectable in comparatively large nerves outside the central organ.

A sufficiently sensitive instrument was forthcoming when the reflecting galvanometer was invented in 1858 by the British mathematician and physicist Lord Kelvin. It had a tiny moving mirror actuated by the galvanometer coils. A light beam was reflected by the mirror to a large measuring scale a few feet away. A small deflection of the mirror was represented by a much greater movement of the reflected spot—as is evident when a hand-held mirror reflects light onto a distant wall. It was a form of amplification; hence, a small current imperceptible on a conventional galvanometer produced a relatively large deflection of the light spot on the scale. In the 1860's a good reflecting galvanometer with an indicator scale one meter away registered a sizable deflection for a microampere (a millionth of an ampere). It had an important place in electrophysiology, but several years passed before it was applied to brain currents.

The instrument was first employed to confirm and strengthen du Bois-Reymond's basic findings, for it provided a clearer look at the electrical activity of nerves, especially at the electrical potential shift called negative variation. One of the early users was a Liverpool physician, Richard Caton, a lecturer in physiology at the Royal Infirmary School of Medicine. He worked in a darkened theater with a reflecting galvanometer that cast the beam of an oxyhydrogen lamp upon an eight- or nine-foot scale. Caton showed his audiences how the instrument could detect the changing potentials of du Bois-Reymond's negative variation in a frog's nerve. And he fascinated onlookers by demonstrating the rhythmic electrical activity involved in the frog's heartbeat.

In the early 1870's Caton was attracted to Fritsch and Hitzig's ESB and, in turn, he wondered if the electricity of sensory nerves might not flow to the brain, where his reflecting galvanometer could pick them up. Caton obtained a grant for this research from the British Medical Association, and in 1875 he reported back to the Association with results of classic significance for understanding the nervous system.

Caton had worked with rabbits and monkeys whose skulls had been opened and the brains exposed so he could touch his galvanometer electrodes to the gray matter. In every case he found evidence of an ever-fluctuating source of natural electricity along the surface of the animal's brain. Most interesting was Caton's report of a sudden potential change occurring in a specific area when an animal turned its head or chewed some food. Even more fascinating was his test of a brain area that Ferrier had related to eyelid movements. Here Caton detected a potential shift when light fell on the eye at the opposite side of the head. It was comparable to the negative variation that du Bois-Reymond had found in nerves.

Caton's report included an offhand note that actually represented a major discovery. Besides placing his electrodes on the exposed gray matter, Caton also tried them on the external surface of the skull, and he detected a flow of feeble currents in "varying directions." Mary A. B. Brazier, a biographer of Caton and a scientist at the UCLA Brain Research Institute, believes the Englishman's comparatively minor reference really reported "the discovery of the electroencephalogram" (EEG), popularly known as "brain waves."

Caton continued his work with a more careful study of the sensory-stimulated electrical activity of the brain. Using rabbits and monkeys, for example, he investigated the natural electrical effects of mastication detected near a small, difficult-to-locate point on the cortex where movements of the jaw could be caused by ESB. When an animal chewed its food, Caton detected negative variations. He noted the same results when an animal was made only to think of food. "If I showed the monkey a raisin but did not give it," said the English physician, "a slight negative variation of the current occurred."

These and other findings were presented by Caton in 1887 at the Ninth International Medical Congress in Washington, D.C. His paper, entitled "Researches on Electrical Phenomena of Cerebral Grey Matter," included a report that, in this electronic age, gives us the paradoxical picture of a man dealing with the vision-related electrical activity of the brain yet having only a flame for a light source. He placed the flame, the only light in the room, before an animal's eyes and watched the galvanometer record negative variations when he interfered with the light passing to the eye.

"If I partially shaded the animal's eye from the light," reported Caton, "the effect on the electric current was diminished. The exact way in which the light produced its effect is not so easy to determine. It may have excited the visual centre especially, or the result may possibly have been due to the heat radiated from the flame acting on the electrodes . . ."

Caton's original discovery of the EEG remained relatively

unknown for many years. He had first asked to present his results to the Royal Society, but changed his mind and went before the British Medical Association, which financed his research. Speaking before the Royal Society, he would have been published in its widely read journal, but the report appeared in the *British Medical Journal* instead, which physiologists seldom consulted. As a result, Caton's discovery of the EEG was repeated and republished by Adolph Beck, a famous Polish scientist who lived from 1863 until his death at the hands of the Nazis in 1939. About fifteen years after Caton's original work, Beck's curiosity about the electrical activity of the brain was aroused by Russia's Ivan M. Sechenov, a physiologist who had studied in western Europe under Müller, du Bois-Reymond, and Helmholtz. Sechenov had detected electrical activity in the spinal cord and part of the brainstem, the medulla oblongata. Beck set out to find electricity in the brain itself, first in frogs, then in rabbits and dogs. His work was summarized in 1890 by a widely read physiological journal, *Centralblatt für Physiologie,* and then fully discussed in his doctoral thesis the following year.

When he applied his galvanometer electrodes to an animal's cortex, Beck reported, ". . . there was a continuous waxing and waning variation taking place, which neither related to the respiratory rhythm nor was it synchronous with the pulse, nor finally was it in any way dependent on movement of the animal, since it was present in curarized dogs." He concluded that it was a "fundamental variation" found in all brain centers.

Like Caton, Beck localized the brain's sensory regions, although his extra thoroughness contributed substantially more to an understanding of the functions. Beck, for example, flashed a burning magnesium ribbon before an animal's eye and located the corresponding electrical activity of the brain. He stimulated the skin of an animal and found where it elicited cerebral activity. He also made a fundamental discovery overlooked by Caton; he recognized that a sensory-induced electrical response at a single point in the brain interrupted the slow, even wave pattern flowing over the entire brain in the resting state. The interruption occurred as the subject's eyes caught a flash of light, the ears heard a clap, or the skin took a small electric shock. Sixty years later, in 1949, the phenomenon was explained by two scientists as they discovered the "reticular activating system," a small but complicated area in the brainstem. When stimulated—as by a signal from sensory nerves—the system, in effect, switches off the slow, rhythmic brain waves present in the resting state.

When Beck's claim to discovery of the EEG was published in the *Centralblatt für Physiologie,* the editor found it subject to challenge. A physiology professor in Vienna, Fleischl von Marxow, immediately wrote a letter to the journal, claiming that a series of his experiments on "different animals" had revealed that sensory stimulation caused electrical activity detectable in the brain by a sensitive galvanometer. Von Marxow had explained the experiments in a sealed letter dated in 1883, and it had been held for him in the vault of the Imperial Academy of Sciences at Vienna. Upon reading the Beck publication, von Marxow had the letter opened and presented to the *Centralblatt,* where it was printed. The second paragraph read:

"If one connects two symmetrically localized points on the surface of the cerebral hemispheres to a sensitive galvanometer . . . one observes little or no movement of the galvanometer. Stimulation of a sense organ, however, whose central projections are located in one of the recording points, causes the needle to turn in a definite direction. Stimulation of this sense organ on the other side induces it to turn in the opposite direction."

The Viennese professor pointed out that the galvanometer even registered electrical activity from the skull, and he prophetically concluded: "Perhaps it will be even possible to observe, by recording from the scalp, currents evoked by various psychological acts of one's own brain."

Beck, however, would not concede that the secret letter established priority for the scientific discovery. But during the ensuing discussion between Beck and von Marxow, the editor of *Centralblatt* received a short letter from England in which the writer, Richard Caton, asked: "Would you permit me to settle their argument?" He then referred to his publications in the *British Medical Journal* and the transactions of the Ninth Medical Congress in Washington. The letter ended the Beck–von Marxow controversy.

Then it turned out that a fourth person had independently discovered the electrical activity of the brain only a year after Caton reported his findings. A Russian, Vasili Yakovlevich Danilevsky, wrote the editor of *Centralblatt* to say that some of his experiments in 1876 had revealed "spontaneous" electrical activity in the brain. Danilevsky's work had been published in his doctoral thesis at the University of Kharkov in 1877, and although he agreed that Caton was first with the discovery, his thesis made it plain that he was a close second.

Still later it was learned that several other Russian investigators had worked with the electrical activity of the brain in the period between Danilevsky's experiments and Beck's work in Poland. A famous physiologist, Nikolai Y. Wedensky, even used a telephone to listen in on the electrical activity of nerves, muscles, and finally the brains of his laboratory animals. When the phone wires were connected to the brain of a dog or cat, the rhythmical flow of electric waves was barely audible. In some cases Wedensky heard "faint roars" and other noises as the brains were stimulated, and negative variations apparently activated the telephone earpiece.

In the closing years of the nineteenth century improved measuring instruments allowed physiologists to take a more and more precise look at the electrical activity of the brain and nerves. The capillary electrometer was developed to measure extremely small currents. The new string galvanometer allowed scientists to do a better job of observing and measuring oscillating currents. Photography was also adapted to record the electrical waves of the brain. The photographic record was made by directing the undulating light beam of a reflecting galvanometer upon a moving strip of film. When developed, it showed an undulating line representing the brain's changing electrical activity charted against time.

Two Russian physiologists pioneered in recording the electroencephalogram photographically. The first was Vladimir V. Pravdich-Neminsky, who, working with dogs, published the first photographic reproduction of brain waves in 1912. In the next few years the same technique was used on dogs and monkeys by Napoleon Cybulski. The two experimenters timed the animals' brain waves at frequencies between eight and twenty-two per second. Pravdich-Neminsky and Cybulski both recognized that brain waves changed patterns with sensory stimulation.

As the nineteenth century ended, physiologists were using their new technical capabilities to enlarge upon the knowledge initially uncovered by men like Galvani, du Bois-Reymond, Fritsch and Hitzig, Ferrier, Beevor and Horsley, and Caton. They were attempting to understand the nature of the electroencephalogram and related activity in nerves. They were making advances with cerebral localization methods to map the brain's sensory functions. And they were benefiting from improved electrical sources and methods for brain stimulation to define the organ's motor functions more precisely.

But in those days most brain research was conducted on laboratory animals: frogs, dogs, monkeys, cats, apes, and others. How could similar experimentation be applied to man? The twentieth century's rapid advances in technology, especially in electronics, finally made it possible. In 1898, there was a preview of things to come—a European experimenter, J. R. Ewald, became the first to conduct brain stimulation experiments on freely moving animals. He drilled a hole in a dog's skull and screwed in an ivory cone through which he inserted an electrode to the animal's brain. Wires from the electrode ran up a leash to a switch and a small battery. As Ewald walked his brain-wired dog, he could observe how the remotely controlled electrical stimulation affected the animal's motor functions.

4

THE NEURON THEORY

In October 1889 the annual meeting of the German Anatomical Society at the University of Berlin was well attended by world-famous scientists, including the renowned Robert Koch, who sixteen years later would win the fifth annual Nobel Prize in Physiology or Medicine for his development of a tuberculosis test. Some of those present thought the 1889 meeting would become famous for Koch's prospective tuberculosis cure, but their speculations proved wrong. Instead, the conference was memorable because of a little-known Spanish histologist, Santiago Ramón y Cajal, who had, in his own words, "gathered together for the purpose all my scanty savings and set out, full of hope, for the capital of the German Empire."

The august conferees found the visitor from Spain something of a curiosity. They weren't accustomed to Spanish scientists, for the country had produced few, and none of note. Cajal's language also set him apart, for he could only converse with the non-Spanish-speaking delegates in poor and halting French.

"It is unnecessary to say that my colleagues at the congress accorded me a courteous reception," Cajal wrote in his autobiography. "There was in it an element of surprise and expectant curiosity. It was a shock for them, no doubt, to meet

49

a Spaniard who cultivated science and had of his own volition entered upon the paths of research. At the conclusion of the reading of papers, to which, on account of my impatience, I devoted little attention, there came the demonstrations.

"From an early hour I was installed in the laboratory devoted to this purpose, where numerous microscopes shone upon large tables before broad windows. I unpacked my preparations; I requisitioned two or three of the magnifying instruments beside my own excellent Zeiss model, which I had brought as a precaution; I focussed them upon the sections which showed the most important facts regarding the structure of the cerebellum [a part of the brain], the retina, and the spinal cord, and finally I began to explain to the curious in bad French what my preparation contained. Some histologists surrounded me, but only a few, for, as happens in such competitions, each member of the congress was looking after his own affairs; after all, it is natural that one should prefer demonstrating his own work to examining that of someone else."

The few who saw Cajal's work included some of the greatest names in histology (the microscopic study of organic tissues), Albrecht von Kölliker, Wilhelm His, and Wilhelm Waldeyer, all of whom had a deep interest in the microscopic anatomy of nerve tissue. "As to be expected," wrote Cajal, "these savants, then world celebrities, began their examination with more scepticism than curiosity. Undoubtedly they expected a fiasco. However, when there had been paraded before their eyes . . . a procession of irreproachable images of the utmost clearness, the supercilious frowns disappeared. Finally, the prejudice against the humble Spanish anatomist vanished and warm and sincere congratulations burst forth."

The Spaniard became the hero of the meeting. He was besieged with questions which he answered "in clumsy French, minutely and patiently."

"The most interested of my hearers was A. Kölliker, the venerable patriarch of German histology," Cajal wrote. "At the end of the session he took me in a splendid carriage to the luxurious hotel where he was staying; entertained me at dinner; presented me afterwards to the most important histologists and embryologists of Germany, and, finally, made every effort to render my sojourn in the Prussian capital agreeable.

" 'The results that you have obtained are so beautiful,' he said to me, 'that I intend to undertake a series of confirmatory studies immediately, adopting your technique. I have discovered you, and I wish to make my discovery known to Germany.' "

A few months later Kölliker had confirmed Cajal's results. The Spaniard had clarified man's conception of the nerve cell and its physical place in the electrical network of the nervous system. This initial work and its subsequent development brought Cajal the Nobel Prize of 1906.

As was true with the electrical activity of the nervous system, an anatomical understanding of the minute nerve cell was tied to technological advances, largely to the improvement of the microscope and the techniques of using it. Good magnification was important, but development of histological preparations was also a key to success. The story began more than two hundred years before Cajal's time.

In the mid-1600's the English scientist Robert Hooke viewed thin slivers of cork with a compound microscope he had helped develop, and he saw rows of holes, like the multiple "cells" of a prison or monastery. He was actually observing only the shrunken remains of fluid-filled structures that had occupied the spaces when the cork was alive. The living structures retained the name "cells," although it was a misnomer. Such visual misunderstanding played an important part in the early history of man's efforts to reveal the secrets of the nerve cell. Hooke's wonderful microscope actually became a frustrating, deceptive tool because of chromatic aberration, a technical problem that remained unsettled until the first half of the nineteenth century. One look at the tiny structural features of nerve fibers seldom matched the next.

In 1761, for example, a German microscopist, Martin Ledermüller, reported that he saw nerve fibers as packets of hollow tubes, which certainly did not support an earlier observation by Anton Leeuwenhoek, who saw nerves as a train of globules. Twenty years later Felice Fontana of Florence said that nerve fibers were transparent tubes filled with gelatinous fluid; he conceded, however, that such microscopic images had to be accepted with caution. In France, an early nineteenth-century microscopist, René Dutrochet, saw globules clinging to the surface of nerve fibers, and when he looked at the brain of a frog, he saw globules packed in rows among comparatively few fibers. Dutrochet decided he was looking at cells, but it would be difficult to say that he was the first to recognize nerve cells.

In the early 1800's, a French mechanic, M. Selligue, found in the microscope that more than a single doublet (a pair of lenses) could solve chromatic aberration, and this discovery led to the development of "achromatic" instruments that made the microscope a much more dependable tool for the biological sciences. It was immediately used by physiologists, one of whom was a Czech professor at Breslau, Germany, Jan Evangelista Purkinje, who reported that he and his students focused the new achromatic microscope upon animal tissue "with real wolf's hunger." His observations were soon productive, for in 1837 Purkinje appeared at a Prague meeting of natural scientists and for the first time presented a good general description of the nerve cells of the brain and spinal cord. His words and drawings revealed that the cells had nuclei and processes—which meant that each had a protoplasm-filled main body enclosing a central body within itself, and a fibrous tail extending out from the main body. The Czech's conception of certain cells in the cerebellar cortex was so accurate that those cells were subsequently named "Purkinje cells."

To Purkinje's credit, his recognition of nerve cells came a year before a German botanist, Matthias Schleiden, elaborated on the cell theory for plants, and two years before a German physiologist, Theodor Schwann, spelled out the cell theory for animals, postulating that the cell is the basic building block of all living things. The Czech professor, however, failed to explain the nerve cells' unusual body and tail, or their relationship to one another or to the brain and nerves.

An explanation soon came from two students in Johannes Müller's laboratory. One was Hermann von Helmholtz, who later determined the speed of the nerve impulse. Helmholtz's microscopic observations of nerve fibers made him think that the fibers were made up of the processes of nerve cells—in many cases, at least, since he wasn't sure about all of them. The second student was a young Dane, A. H. Hannover, who tried for a prize the Royal Society of Science of Denmark was offering to the person who could best illustrate the benefits to physiology from microscopic research on the nervous system. Hannover prepared nerve tissue with a solution of chromic acid and under the microscope found that the elongated processes of nerve cells were much longer than previously realized. This finding supported the idea that the processes might be the fibers of nerves.

But the evidence told little about the function of nerve cells. What, if anything, did they have to do with the nervous system's electrical activity, being defined by men like du Bois-Reymond? Were the elongated processes of nerve cells connected? Were they continuous or contiguous? Such were the most difficult questions facing microscopists at the middle of the last century. "The anatomy of the intimate structures of the brain," said a Vienna anatomist in 1846, "is and remains apparently a book sealed with seven seals and written moreover in hieroglyphics."

The problem was now to find new histological preparations that could be better observed with the achromatic microscope. For the sake of visual integrity microscopists needed ways of preserving or "fixing" dead tissue so it could be observed in a state as lifelike as possible. For clarity's sake the tissue had to be cut into sections thin enough for the viewer to see individual cells rather than a confusing pile of cells superimposed on one another, and the cells had to stand out from the surrounding material if viewers were to understand their intimate structures. Reaching these goals took most of the remaining years in the nineteenth century.

Fixing was slowly improved by trying various chemical solutions on the tissue. In 1851, for example, an English experimenter, Lockhart Clarke, reported on fixing a spinal cord with acetic acid and alcohol, which allowed him to slice it into thin sections with a sharp knife. Before mounting the sections on glass he treated them with turpentine and Canada balsam.

The hand-held knife, regardless of its edge, had obvious drawbacks for cutting an extremely thin, even section of tissue, so microscopists welcomed the development of the microtome around mid-century. It was like a miniature guillotine, with a thin, sharp blade in a guide that carried the cutting edge evenly and precisely down through the fixed tissue secured to the base of the device. Purkinje was one of the earliest users of the microtome.

Although fixing and sectioning were being improved, neither solved the visual problem arising from the tissue's low contrast. One of the best solutions was found when microscopists turned to a process dating back to 1770. An English doctor, scientist, and essayist, Sir John Hill, had then hit upon a method for improving the contrast of wood fibers for viewing through a microscope. He had soaked sections of wood in carmine and found that different parts of the wood absorbed the dye at different rates, making them more contrasting to the eye. About 1854 a German histologist, Joseph von Gerlach, employed a centuries-old embalming technique to inject carmine into blood vessels, and he found that it stained nearby tissues, increasing the contrast for microscopic observation. Gerlach applied the same carmine solution directly to sections of tissue cut from an animal's central nervous system, but the results were disappointing—until he accidentally left a section in a diluted solution of the dye overnight and found that the tissue's various parts had been beautifully set off against each other. Carmine became a standard stain for histologists investigating the nervous system, although it was far from perfect and scientists were still far from clear about what they could see through the microscope.

By the 1850's and 1860's experimenters pretty well agreed that each nerve cell sent out one main process, and bundles of these fibers formed the nerves that men had seen for centuries. The agreement, however, ended when scientists tried to describe the exact physical relationship between the cells. Here they divided into two camps, the "reticularists" and the "anti-reticularists." The first group adhered to a reticulum theory originally set forth by Gerlach, who decided that nerve cells were connected by an independent network of fibers. He pictured the network as a kind of trellis stretching between the long processes of nerve cells, and he suggested that it was the conductor of impulses from cell to cell. The theory had much more support than the anti-reticularists could muster, although in 1887 they received encouragement from two well-known European scientists, Wilhelm His and Auguste Forel, who proposed that nerve cells might not be connected, that the branchings from any given cell really had free endings in the gray matter of the central nervous system. But His and Forel's case lacked the strength of good clear microscopic observations, which seemed to have supported the opposite point of view, propounded by a well-known Italian anatomist and physician, Camillo Golgi.

Golgi had discovered a new and improved stain for central nervous system tissue. The staining process required most of a week to complete. The tissue was hardened several days in solutions of osmic acid and potassium dichromate, and then placed in a silver nitrate solution for another day or two. Finally it was treated with dehydrated alcohol, oil of clove, and oil of bergamot, after which the tissue was washed and mounted for viewing. Under the microscope the nerve cells stood out as if they were silver and black etchings. The stain reaffirmed that a nerve cell has one long cylindrical extension (the axon). Moreover, Golgi's stain also revealed that a cell has many smaller processes (dendrites). The Italian, however, still could not explain exactly how these appendages were involved in the disputed cell-to-cell relationship, but he sided with the reticularists and became their leader.

Nevertheless, Golgi's stain was not good enough. He was soon frustrated trying to unravel the unimaginably complex arrangements of nerve cells, and he left the field, concluding it was a fruitless pursuit. He became famous for a treatment of malaria, but more famous when he shared the Nobel Prize of 1906 with the Spanish histologist Cajal, for work on the nerve cell. Both men, however, did not share the same ideas on the structure of the nervous system. Cajal, by now, was the main exponent of the anti-reticularists.

Santiago Ramón y Cajal was a poor and sickly Spanish anatomist who had become enthralled by microscopy around 1877. He saw it as an avenue to new, exciting worlds of science and decided on histology as a career. It was a field practically unknown in Spain, and the selection ensured his continuing poverty. While supporting his family through teaching, Cajal invested any extra money in his microscope and laboratory. They became the master of his time and monopolizer of his thoughts. It is said that at a single sitting he once spent twenty hours watching a white corpuscle escape from a capillary.

"Come with me to the laboratory," wrote Cajal in a popular Spanish magazine. "There upon the stage of the microscope, tear up the petal of a flower, forgetting for a moment its beauty and fragrance. Then take a bit of animal tissue; tear it apart without compunction even though it pulsates and trembles at the touch of the needle. Then look through the window of the eyepiece, and the leaf of the plant and the tissue of the animal will reveal to you in every part the same structure—a sort of honeycomb built up of little cells and more little cells, separated by connective substance, and harboring in its cavities, not the honey of the bee, but the honey of life in the form of semisolid, granular material, encircling a tiny corpuscle, the nucleus."

This devotion to the "stage of the microscope" eventually brought Cajal to the nerve cell, which he called ". . . the aristocrat among the structures of the body, with its giant arms stretched out like the tentacles of an octopus, to the provinces on the frontiers of the outside world, to watch for the constant ambushes of the physical and chemical forces. . . ." The Spanish anatomist thought he might help explain the physical basis for thought and will. Psychology, then emerging as a science, was already demanding a sounder understanding of physical processes behind the discipline. "To know the brain," said Cajal, "is the same thing as knowing the material course of thought and will, the same thing as discovering the intimate history of life in its perpetual duel with eternal forces, a history summarized and literally engraved in the defensive nervous co-ordinations of the reflex, the instinct, and the association of ideas."

Cajal's remarkable work that emerged at the 1889 meeting in Berlin depended on the Golgi stain, which the Spaniard learned about during a trip to Madrid and talks with Luis Simarro, a psychiatrist and neurologist. Simarro was interested in the way brain cells degenerated with certain mental diseases, and he showed Cajal microscopic slides of brain tissue prepared with the Golgi stain. The visitor returned home and put the stain to work. He encountered the limitations that had frustrated Golgi but refused to accept them. Instead, he painstakingly experimented with variations on the Golgi stain and eventually improved it.

Cajal then turned to experimentation that had already

been tried and abandoned by other scientists, including Golgi. They had assumed that much could be learned about the nerve cell if it was observed during its early stages of life, but this was a task too complex and delicate for most investigators. Cajal, however, applied his microscope and improved stain to the embryonic nerve tissues of birds and small mammals, and he found that success depended on carefully applying the stain at certain periods of development. The methodical applications provided him with an amazingly clear view of the tiny nerve cells, and for the first time the persistent histologist sensed the true relationship between them.

The little-known Cajal was doing these experiments in the late 1880's, when he was having trouble communicating his findings to the world. He tried solving the problem by publishing his own journal, the *Trimonthly Review of Normal and Pathological Histology*, of which he could afford to print and mail only sixty copies to scientists of other countries. It was largely ignored. For the few who did pay attention, it challenged too many well-accepted ideas about nerve cells, and the Spaniard was dismissed as a victim of his own imagination. But, confident that he had important contributions to make, Cajal decided on a direct, personal confrontation with the continent's most important scientists to present his histological evidence. He joined the German Anatomical Society and proceeded to the next meeting, the Berlin conference where he surprised Albrecht von Kölliker and other famous figures. Henceforth the name of the Spanish histologist was anything but obscure.

In clarifying how nerve cells relate to one another, Cajal revealed that each is a self-contained unit with an axon that reaches out to, but is not continuous with, another cell. Nerve fibers are definitely made of these processes, said Cajal, but, more important, the cells are the communicating links of nerve tissues, with the axon of one cell reaching out to the dendrites or the body of the next. The elongated processes, explained the Spaniard, are insulated from one another except at the far end of each axon, where it makes contact with the next cell. The arrangement, in a rough sense, forms the insulated electric cables of the nervous system. In explaining these relationships, the Spanish histologist offered a basis for the "neuron doctrine," or "neuron theory." The name was actually coined by a Berlin professor, Wilhelm Waldeyer, who, as shown earlier, was one of the surprised witnesses to Cajal's presentation at the 1889 conference. Because he named the theory, Waldeyer was often mistakenly credited with having established it. In a footnote on a monograph written just before his death in 1934, the Spanish histologist said: "Professor Waldeyer, to whom poorly informed persons attribute the neuron theory, supported it with the prestige of his authority but did not contribute a single personal observation. He limited himself to a short, brilliant exposition (1891) of the objective proofs . . ., and he invented the fortunate term of *neuron*."

The presentation of Cajal's work in 1889 was substantial support for the ideas set forth two years previously by His and Forel, and it provided reason enough to abandon the reticulum theory, which, however, suffered a long, lingering death. Indeed, it was still a matter of controversy as late as the 1930's. Golgi clung to his theory and refused to endorse Cajal's work. His coolness was evident when the two men shared the 1906 Nobel Prize. When the awards were presented in Stockholm, Golgi's address, preceding Cajal's, left many of the audience in dismay. The speech, which would ordinarily review work related to the prize, was an obvious affront to the co-winner, for Golgi tried to revive the disproven reticulum theory. Cajal's address, a review of his work on the nervous system, only added evidence that the neuron doctrine rested on the strength of research capable of maintaining the doctrine far into the future.

After 1889 and his dramatic introduction to the scientific world, Cajal continued adding to the knowledge of nerve cells. Most of his accomplishments, as in the past, came from improvements in staining methods.

"For the biologist," said Cajal in those years, "every advance in staining technique is like gaining a new sense with which to explore the unknown. As if Nature were determined to keep hidden from our eyes the marvelous structure of the cell, this magnificent protagonist of life is obstinately concealed in the double invisibility of smallness and homogeneity. Structures of amazing complexity appear under the microscope colorless, uniform, and as simple in architecture as a mass of jelly."

In the 1890's Cajal made another of his memorable contributions by helping to establish the direction of flow of the nerve impulse in relation to the nerve cell. With tissue from birds and small mammals, the Spanish histologist studied the visual and olfactory apparatuses, where he knew the cells transmitted sensory signals from the outside world toward the brain. He determined that, in the neuronal arrangement leading back to the brain, each cell fell into a common pattern. Its dendrites always pointed toward the outside world and the incoming sensory signals, while its axon pointed inward with the flow of signals toward the brain. Thus Cajal deduced that the direction of electrical activity between two nerve cells was from the axon of the first cell to a dendrite of the second cell. In the early stages of life, when cells grow into place, Cajal decided, the orientation of their processes lined up with the flow of electrical impulses. He named this the principle of "dynamic polarization."

Before the turn of the century the Spanish scientist established other important points about nerve cells. He recognized that in moving up the scale from lower to higher vertebrates, with a coincidental growth in intellectual power, an increase occurred in the number of connections between nerve cells. He also felt there were indications of changes in nerve cell connections resulting from acquired skills. He believed, for instance, that when a person learns a musical instrument, becomes adept at drawing, or acquires any special skill, nerve pathways are enhanced in the involved parts of the nervous system. He envisioned the change as an added richness of connections between existing cells, not as an increase in cells.

In 1896 Cajal tried a methylene blue stain recently developed by a German scientist, Paul Ehrlich, who became the founder of modern chemotherapy. The stain was not lethal, like the Golgi preparation, so Cajal repeated many of his earlier studies on living tissue. Besides strengthening and confirming his original findings, he further disproved the reticulum theory.

After the turn of the century Cajal developed another remarkable stain for nerve tissue, which depended on heating a solution of silver nitrate for several days along with the tissue to be observed. It made the cells practically transparent and enabled the Spanish histologist to add more detail to the facts he had already provided. From Cajal's research came an increasing number of publications and some comprehensive textbooks, all of which added to his fame. As his works spread over the world, they brought back the greatest of international honors in science and medicine. He was invited to London by the Royal Society to give the 1894 Croonian Lecture, which had been presented since 1749 by Europe's most famous scientists. Five years later—when the Spanish-American War had cooled relations between the United States and Spain—Cajal received and accepted a surprise invitation to join four other famous European scientists at Worcester, Massachusetts, for the tenth anniversary celebration of Clark University. But none of the honors surprised him as much as the announcement that he was to share the 1906 Nobel Prize.

In the late 1940's the venerable English scientist Sir Charles Sherrington summed up what Cajal had accomplished for the neurological sciences: "He solved at a stroke the great question of the direction of nerve-currents in their travel through brain and spinal cord. He showed, for instance, that each nerve path is always a line of one-way traffic only, and that the direction of that traffic is at all times irreversibly the same. The so-called nerve networks with unfixed direction of travel [the reticulum theory] he swept away. The nerve-circuits are valved, he said, and he was able to point out where the valves lie—namely where one nerve cell meets the next one."

5

LIFE WITHOUT MIND

In December 1932 Professor G. Liljestrand of the Royal Caroline Institute in Stockholm delivered the presentation speech for that year's Nobel Prize in Physiology or Medicine, awarded then to two English scientists, one of whom was Sir Charles Sherrington, Waynfleet Professor of Physiology at Oxford. In reviewing Sherrington's work, Professor Liljestrand said: "Of fundamental importance for our knowledge of the workings of the nervous system was the discovery that an external influence, a so-called stimulus, can, without the cooperation of the will, call forth a definite response, such as the contraction of certain muscles. A well-known example is presented by the involuntary blinking at a loud and unexpected noise. The external influence is, so to speak, thrown back or reflected, from which the phenomenon received the name 'reflex.' For every one of our movements, even under the influence of the will, for numerous processes in the interior of the body, and in all probability also for mental life itself in its various forms, the reflexes play a highly important role. . . .

"Sir Charles Sherrington has made extraordinary contributions to our knowledge of the reflex phenomena . . ."

The career of this Nobelist, who lived from 1861 to 1952, covered a most significant epoch in a long search for answers to the mysterious phenomenon of the reflexes.

For centuries it had been recognized—indeed, by every cook who cut off a chicken's head—that life mysteriously persisted in animals whose brains were suddenly removed. Leonardo da Vinci wrote perceptively of the phenomenon nearly four hundred years before Sherrington's time. He said: "The frog retains life for some hours when the head, heart and bowels have been taken away. And if you prick the said [spinal] cord, the frog instantly has convulsions and dies. All the nerves of the animal derive from here: when this is pricked it instantly dies."

The pioneer description of the function of reflex actions was written more than two hundred years before Sherrington by the famous French philosopher René Descartes, who grasped the principle of reflexes without benefit of experimental evidence. Descartes saw the body as a machine, which in an animal was no more than a machine, but in man was influenced by the rational soul (*l'âme raisonnable*). Laboring under the ancient Galenic theory of animal spirits, the French philosopher envisioned these spirits flowing down from a reservoir, namely the brain, through the nerve tubes to the muscles, whose shape could be changed by the spirits to enable the machine to run.

Descartes drew an animated analogy between the body and a waterworks, which, in his time, was like an amusement park with grottoes, fountains, and gardens. The flow of animal spirits from the brain was compared to the flow of water from the waterworks' reservoir in sufficient force to operate various machines: ". . . even to make them play several instruments or pronounce words, according to the varied disposition of the tubes which conduct the water," explained Descartes. The rational soul seated in the human brain, he said, was like the waterworks' engineer or fountaineer, "who ought to be in that part of the reservoir with which all the various tubes are connected, when he wishes to quicken or slacken, or in any way alter" the machines.

In the same description, Descartes discussed how outside influences affect the waterworks' machinery independent of internal controls, and the passage is now considered to be the first conceptualization of reflex functions. He speculated that in the body innumerable trigger mechanisms are constantly set off by the events of its ambient universe. The French philosopher, speaking in terms of his waterworks analogy, put it this way:

"External objects which, by their mere presence, act upon the organs of sense; and which by this means, determine the machine to move in many different ways . . . may be compared to the strangers who, entering into one of the grottoes of these water works, unconsciously themselves cause the movements which they witness. For they cannot enter without treading upon certain planks which are so disposed that, if they approach a bathing Diana, they cause her to hide among the reeds; and if they attempt to follow her, they see approaching towards them a Neptune, who threatens them with his trident; or if they pass in another direction they cause some sea-monster to dart out who vomits water into their faces; or like contrivances, according to the fancy of the engineers who made them."

This account was eighty-seven years old when Descartes' ideas were experimentally supported by an Edinburgh neurologist, Robert Whytt, whose study of nervous functions was remarkably advanced for the middle of the eighteenth century. He had already learned the relatively modern technique of extirpation, i.e., he removed known parts of the central nervous system in animals and observed the results. Some of his extirpative work was designed to locate the source of what Whytt called "vital motions," although, from his descriptions, it is now evident that he was talking about reflex actions. Whytt explained that "the motions excited by any pain, or irritation, are so instantaneous, that there can be no time for the exercise of reason, or a comparison of ideas in order to their performance; but they seem to follow as a necessary and immediate consequence of the disagreeable perception." He decided that the source of vital motions was related to the spinal cord, for when parts of the cord were cut away, certain motions ceased. Whytt, for example, recognized the eye's familiar pupillary response to light as a vital motion, and by extirpation he traced its functional source to a part of the central nervous system called the corpus quadrigemina.

In 1763 Whytt demonstrated his advanced thinking about reflexes when he described an important phenomenon, now called the "stretch reflex," which was to escape the attention of future investigators until the 1920's. As a muscle is stretched, it sets up reflex signals that lead to the contraction of the same muscle in a direction opposing the stretch. Without the stretch reflex, muscles, offering no resistance, become flaccid. This crucial reflex—it allows us to keep our balance, for example—was recognized and briefly described by Whytt as follows:

"Whatever stretches the fibres of any muscle so far as to extend them beyond their usual length excites them into contraction about in the same manner, as if they had been irritated by any sharp instrument, or acrid liquor. The motion of stretching the fibres will be greater or less, as the muscle is more or less stretched; unless it be so extended as quite to lose its tone and become paralytic."

Shortly after Whytt's death in 1766 a brilliant Viennese anatomist, Georgius Prochaska, was writing and lecturing on the "sensorium commune," which contained his conceptualization of reflex functions. The sensorium commune, said Prochaska, was a place at which the nerves of sensation met and communicated with the nerves of motion. In this place, explained the anatomist, impressions received by the senses are transformed into action. Prochaska did not place his sensorium commune in the main, upper part of the brain, but suspected it was in the lower parts of the organ and in the spinal cord. This was evident, he said, in a decapitated animal, for the reactions between senses and motion continue despite the loss of the brain. Prochaska saw that, wherever its location, the sensorium commune was essential to our preservation, for it transformed sensory impressions into motor actions that allowed one to avoid injury. Furthermore, when the senses received impressions of beneficial elements, the sensorium commune produced actions to enhance and continue those benefits. Prochaska illustrated the process with descriptions of what were later defined as reflex actions.

"Many examples certainly prove this general law of the reflections of the sensorium commune," he wrote, "of which it will be sufficient to adduce a few. Irritation of the internal membrane of the nostrils excites sneezing, because that impression, made by irritation of the olfactory nerves, is by them carried to the sensorium commune, is there reflected, according to a certain law, upon motor nerves going to the muscles appropriated to respiration, and, through these, produces a forcible expiration through the nose, in which, by the air forcibly passing, the irritation is removed. So it happens when any irritation is caused to the wind-pipe by a crumb of bread or a drop of liquid falling into it: this irritation, carried to the sensorium commune, and thence reflected upon the nerves appropriated to respiratory motion, excites a forcible cough, the most apt remedy for expelling the irritant. . . . If a friend approaches our eye with his finger, although we are persuaded that no harm will be done to us, yet that impression carried by the optic nerve to the sensorium commune, is in the sensorium so reflected upon the nerves appropriated to the motions of the eyelids, that the palpebrae [eyelids] are involuntarily closed so as to avoid the contact of the finger. These and innumerable other examples that might be adduced, show manifestly how much the reflection of sensorial into motor impressions by the sensorium commune regards the preservation of our body."

Although the principles of reflex functions had been remarkably well described by Descartes, Whytt, Prochaska, and others, the phenomenon was treated as little more than a curiosity well into the nineteenth century, when reflexology was finally put on a firm scientific base by an unusual English physician from Nottingham, Marshall Hall. A prolific though verbose writer, Hall published over 150 papers and 19 books covering subjects that ranged from the diseases of women to bloodletting (which he opposed), to artificial respiration, to the injustice and inhumanity he saw accorded Negroes when he visited America in 1853. He was also a tireless experimenter who, toward the end of his career, claimed to have devoted 25,000 hours to the study of the spinal cord. With such devotion, said one historian, Hall became "the father of reflex action as a clinically discernible and meaningful fact, rather than a purely laboratory or experimental phenomenon."

Despite the distinction, the English physician appeared ill-informed on both the background and current status of his subject. Indeed, Hall may actually have rediscovered reflex actions for himself. He was apparently unaware of Whytt's and Prochaska's findings. He revealed little knowledge of current scientific events related to the nervous system, the work of du Bois-Reymond and Purkinje, for example. And he seemed oblivious of current experimental work on reflexes that came very close to what he was doing. For example, a contemporary French anatomist, Pierre Jean Marie Flourens, had reported on removing the cerebrum of a healthy chicken and keeping the bird alive ten months—which might have been longer had the scientist not been forced to leave his Paris laboratory and the experiment. Flourens said the brainless chicken had lost its sight, hearing, and volition, but was otherwise normal, being able to stand in a fixed position until given a push or thrown in the air, in which event it walked or flew a short distance.

Hall's experiments were something like Flourens'. One of the Englishman's papers tells of his decapitating an experimental animal "in the manner usual with cooks, by

LIFE WITHOUT MIND   69

means of a knife, which divided the second and third vertebrae." He went on to say that he placed the head on a table for observation and noted that the mouth continued to open and close as it might in breathing. "I now touched the eye or eyelid with a probe," said the English physician. "It was immediately closed: the other eye closed simultaneously." He continued touching his probe to other parts of the head while noting reflex actions, and then he turned to the lower parts of the decapitated animal: "The limb, the tail, were stimulated by a pointed instrument or lighted taper. They immediately moved with rapidity. The sphincter was perfectly circular and closed: it was contracted still more forcibly on the application of a stimulus. The limbs and the tail possessed a certain degree of firmness or tone, recoiled on being drawn from their position, and moved with energy on the application of a stimulus."

In both instances, explained Hall, the reflex actions were stopped by removal of the central nervous system. In the head, they were ended by withdrawing the medulla, a lower part of the brain. In the body, he ended the reflexes by withdrawing the spinal cord marrow. "The limbs were no longer obedient to stimuli," said Hall of the spineless animal, "and were perfectly flaccid, having lost all their resilience. The sphincter lost its circular form and its contracted state, becoming lax, flaccid and shapeless. The tail was flaccid and unmoved on the application of stimuli. . . ."

While Hall's observations were unusually thorough, they hardly produced much new learning on reflexes. Actually he gained fame by going beyond other scientists in attributing the main functional site of reflexes to the spinal cord. Until his time, the cord was assumed to be essentially a bundle of nerves acting as communication lines between the brain and various parts of the body. Hall agreed to this role, but also recognized in the spinal cord the characteristics of another brain, largely independent of the real brain at the top of the cord. He may even have thought that the "spinal brain" was superior to the real brain, for he noted that the spinal cord was always awake and alert, whereas the brain needed sleep.

Remarkably, the doctor from Nottingham recognized the "spinal brain" as a long, integrated unit rather than a series of unrelated segments, as the articulated vertebrae had led some people to think. He reached this conclusion while observing the writhing of a beheaded snake and deciding that as any point on the body moved, the stimulus of skin rubbing the ground was transmitted via the spinal cord to a second point, causing it to move—the action repeating itself over the entire length of the snake. Thus, concluded Hall, a headless serpent wriggles until death stills the repetitive action. To prove his point, Hall showed that a live but decapitated snake could not wriggle when its body was suspended free of any skin-to-ground contact.

The Englishman's concept of the spinal cord stirred so much opposition that it turned him into one of the century's more controversial scientists. Most of the medical press, with one exception, the famous Lancet, denounced Hall and his supporters. The animosity was probably related to the theological questions raised by his dualistic idea of the spinal cord. By Hall's time the dominance of the brain as the seat of the soul had become widely accepted, but now he was indicating that man had two brains, one in the head and one in the back, and when the former was removed, the latter remained in control of the still-existing life. But what happened to the soul? The question was an inflammatory one for men who had the soul comfortably settled in the main organ of the head, and it ignited a controversy that continued for years. Some argued that the soul was removed when the brain was withdrawn and that the remaining reflex actions were nothing but soulless, mechanical acts. Others felt that there could be two souls, one for the brain, one for the spinal cord. Of course, the question was unresolvable.

Hall, an egotist who thrived on controversy, continued writing and talking with vigor about his idea of the spinal brain. Meanwhile, he was banned from publishing his works in the *Philosophical Transactions of the Royal Society* because the men in editorial control felt the controversial doctor had become the exponent of theories too absurd for serious science. Such accusations only fired Hall to fight his detractors and, according to one biographer, his emotions led him "to take an embarrassingly active part in the discussion [about himself] . . ." However, the animosity toward Hall slowly gave way to more sober thoughts, and his ideas were found worthy of consideration in high places. In 1850 he was invited to give the honored Croonian Lectures, which he delivered under the title: "The Diastaltic Action of the Spinal Cord." "Diastaltic" pertained to a style of melody in ancient Greek music designed to exalt or expand the mind; Hall adopted the word for his own purposes in saying that the spinal cord's reflex functions made it a brain in its own right. By the time of his death in 1857 it was well established that the doctor from Nottingham had offered a theory of reflex actions that was to spur others toward a fuller comprehension of the fascinating phenomenon.

While Charles S. Sherrington, who was born four years after Hall's death, was growing up and receiving his extensive education in physiology, the field of reflexology was comparatively static. Textbooks talked about reflexes superficially, for they were unable to provide functional information. Authors were limited mostly to giving examples of reflex actions such as sneezing, coughing, vomiting, and recoiling from pain. By 1891, when Sherrington set his mind to the study of reflexes related to the spinal cord, he had worked with, or met, most of the leading men in the neurological sciences. He had studied under Sir Michael Foster, the first occupant of the newly created chair of physiology at Cambridge. He had spent a winter in the Strasbourg laboratory of Friedrich Goltz, then engaged in some famous experiments wherein he was removing large portions of dogs' brains yet keeping them alive for extended periods. And on a mission to Spain to study a cholera outbreak, Sherrington met Cajal, who was yet to become famous for his work in nerve histology. All these experiences were important to the efforts that were to make the English scientist famous.

He soon recognized that if he was to add to the existing knowledge of reflexes, he would have to undertake a painstaking, detailed anatomical investigation of the structures of the nervous system that seemed to be functionally involved with reflexes. It literally meant untangling and identifying the unimaginably complex maze of nerves leading to and from the spinal cord and the brainstem, which lies above the cord. The anatomical investigation took most of the 1890's. The results and some of Sherrington's subsequent accomplishments were summed up in 1906 at Yale University, where the Englishman was visiting to present that year's Silliman Lectures. The ten-lecture series was promptly published in a book, *The Integrative Action of the Nervous System*, whose prose, often beautifully composed, revealed that the scientist was also a humanist with an impressive understanding of classical language, literature, and art. The book, now a classic in neurophysiology, was republished in 1947 and again as a paperback in 1961.

As with many other great scientists, Sherrington's strength grew from an immense capacity for attention to detail. This was illustrated by his animal "preparations," which were considered masterpieces of experimental technique. An important example is found in some of Sherrington's most basic work, which required a "decerebrated preparation" to bring about a condition known as "decerebrate rigidity." It demanded the skilled development of extra-precise surgical methods to remove the upper parts of an animal's brain so as to rob it of volition but not life. When the procedure was successfully completed, the animal's muscles controlled by the lower part of the brain and spinal cord held it in a fixed, rigid position. The brainless beast could then be stood on its feet, as motionless as a statue. The same experiment had been performed with birds for decades —as we learned earlier in reference to Flourens' experiments—but in mammals serious hemorrhaging following the brain surgery had brought rapid death and prevented any meaningful experimentation. Sherrington overcame the problem by skillfully tying off certain arteries and blocking the blood flow from others by enhancing the formation of clots. Eventually he learned to prepare animals that would remain perfectly rigid and alive for as long as four days. The basis for these skills undoubtedly came from Goltz, whose dogs after excision of large parts of their brains still retained surprising degrees of sensibility and mobility. Some of the dogs were kept alive for weeks and, in one case, for eighteen months. Sherrington's first scientific paper, published in 1884, was about one of the Goltz dogs.

In his eighth Silliman Lecture Sherrington described a decerebrated monkey that had been suspended on strings. The arms, with the palms of the hands turned inward, were straightened out and thrust backwards. The same was done to the legs. The long tail was extended and, despite its weight, remained horizontal, or even curled slightly upward. The head was tilted back, and the jaw, tightly closed, was lifted upward against the pull of gravity. If someone tried to move a limb, he encountered resistance from the muscles, and if it were forced out of place, it instantly flew back into position when released. If small amounts of ether or chloroform were administered to the monkey, the rigidity disappeared until the effects wore off.

In the foreword of the 1947 edition of his classic book Sherrington said his decerebrated animals were modeled on Descartes' view of all animals: ". . . wheelwork animals geared into the turning universe . . ." with ". . . no thoughts, no ideas; they were trigger-puppets which events in the circumambient universe touched-off into doing what they do . . ." But Sherrington, musing that Descartes must never have owned a pet, said that the decerebrated animal ". . . is found to be a Cartesian puppet: it can execute certain acts but is devoid of mind. That it is devoid of mind may seem a dogmatic statement. Exhaustive tests, however, bear the assertion out. Thoughts, feelings, memory, percepts, conation, etc.; of these no evidence is forthcoming or to be elicited. Yet the animal remains a motor mechanism which can be touched into action in certain ways to exhibit pieces of its behavior."

Sherrington recognized that decerebrate rigidity provided the opportunity to experiment with a live, healthy, un-anesthetized motor mechanism directed solely by the brain-stem and spinal cord without the natural interference created by the thoughts of a whole brain above. Thus he referred to the preparations as "spinal animals." For years the English scientist prepared decerebrate monkeys, dogs, and cats to study nerve circuits flowing to and from what remained of their central nervous systems. To focus his research on particular reflex functions, Sherrington eliminated uninvolved peripheral nerves by removing them or tying them off. Through this complex, tedious procedure, repeated again and again, he learned the anatomy and physiology of reflexes. The evidence allowed him to speak on the three-way system of simple reflexes.

"From points within and on the surface of the animal," explained Sherrington, "nerve-threads run to its muscles, but in their course thither are engaged by the central organ [spinal cord] and are there relayed; the central organ becoming a sort of switchboard where muscles can be switched on or off."

Thus Sherrington offered a basic description of the "reflex arc," which is of fundamental importance to any understanding of the nervous system. Indeed, a single reflex arc seems to exhibit all the fundamental modes of operation of the nervous system. Like the system on a larger scale, the

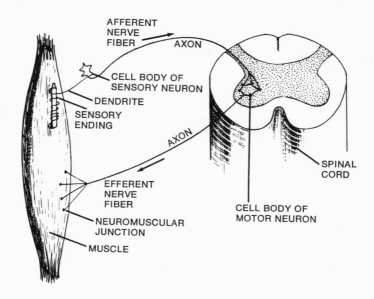

AFFERENT
NERVE
FIBER
AXON
CELL BODY OF
SENSORY NEURON
DENDRITE
SENSORY
ENDING
AXON
SPINAL
CORD
EFFERENT
NERVE
FIBER
CELL BODY OF
MOTOR NEURON
NEUROMUSCULAR
JUNCTION
MUSCLE

Schematic drawing illustrating principle of simple reflex arc. Sensory ending is stimulated when muscle stretches, and impulses go to spinal cord and synapse with motor neuron. Motor neuron fires, sending impulses back to muscle, causing contraction to counteract stretch.

single arc gathers sensory signals and passes them through the decision-making central nervous system, which reacts by turning related muscles on or off.

The ends of nerve fibers that collect sensory signals for the multiple reflex arcs of the nervous system are not all alike, explained Sherrington, but are designed to sense different kinds of stimuli. One may sense heat but not light, while one for light ignores heat. With its many types of sensors, a living organism can react to a wide variety of external and internal stimuli by way of the reflex arcs operating around the lower part of the brain and spinal cord.

But as Sherrington pointed out in his Silliman Lectures, it would be a gross oversimplification to think that a reflex arc ever operated as a separate and independent system; it should only be considered as such to aid in the explanation of the principle behind it. In truth, the English scientist observed, thousands of reflex arcs might work together in a coordinated system of systems, as was evident in the way a decerebrated animal's machine-like acts always occurred as part of an integrated pattern of acts.

From this observation came one of Sherrington's fundamental contributions to the neurological sciences—the concept of the "common path." He explained that while the input side of an arc has a privately held sensory receptor cell with a specific mission, the output side leading to a muscle is likely to be an efferent nerve shared by many arcs with many different kinds of sensory inputs. Thus these many and varied arcs converge upon a common path. Sherrington added that while the path may receive from multiple arcs, it still handles a single message at a time. The message, however, may be a summation of signals from the several sources, now reinforcing, now inhibiting, and now excluding one another.

For an example of a common path in action Sherrington cited the hip flexor muscle, which bends the leg and plays a major role in standing and walking. He said that the efferent nerve forming a common path to this muscle could, in any given period of time, receive messages from widely distributed sensory receptors, each designed to sense a specific stimulus, like heat, cold, sound, light, or smell. Therefore, the signals regulating the flexor at one moment come from some relatively distant point on the skin, then from the opposite foot, next from the eyes, then from the foot of the same leg, from a hand, an ear—and on and on as the muscle is regulated to apply the mechanical forces necessary to maintain the body upright, move it in a desired direction, lead it away from danger, and accomplish endless other missions throughout the individual's life. And here Sherrington was speaking of only a single common path of a great many, all linked to thousands of reflex arcs working together in giving the moment-by-moment directions that create an integrated, living organism from a complex collection of tissues.

"The animal mechanism is thus given solidarity by this principle which for each effector organ allows and regulates interchange of the arcs playing upon it," said Sherrington, "a principle which I would briefly term that of 'the interaction of reflexes about their common path.'"

The English physiologist arrived at such an involved comprehension of the nervous system through many ingenious experiments and observations. For one of his best-known series of experiments he devised an artificial flea with a fine entomological pin energized by a feeble electric current. The pin could be inserted into the outer hair-bulb layers of a decerebrated dog's skin without mechanically stimulating the nerve endings, but when the current was turned on, the results were comparable to a flea bite. To relieve the irritant the mindless, rigidly fixed animal would lift a leg and groom its fur with the rhythmic action common to all dogs. The physiologist employed his electric flea for an exhaustive study of the "scratch reflex." At the same time he learned a great deal about reflexes in general.

On the simplest level he found that the scratching leg of the mindless dog could follow the flea when it was moved to different points on the animal's skin. If the flea was inserted near the ear, the scratching foot would locate the spot, and then move back if the flea was subsequently applied near the groin. When Sherrington inserted two fleas a distance apart, the scratching action would alternate from one site to the other, depending on which flea was energized at the moment.

On a more complex level electric fleas were used with a recording myograph to analyze the motions of the dog's leg and the neural communication system involved in the scratch reflex. Sherrington first noted that a single flea bite did not produce a scratch; a continuing series of bites was required. He also applied bites at a changing frequency to see if they altered the scratch frequency, but, regardless of the rate of bite, he found the scratch remained essentially the same, except when slowed by fatigue. Such experiments led to the conclusion that nerve circuitry from the irritated skin was involved in the summation of a flea's multiple acts, not in individual bites or in the rate at which bites occurred. However, Sherrington found that the intensity of bites was a factor in the elicitation of scratching. Simulated bites with a low electrical level were ignored, but when the current was increased to a certain point, the scratching began.

Continuing experiments with artificial fleas led Sherrington to other fundamental conclusions about the nerve circuitry of the scratch reflex. He concluded that when enough bites warranted a scratch, the process of summation occurred, not near the skin where the stimulus was received, but in the nerve mechanism leading to the muscles of the scratching leg. Sherrington also learned that once the proper summation of bites had led to a scratch, the same reflex system was more easily triggered into action by a second series of bites. And he recognized that different kinds of reflexes impose a system of priorities on themselves. For example, he found that the scratch reflex will cease functioning in deference to the higher-priority flexor reflex, the one involved should a person be forced to catch his balance on one leg after he has stepped on a tack with the opposite foot.

Sherrington's decerebrated animals were employed to study many other reflexes besides the scratch reflex, as is indicated in the following passage drawn from the foreword to the 1947 edition of his famous work:

"The list of such purposive movements [reflexes] is impressive. If a foot tread on a thorn that foot is held up from the ground while the other legs limp away. Milk placed in the mouth is swallowed; acid solution is rejected. Let fall, inverted, the reflex cat alights on its feet. The dog shakes its coat dry after immersion in water. A fly settling on the ear is instantly flung off by the ear. Water entering the ear is thrown out by violent shaking of the head. An exhaustive list would be much larger than given here. . . . But when all is said, if we compare such a list with the range of situations to which the normal cat or dog reacts appropriately, the list is extremely poverty stricken as a conspectus of behaviour. It contains no social reactions. It evidences hunger by restlessness and brisker knee-jerks; but it fails to recognize food as food: it shows no memory, it cannot be trained or learn: it cannot be taught its name. The mindless body reacts with the fatality of a multiple penny-in-the-slot machine to certain stimuli, all of them, as in the case of the penny-in-the-slot machine, physical, and not psychical."

As he looked at the integrated whole of the nervous system, Sherrington may have seen it as an inverted pyramid, with the reflex arc at the pointed bottom and the entire system across the broad top. Within this structure of little systems piled into larger, more complex systems, the English physiologist recognized and described for the first time some extremely basic functions, any one of which was important enough to have brought scientific fame to its discoverer. Two of his most important contributions in this area were the "proprioceptive system" and the "stretch reflex."

In 1906 Sherrington added the Latin combining form "proprio" to "ceptor" to describe an important area of nervous system action. He decided that under the vast sheet of closely placed receptor organs designed to pick up various stimuli at the skin's surface, an equally vast number lie within the body's deep tissues. "The deep receptors," he explained, "appear to be very usually adapted to mechanical stimuli of certain kinds. Thus they seem adapted to react to compressions and strains produced by muscles, and an important adequate agent for them seems to be mass acting in the modes of weight and inertia, involving mechanical pressures and mechanical stresses."

These deep receptors, decided Sherrington, provide muscles with the capability of sensing their own movements and positions for relay of the information to the central nervous system. This kind of muscle sense had long been evident but a puzzle to scientists. Originally they assumed that the guiding signals for movement and posture came from external stimuli, like pressure upon the soles of the feet, but the renowned French physiologist Claude Bernard opened the assumption to question with a few simple experiments. After removing the skin from the legs of a frog, thereby cutting away its external sense receptors, he found it could still leap and swim normally. Next he severed all the nerve connections between a dog's leg muscles and spinal cord, but left those leading to the pads of the feet. The French physiologist then observed that the animal could not stand. It had apparently been robbed of some internal sensing facilities necessary to the positioning of the legs. Sherrington in a way reversed this experiment to support his proprioception theory. He severed the sensory nerves that provided feeling in a cat's paws, then enticed the animal to walk from rung to rung on a ladder suspended horizontally—which it was able to do in normal fashion. The experiment reinforced Sherrington's theory that proprioceptors in voluntary muscles provide us with the important sensations of physical being. It was a key concept for understanding the nervous system's complex informational network. Equilibrium is maintained, for example, with the guidance of the deep sensors working with the brain's cerebellum. Coordinated voluntary movements, such as those involved in driving a car or typing, depend upon proprioception.

Sherrington's understanding of this principle was obviously a step toward his definition of the stretch reflex. It evolved from his long-time interest in the knee-jerk phenomenon that is routinely checked in physical examinations. The knee-jerk was first considered scientifically in the 1870's. Sherrington wrote about it around 1890, but failed to find an explanation until 1924, when he and another English scientist, E. G. T. Liddell, outlined the stretch reflex to the Royal Society. The answer had been supplied by painstaking anatomical studies which led the two men to realize that the knee-jerk is the product of a reflex system triggered when proprioceptors are stimulated by the stretch of a certain muscle. They explained the phenomenon as follows.

The familiar kick occurs when a tap on the knee causes the patellar tendon to pull and thereby stretch the quadriceps femoris muscle of the thigh. But actually a contraction, not a stretch, of this muscle causes the immediate outward kick of the leg. Therefore the question arises: How does the stretch produce the contraction? The answer came when the English scientists recognized that a sudden stretch of the thigh muscle stimulates proprioceptors that send an inward (afferent) signal to the spinal cord, where a reflex mechanism returns an outward (efferent) signal to the same muscle, causing it to contract. This system, which feeds back upon itself, is the stretch reflex.

The Sherrington-Liddell explanation, applicable to all muscles, was a fundamental contribution to the neurological sciences. The stretch of any muscle, it turns out, is promptly accompanied by a contraction triggered by reflex nerve circuitry of the kind responsible for the knee-jerk. This neural mechanism that provides a push for every pull makes living muscle resilient; it gives the tissue tonus. If the nerves of the stretch reflex are destroyed, the related muscles suffer from flaccid paralysis. The mechanism is at work night and day, even during periods of deep relaxation, providing muscles with the small amount of tension always evident in life and absent in death. But more than providing muscle tonus, the stretch reflex constantly maintains all the counterforces necessary for posture and equilibrium. When a misstep forces a person to catch his balance, the stretch reflex reacts without conscious direction to right the body. And, incidentally, when the stretch reflex, for reasons unknown, is set off while one sleeps, the result is a falling sensation that often awakens the victim in a fright.

Sherrington's remarkable accomplishments were closely related to his recognition and adoption of the neuron theory at a time when it was not yet completely accepted. His respect for the theory was in turn related to his close friendship with Cajal, which began during the English scientist's visit to Spain in 1885. When Cajal went to England to deliver the Croonian Lectures of 1894, he lived with the Sherringtons, and for a time secretly pursued his microscopy in their guest bedroom. The Spanish histologist's work was of fundamental importance to Sherrington's comprehension of the spinal reflexes. In the first sentence of his Silliman Lectures, Sherrington paid respect to the neuron theory:

"Nowhere in physiology," he said, "does the cell theory reveal its presence more frequently in the very framework of the argument than at the present time in the study of nervous reactions." The lecture continued with a description of the nerve cell as the nervous system's phenomenal basic building block with a life of its own and the unique ability "to spatially transmit (conduct) states of excitement (nerve-impulses) generated within them." But the most important feature, said Sherrington, was the cell's remarkable capability for providing the multi-cellular animal with ". . . nervous reaction which *par excellence* integrates it, welds it together from its components, and constitutes it from a mere collection of organs an animal individual."

As they have studied the nerve cell, most of this century's biology and psychology students have undoubtedly been exposed more to the name of Sherrington than Cajal, for the former coined a well-remembered term for nerve physiology: "synapse." He first used it in an 1897 textbook to identify the "nexus" between two cells, the junctions where Cajal revealed that "nerve-circuits are valved." For the new name, "synapse," Sherrington adapted a Greek word, meaning "to clasp."

In his ninety-one years Sherrington produced an immense output of writings that ranged from his scientific books and papers to a small volume of verse, *The Assaying of Brabantius and other Verses,* which caused one reviewer to wish that more verse could be published by "Miss Sherrington." From all of Sherrington's highly productive years, said the late John Fulton, the famous medical historian at Yale University, "emerged the vast sweep of present-day knowledge of neurophysiology. . . ."

6

REFLEXES OF THE BRAIN

On June 9, 1866, the official Censors' Committee of St. Petersburg presented an indictment against a Russian physiologist, Ivan M. Sechenov, for attempting to publish a small book, *Reflexes of the Brain,* which a magazine had already printed in 1863. The Committee attacked the theme of the book as follows:

"This materialistic theory reduces even the best of men to the level of a machine devoid of self-consciousness and free will, and acting automatically; it sweeps away good and evil, moral duty, the merit of good works and responsibility for bad works; it undermines the moral foundations of society and by so doing destroys the religious doctrine of life hereafter; it is opposed both to Christianity and to the Penal Code, and consequently leads to the corruption of morals."

The indictment, as it turned out, was dropped, and the book was published when Sechenov's friend, the Minister of Justice, interceded for him. *Reflexes of the Brain* quickly made an impact on Russian intellectuals and students, and the latter adopted it as their handbook for the 1860's and 70's. One was eighteen-year-old Ivan Pavlov, who was deeply influenced by the book.

Sechenov was a physiologist who, in keeping with tradition, visited western Europe as part of his early education.

On his first of two trips he studied with such eminent scientists of the German school as Emil du Bois-Reymond and Hermann von Helmholtz, who, at the time, were in revolt against the vitalism of their common teacher, Johannes Müller, nearing the end of his long, distinguished career. Helmholtz and du Bois-Reymond had become strong proponents of a mechanistic, materialistic approach to the understanding of living things. They felt that living organisms could be studied in parts, as one would investigate a machine, to determine the physical and chemical facts underlying life. Impressed by this philosophy, Sechenov returned home with equipment developed by du Bois-Reymond, and he introduced electrophysiology to the leading Russian universities.

In a few years the physiologist was back in western Europe working and studying in the Paris laboratory of Claude Bernard, another of the nineteenth century's great physiologists. There Sechenov encountered the deterministic philosophy prevalent in the French school of physiology. It emphasized performance as a whole, as opposed to the German idea of focusing on the parts of a living organism. The French concept was illustrated in Bernard's description of what he called the *milieu intérieur*. He noted that despite its ever-changing exterior environment, a higher animal has an independent, stable interior environment around the organs, tissues, and their elements. ". . . each one," he said, "is surrounded by this invariable *milieu* which is, as it were, an atmosphere proper to itself in an ever-changing cosmic environment. Here we have an organism which has enclosed itself in a kind of hot-house. The perpetual changes of external conditions cannot reach it; it is not subject to them, but is free and independent." Bernard concluded that ". . . the nervous system is called upon to regulate the harmony which exists between all these conditions."

Soon after returning to Russia from the Paris laboratory, Sechenov wrote *Reflexes of the Brain*, which synthesized the philosophies he had encountered in both the German and French schools. The treatise was first published by a magazine in serial form, then in book form, following a three-year struggle with Russian censors. The little volume proposed that reflexes are the basis of conscious and unconscious life, and that psychical life is tied directly to our environment as perceived by the nervous system. This involved a three-part reflex process, said Sechenov. First the body's various sensory receptors monitor the environment and carry the signals along inward-bound (afferent) nerve circuits. Second, the signals pass through a central control process, or "arc," whose operation is describable in physical terms. This process does not necessarily, as often assumed, operate within the brain, but in the confines of the brainstem and spinal cord. Finally, the central arc initiates signals along outgoing (efferent) nerve circuits, which produce muscular contraction. Sechenov proposed that this three-way circuit was an electro-mechanical system that, in the final analysis, guides a living organism in all of its thoughts and actions.

He continued by saying that controls could be applied to the three-way system by higher brain-center signals modifying those that flow through the central arc. The flow might be enhanced or inhibited at the arc, as though it were a valve actuated by the mind to regulate one's constant, inevitable interaction with his environment—in other words, controlled behavior. The valve, in Sechenov's way of explaining the arc, is opened by our more emotional, less rational mental activities. Inhibitory control, on the other hand, depends upon the exercise of learned, rational thought, and the degree of learning thus applied is an index of maturity. Regardless of control, said the physiologist, the results of all that we do and think are evidenced through some form of muscular expression.

"The infinite diversity of external manifestation of cerebral activity can be reduced ultimately to a single phenomenon—muscular movement," stated the author. "Whether it's the child laughing at the sight of a toy, or Garibaldi smiling when persecuted for excessive love of his native land, or a girl trembling at the first thought of love, or Newton creating universal laws and inscribing them on paper—the ultimate fact in all cases is muscular movement.

". . . the reader will readily grasp that absolutely all the properties of the external manifestations of brain activity described as animation, passion, mockery, sorrow, joy, etc., are mere results of a greater or lesser contraction of definite groups of muscles, which, as everyone knows, is a purely mechanical act. Even the confirmed spiritualist cannot but agree with this. Indeed, how can it be otherwise, when we know that in the hands of the musician a soulless instrument produces sounds full of life and passion, that stone becomes animated under the hands of the sculptor? The life-giving hands of musician and sculptor perform purely mechanical movements, which, strictly speaking, can be subjected to mathematical analysis and expressed by formulas. How, then, could they express passion in sounds and images, unless the expression were a purely mechanical act? In view of this, the reader will agree that the time will come when men will be able to analyse the external manifestations of the functioning of the brain as easily as the physicist analyses now a musical chord or the phenomena of a freely falling body."

Sechenov based *Reflexes of the Brain* on some comparatively minor experiments conducted in Bernard's Paris laboratory, where he worked with decapitated frogs while their bodies were still alive and reacting to such stimuli as pain. Mainly he dipped the toe of a brainless frog in acid and timed the withdrawal of the leg with a metronome. He noted that he could vary the time by touching different points of the frog's exposed spinal cord with a salt crystal. The action of the salt, decided Sechenov, was comparable to that produced by inhibitory signals coming from rational thoughts in the brain. His controversial book looked far beyond this slender research to develop his broad concepts relating physical and psychical life. While it stirred controversy, he continued his laboratory investigations and provided a firmer scientific basis for the central inhibition of reflex activity, which he is now credited with discovering. To illustrate how far advanced was Sechenov's work on central inhibition, the American scientist Horace B. Magoun describes how he and his colleagues found in the 1940's that stimulation of a part of the brainstem inhibits certain motor activities related to the spinal cord. For years Magoun assumed that they had found this inhibitory mechanism for the first time, but then in the library of Washington University he came across the collected works of Sechenov and learned to his surprise that the same observation had been made in the last century by the Russian physiologist.

As an author of the 1860's, Sechenov added little tranquillity to his homeland when *Reflexes of the Brain* proclaimed that life and all that goes with it is purely a mechanical act resulting from the contraction of muscles. Once past the censors, the small volume triggered a heated public controversy that lasted for many years, and to the end of his life the author remained under surveillance by the Tsarist government, whose Minister of the Interior portrayed Sechenov as "a propagandizer of extreme materialism and the greatest theoretical popularizer in nihilistic circles" of whom everyone should be "continuously watchful." But the Russian physiologist was a man of personal strength and courage, and he continued writing and saying what he believed. When his book was under investigation by the courts, a friend asked Sechenov why he did not seek the counsel of an attorney—to which he answered: "Why should I need a lawyer? I shall take a frog with me to court and perform my experiments in front of the judge; then let the State's attorney refute me."

Meanwhile the ideas expressed in his book made him a hero of Russia's progressive thinkers and students. At the time his volume was being published, Sechenov held a professorship at the Medico-Chirurgical Academy in St. Petersburg, and his lectures became popular with young people, including young women whose only way to gain entrance was to come disguised as men. This popularity made him all the more controversial, but then Sechenov resigned from the Academy over a matter of principle, although the police maintained that the government had "deigned to dismiss" the scientist because of his "popularity among the students." The position went to one of Sechenov's former students, I. F. Cyon, who had become known for his reactionary thinking and had obtained the post with the help of a high-ranking government official. The students responded with "riots," and Cyon sought and obtained police protection for his lecture hall, but with the students' continuing pressures, he quit the post. Pavlov, who had become Cyon's assistant, also resigned.

The controversy and the leading participants offered some interesting parallels to another public flap that had just occurred over the novel *Fathers and Sons*, by Ivan S. Turgenev. In the 1860's Turgenev had become the target of the press because of his fictional character, Bazarov, a science student portrayed favorably as an agnostic and materialist. Sechenov, it has been said, served as the model for Bazarov. However, Turgenev, as the butt of criticism, was not as durable as Sechenov, and he left Russia.

Until the end of his life Sechenov continually had to defend his revolutionary ideas about the physical basis of the psyche. In general his critics felt that Sechenov, as a physiologist, was intellectually unprepared to apply his work to psychology, and they felt that the outlandish ideas in his book were proof enough. At one point Sechenov answered them with an essay entitled "Who Must Investigate the Problems of Psychology and How?" in which the answer turned out to be the physiologist. More than a decade after *Reflexes of the Brain* had been published it was still fueling the verbal fires of critics who clung to their hopes of incinerating the author. In 1877 Dostoyevsky wrote a friend, saying: "Sechenov knows nothing about his opponents (the philosophers), and thus he does more harm than good with his scientific conclusions."

Dostoyevsky's conclusions, however, were most unprophetic, for Sechenov was to become the father of Russian physiology and to be recognized as a leading pioneer in the neurological sciences, especially in reflexology. Most references in Western scientific histories name Sechenov as the discoverer of central inhibition, but neglect to say that he independently recognized a number of nervous principles, the discoveries of which have been attributed to other scientists.

For example, Sherrington (with his artificial flea experiments) is credited with first explaining that a summation of several stimuli was required to elicit a reflex reaction and that as long as the strength and the frequency of the stimuli remained constant, they continued to prompt the reaction. A letter written by Sechenov indicates that he had recognized this principle when Sherrington was only seven years old.

"I yesterday wrote to you," he said in a letter to his wife dated February 4, 1868, "that the effects of successively switching on and off a direct current applied to a sensory nerve are cumulative. Today I arranged the experiment thus: a direct current A is switched on and off any number of times per minute by means of a metronome; this makes it easy to count the number of times the current has been switched on and off. As a result I found that for a given strength of current the frequency of clicks necessary to elicit movement remains approximately constant. Consequently by this method perhaps it will be possible to measure a property of the nerve centers that has not been understood thus far, to add up individual excitatory shocks. This opens up a broad field of investigation: the study of the variation in this property under the most various conditions. I am simply getting dizzy from the vast accumulation of facts requiring explanation."

Two years before this letter was written Sechenov apparently recognized the principle of proprioception credited to Sherrington's work a quarter of a century later. The Russian talked about ". . . the role of the muscle sense in the analysis of the measurement of space and time" after making clinical observations of ataxic (uncoordinated) patients with the help of another great physiologist, Sergei P. Botkin.

In the same year, 1866, Sechenov discussed another principle of nervous action that was to be confirmed in the following century when it was recognized that the transmission of the nerve impulse is a chemical function. The Russian noted that the excitability of nerves was dependent on the blood supply reaching them, and without it the electrical activity and the life of the nerve cease. "This clearly indicates," he said, "the close link between chemical acts in the nervous tissue and the physiological property under study." He concluded that when the nerve moves from a state of rest to excitability, it is "related to chemical upheavals within the nerve." He was right, but could hardly prove it at the time, since a great deal more had to be learned about the neuron and its role in the nervous system.

In the closing years of his life, Sechenov put his physiological findings to work in a study of the working and resting habits of man. One of the most famous photographs of the scientist shows him seated in a chair mounted on a table where he is using his hands to actuate a contraption of cords, pulleys, and levers. Through such experiments, with Sechenov acting as his own subject, he arrived at some important conclusions regarding the nature of fatigue and its relationship to the nervous system. He concluded that man, employed or unemployed, required eight hours of sleep per day, and that waking activities should not occupy more than sixteen hours.

Despite Sechenov's laboratory work, remarkable for its originality and advanced look toward basic neurological principles, his most important contribution to the science was probably the small volume *Reflexes of the Brain*, based on a minimum of laboratory effort. It provoked important new lines of thought about the relationships between the nervous system and behavior, and it attracted the attention of Russia's best students and thinkers, thereby stimulating important neurological research that left marks on the futures of both physiology and psychology. His influence spread by way of men like Ivan R. Tarkhanov, an electrophysiologist who is remembered for basic work in reflexology and cutaneous sensations; Vasili Y. Danilevsky, who independently discovered the electrical activity of the brain, which had just been recognized in England by Richard Caton; Nikolai Y. Wedensky, whose basic work on the properties of nerves included listening to the electrical activity with a telephone; and Vladimir M. Bechterev, a famous physiologist and psychiatrist.

Oddly enough, Sechenov, according to one Russian scientist-historian, never met or corresponded with the man through whom his ideas would gain their greatest influence. Throughout a long, fruitful career that made him the giant of all Russian physiologists, Ivan Petrovich Pavlov looked up to Sechenov as a spiritual master whose "teaching of the reflexes of the brain is, in my opinion, a sublime achievement of Russian science." He continually paid tribute and gave credit to Sechenov as a guiding force in his own work on the nervous system. For example, in 1906, one year after Sechenov's death and two years after Pavlov won the Nobel Prize, he delivered a public address on the subject that was to bring him his greatest fame, conditioned reflexes, and there he credited his mentor with having prompted the work. "The beginnings of our investigations date back to the end of 1863," he said, "when Sechenov's famous essays Reflexes of the Brain were published."

Pavlov's career had three parts, one comparatively minor, two decidedly major. His first scientific paper, published in the late 1870's, was entitled "Experimental Data Concerning the Accommodating Mechanism of the Blood Vessels." He was then interested in the physiology of blood circulation, and it led to his independent discovery of the heart's trophic nerves, which, unknown to the Russian, had already been identified. Soon he turned to the first of his two major endeavors, the study of digestion, which was to bring him the Nobel Prize. In the last quarter century or more of his life Pavlov engaged in his most important scientific pursuit. Following Sechenov's lead he developed the fundamentals of conditioned reflexes. These three changing interests were all related; the earlier work stirred his interest in the final undertaking, for which Pavlov is best remembered. In fact, many people believe that it was his work with conditioned reflexes that led to the Nobel Prize, but actually the award came as this phase of his research was just getting underway.

As a young man, Pavlov read and admired the British philosopher and literary critic George Henry Lewes, whose works included popular writings in science. Among them was the *Physiology of Common Life,* and Lewes's final work, *The Problems of Life and Mind.* Pavlov's interest in digestion was reportedly inspired by Lewes's work on physiology, in particular by a complex illustration of the digestive tract that the author had obtained for the book from Claude Bernard. Lewes's final work undoubtedly had its influence on Pavlov's later career, for it discussed among other views on psychology the relationship of biological facts and an understanding of mental functions.

Following his early work in circulation and the completion of his doctoral thesis in 1883, Pavlov spent two years in Germany, where he worked in the laboratories of two well-known scientists, Rudolf Heidenhain in Breslau, and Carl Ludwig in Leipzig. The latter was interested in the secretory glands and their nerves. He revealed, for example, that the salivary glands could be made to secrete by stimulating the attending nerves, even though the animal had been decapitated. The experiment played a role in Ludwig's rejection of the vitalistic assumption that life was an entity apart from biological laws. Heidenhain was interested in gastric secretion and at the time of Pavlov's visit was experimenting with a gastric pouch he had developed. The German scientist had surgically altered an animal's stomach to form a pouch (or fistula) apart from the original stomach and accessible to the experimenter through an opening in the abdominal wall. With this arrangement, Heidenhain proposed to measure gastric secretion.

Upon returning home Pavlov began his study of digestion by improving the Heidenhain pouch. He believed it could not provide a true measure of gastric juices because the preparation severed the vagus nerve, so important to the control of secretion. Moreover, the pouch, as originally conceived, provided a mixture of secretion and food, making it difficult to analyze the former alone. The Russian scientist set out to isolate part of the stomach from the incoming food, but to maintain the secretory mechanism. He accomplished it by a delicate, complicated operation on a dog after many trials. Avoiding the crucial nerves and blood vessels, Pavlov made an incision along the stomach wall to open up a small flap, which was then formed into a tube and sutured so as to extend from the stomach out through the abdominal wall. To prevent food from entering the tube, the scientist drew together and stitched the internal mucosa (membrane) where the tube left the stomach. The result was a cul-de-sac closed to the stomach at the upper end and opening through the abdominal wall at the lower end. At the same time secretory mechanisms within the cul-de-sac functioned along with those in the stomach above. When the dog ate, food entered the main stomach, but not the artificially made "small stomach." Here the secretion, free of food, could be gathered through a cannula (a tube inserted from the outside) for analysis.

"I remember my enchantment with Pavlov's daring and faith in the correctness of his surgical plan," wrote one of his laboratory associates in later years. "At first the operation was unsuccessful, about 30 dogs were sacrificed, much effort and time, almost six months, were expended without results, and the faint-hearted were losing their courage. I remember that some professors in related disciplines asserted that this operation cannot and will not be successful because the location of the blood vessels of the stomach contradicts the idea of such an operation. Ivan Petrovich just roared with laughter at such statements the way only Pavlov can laugh; a few more efforts and the operation was a success." Another of Pavlov's colleagues wrote a dissertation on the intricate surgical technique, and the paper used four pages of fine print to explain the step-by-step procedure that lasted four hours and required two hundred stitches.

When Pavlov's technique was finally successful, the dog not only had an artificially created "small stomach," but was also a completely healthy animal that would remain alive indefinitely. One of the first dogs to survive the surgery was named Druzhok, meaning "little friend."

Pavlov's development of the small stomach demonstrated his reverence for a concept that he held crucial to all physiological investigations, and it in turn became an important factor in shifting his interest away from digestion to conditioned reflexes. He was an advocate of the chronic, as opposed to the acute, experiment. Pavlov believed it was an invitation for grave errors to observe or experiment upon an isolated organ of a complex, ongoing organism. Besides, he felt that during experimentation the health of the organ of interest, as well as the entire animal, should remain as nearly perfect as possible in order that (1) the results and the chances of reproducing them would not be influenced by malfunctions, and (2) the work could continue over a sufficient length of time to reveal any changing results. His penchant for dealing with the whole and healthy animal often made it appear as though Pavlov were engaging in anthropomorphism. For example, he was one of the first scientists to observe asepsis in both the care and surgical treatment of experimental animals. Before one of his famous dogs arrived in the operating room, it was held briefly in each of a series of pre-operating rooms where it was bathed, shaved, and otherwise prepared for surgery. Pavlov and his colleagues also personally observed the typical scrubbing routine that surgeons accord human patients. During the operations the scientists used the appropriate anesthetics, and after the surgery the wounds were thoroughly cared for until healed and the animals were kept in immaculate quarters. The results were described by Pavlov as follows:

". . . our healthy and happy animals did their laboratory work with real gusto; they always eagerly moved from their cages to the laboratory and readily jumped onto the tables where our experiments and observations were conducted. Believe me, I am not exaggerating. Thanks to our present surgical methods in physiology we can demonstrate at any time almost all phenomena of digestion without the loss of even a single drop of blood, without a single scream from the animal undergoing the experiment."

Another experiment, "sham feeding," was particularly important to the future of Pavlov's work. It involved severing a dog's gullet, turning the cut ends downward, and sewing them to two holes in the skin of the neck. Thus the top half led from the mouth to the top hole and the outside, and the lower half led from the outside via the bottom hole to the stomach. When the dog ate, food moved from the mouth down the gullet as usual, but partway it dropped out of the top opening. To keep the dog alive, food was introduced through the bottom opening into the lower part of the severed gullet and thence into the stomach, or it was offered directly to the stomach via a metal tube entering by way of the abdomen. The dogs thus fed often survived seven or eight years.

With sham feeding the Russian scientist was able to study the secretion of gastric juices as the result of stimuli occurring solely in the higher regions of the digestive system, or as the result of stimuli produced by food entering the stomach directly. In preparation for these experiments, a dog would be made to fast for several hours, and its stomach would be carefully washed out. Then it would be fed in the normal fashion—except, of course, that the food would drop out of the hole in the neck. However, gastric juices would soon flow from the metal tube leading out from the stomach, and they would continue to do so during the sham feeding and for some time after. Several hundred cubic centimeters of the pure juices could often be collected from a dog's stomach during a sham feeding.* In other experiments on the same dogs, different kinds of food introduced directly into the stomach also caused gastric juices to flow. To test whether the flow was produced by mechanical pressure or chemical action of the food on sensory endings in the mucous membrane, Pavlov applied purely mechanical stimuli to the stomach walls and noted that they did not release the secretions prompted by food.

His experiments revised the general beliefs of the day about the mechanics of digestion. It had been thought that the nervous system was not related to the digestive system, that the latter was a mechanically actuated affair somehow triggered by the physical contact of food. Pavlov proved otherwise by showing that it was linked to the nervous system by way of reflexes that automatically controlled the chemistry and motility of the digestive system. He explained it in simple terms:

"Food excites the gustatory apparatus; the excitation is transmitted by the gustatory nerves to the medulla [in the brainstem], from which it is conducted by the vagus nerves to the gastric glands; in other words, a reflex is produced

* Gastric secretion from Pavlov's dogs provided a needed financial benefit for his work. The juices were sold in Russia as a remedy for people suffering from the failure of their gastric glands to secrete sufficiently for proper digestion.

which travels from the oral cavity to the gastric glands."

Pavlov found that his point could be proven experiment-ally. He learned how to sever nerves behind the secretory mechanisms without incurring damage fatal to the dog. The animal would continue to eat, but would fail to produce the gastric juices so important for turning food into bodily nourishment.

The most interesting of Pavlov's findings were those on the specific excitability of the mucous membranes of the diges-tive system. It had already been recognized that the nervous system reached out to different kinds of sensors—to cells sensitive to light, in the eye, for example, or sound vibra-tions, in the ear, or pressure, on the skin—and now Pavlov revealed that another intricate sensory system had an amazing facility for gathering information along the tracts of the digestive system. These internal sensors, and the nervous mechanisms behind them, seemed to have the re-markable ability to test, judge, and decide on the disposition of whatever entered the digestive process. The system first decided whether a substance was to be rejected or retained. In the case of retention, it set the digestive mill into motion, with an uncanny sense of exactly how to treat various ma-terials to enhance the process.

"In our observations on dogs," said Pavlov in his Nobel address of 1904, "we soon noticed the following fundamental fact: the kind of substances getting into the digestive canal from the external world, i.e., whether edible or inedible, dry or liquid, as well as the composition of food determined . . . the onset or else absence of the work of the digestive glands, the peculiarities of their functioning in the former case, the amount of reagents produced by them, and their condition."

In other words, Pavlov was saying that his research had found the nervous control of digestion to be an extremely purposeful system. When edible substances were introduced into the mouth, thick, viscous saliva flowed with the proper chemical agents to prepare the food for its trip down the gullet to other stages of digestion. On the other hand, if pure salt, acid, or mustard were placed in the mouth, the saliva flow, while still in quantity, had a very different consistency. It was much more fluid and watery, for the purpose of neutralizing the taste and washing out the oral cavity. Bread, Pavlov noted, produced more secretion than meat in a dog's mouth, although one would think the opposite true since the animal would prefer meat. But purposefulness of the secretion was the key, the Russian scientist found. The bread required more saliva, first to moisten it to help the processes of tasting and testing the food, and second to lubricate the comparatively dry material for its descent to the stomach via the gullet. The more Pavlov and his associates experimented, the more remarkable the purpose-oriented system appeared. Regardless of what was dropped into a dog's mouth, the secretory glands were capable of assessing the material and providing the right juices. Pavlov pointed out that quartz pebbles placed in a dog's mouth prompted no salivation while the animal moved them around and then spat them out. But the same pebbles ground into sand and placed into the dog's mouth caused a liberal flow of watery saliva to help the animal eject the fine particles and clean his mouth. The system was so remarkably purposeful that it seemed "to imply intelligence" in the involved glands, said Pavlov.

Much of this experimental work was covered in Pavlov's Nobel address. By that time, however, he had shifted his focus from the workaday reflexive controls of digestion that he had originally outlined in a famous presentation seven years before. Moreover, the general scientific interest in digestion had moved away from the nervous control of the system, which until 1902 had been considered the sole activating force. That year two English physiologists, William Bayliss and Ernest Starling, had discovered that hormones were also involved, a fact that Pavlov subsequently confirmed in his laboratory. While the thrust of the science turned toward the study of hormonal controls, Pavlov's interests remained strongly committed to the nervous system, where they took an unusual and controversial turn in the opening years of the twentieth century.

He became interested in an unexplained phenomenon observed for ages by laymen and scientists alike when their mouths watered at the smell, sight, or even the thought of a delicious meal. The French physiologist Claude Bernard had noted that the gastric juices of a horse began to flow when the animal had no more than caught sight of a bundle of hay. Pavlov saw the same phenomenon in his dogs prepared for sham feeding. The mere sight or smell of food kept at a distance prompted salivary and gastric secretions. The scientist called the action "psychic secretion," and it became the subject of Pavlov's most intense experimentation.

At this juncture in his career, however, the Russian physiologist encountered some sharp disagreements over the turn he was taking. They came from as far away as Sherrington's laboratory in England, but most surprisingly they occurred in his own laboratory, where one of his closest collaborators, A. T. Snarsky, decided that Pavlov was overstepping the bounds of science to tamper with spiritual matters. The disagreement was later described in a speech by Pavlov, who said:

"He [Snarsky] displayed a quick mind susceptible to the joys and triumphs of investigative thought. How great then was my astonishment when this loyal laboratory friend became truly and deeply indignant when he first heard of our plans to investigate the psychic activities of the dog in this same laboratory and with the same means that we had been using for the solution of various physiological problems. No amount of persuasion could affect him; he predicted and wished us all kinds of failures. And all that, as we could understand him, because in his eyes the sublime and unique phenomena which he assumed to lie in the spiritual realm of

man and higher animals could not be investigated successfully and, furthermore, the crudeness of procedures in physiological laboratories was almost insulting. Admitting that
this particular presentation contains an element of exaggera-
tion, it appears to me however not devoid of the characteristics of certain typical attitudes. We cannot close our eyes
on the fact that a genuine and consistent scientific approach
towards the last boundary of life will not occur without
considerable misunderstanding and resistance on the part
of those who since time immemorial have had a different
approach to this field of natural phenomena and have considered their viewpoint the only acceptable and legitimate
one in this particular case."

Pavlov and Snarsky decided to end their working relationship, as the former explained many years later: "I, astonished
by the fantastic nature and scientific sterility of such an approach to the problem at hand [Snarsky's subjective ap-
proach], sought another solution to this most difficult
situation. After persistent deliberation and a most difficult
mental struggle I finally decided to remain in the role of a
pure experimenter with regard to this so-called psychic excitation and to deal exclusively with external manifestations
and relationships. To carry out this decision I took on a new
collaborator, Dr. I. F. Tolochinov, and our work went on for
20 years with the participation of many of my dear collaborators."

During that period Pavlov worked largely with psychic
secretion evident in his dogs' salivary glands (the submaxil-
lary and the parotid). In most experiments, fistulas were
surgically prepared to intercept the ducts that lead the
juices from the glands to the mouth. Special glass funnels,
cemented to the outer ends of the fistulas, allowed experimenters to count the drops of secretion as they were collected for analysis. Pavlov saw the salivary glands as
beautifully direct, uncomplicated indicators of the animals'
reactions to the external world, at least as they pertain to

food. However, he continued to rely on his earlier techniques —the small stomach, sham feeding, and others—to investigate psychic secretion. His new research soon revealed that he was dealing with a complex, elusive, sometimes paradoxical process, extremely difficult to treat on a sound scientific basis. A few examples may reveal why.

The sight of a piece of beef at a distance would cause a hungry dog's mouth to water—as everyone knew—and it was easy to assume that the salivation would continue, and perhaps increase, the longer the animal was teased with the sight of the meat. But Pavlov's tests proved that repeatedly teasing the hungry dog caused the secretion to decrease gradually until it stopped. The psychic secretion, however, could be restored immediately by feeding the dog a piece of meat; then, upon being teased repeatedly with another piece, the dog would again salivate in decreasing amounts until the secretion had stopped completely.

As he proceeded with these carefully tested observations, the Russian scientist found more tantalizing facts about salivation. For instance, a dog that might have been teased with meat until its psychic secretion for that substance was reduced to zero would salivate very strongly on seeing something else it liked, bread perhaps. Next, teasing with bread would slowly remove the secretion to it. The same was true for milk. One at a time, various foods enjoyed by the dog could be wiped out as stimuli for psychic secretion through the teasing process. But, then, in a moment's time the psychic reaction to the meat, bread, milk, and other foods could be restored simply by feeding the dog one of the substances, or, for that matter, any other food it liked.

The experiments were undoubtedly replete with meaning that might be drawn from an understanding of the underlying mechanisms, but the effort to learn about them was often thwarted by difficulties indigenous to the research itself. First, it was hard to subject the results to valid scientific analysis. Furthermore, evidence was not easily verified through the usual scientific means of reproducing it.

Early in the psychic experiments Pavlov was distressed because he and his workers were so easily inclined to disregard that hallmark of science, objectivity, and to slip into an anthropomorphic approach for explaining secretion. He once said: ". . . we consciously endeavored to explain our results by imagining the subjective state of the animal. But nothing became of this except sterile controversy and individual views that could not be reconciled. And so we could do nothing but conduct the research on a purely objective basis; our first and especially important task was completely to abandon the very natural tendency to transfer our own subjective state to the mechanism of the reaction of the animal undergoing the experiment and to concentrate instead on studying the correlation between the external phenomena and the reaction of the organism."

The problem of duplicating the experiments arose from the fact that the stimulus of psychic secretion—food at a distance—was extremely difficult to isolate as a single, pure activator that could be easily reproduced. Such a stimulus was partly the product of the stage setting around it, and the animal recipient in turn was an audience modulated by a thousand experiences from the past. The food acted via the dog's eyes, ears, nose, and other sensory inputs. The change of a dish could alter the nature of the secretion. Or salivation might result from the sound of a feeder's footsteps in a hall, even though the person was not arriving with food but actually leaving for the night. The sight of a man offering bread could produce the secretion for meat if the person had previously fed the dog meat. Such environmental factors became accessories to the results, and they had to be considered if the evidence was to be reproduced accurately.

To control the stimulus and its environmental influences Pavlov developed some unique testing cubicles. They were double compartments, one for the dog, the other for the investigator. The animal, standing on a platform in its compartment, was held in a fixed, upright position by a harness. Flexible tubes from the dog's fistulas led into the experimenter's compartment, where he could collect, measure, and analyze the secretion. The compartments were arranged so that the dog could be subjected to a number of stimuli remotely controlled by the scientist. A movable shelf could be swung into view of the dog to present it with the sight of various foods. There were also provisions for several other sensory stimuli. A light could be flashed into the animal's eyes. A bell controlled by the experimenter was mounted within earshot of the dog. Scented vapors could be released. And a metronome was available to produce sounds at selected beats.

This arrangement was a model of scientific control, but still Pavlov's work was plagued by extraneous sounds and other environmental factors that infringed upon the experimental results. They came from within and without the building and were finally recognized as uncontrollable unless drastic steps were taken to eliminate them. To meet the problem Pavlov designed a special laboratory building in 1910, although the structure remained unbuilt for several years, until after the coming of the Soviets, who granted Pavlov whatever his research required. The building was constructed in Leningrad, and because of a silo-like appurtenance on one of the four sides, the laboratory became known as the "Tower of Silence," although the tower part of the structure accommodated only a spiral staircase. The building had three floors, the two upper ones resting on steel beams with the ends embedded in sand to dampen vibrations. The walls were exceptionally thick, the heavy plate-glass windows were small, and the hermetically sealed doors were double. The foundation was surrounded by a moat packed with straw to isolate the building from surface vibrations. When completed, the laboratory offered what seemed like the best possible environmental control of temperature, light, sound, and odor for Pavlov's dogs. Indeed, it was even too perfect at times, because the sterile environment itself could become an undesirable stimulus.

In his years of experimentation with the complex subject of psychic secretion, Pavlov provided a sounder scientific basis for the ideas set forth more than a half century earlier by his spiritual master, Sechenov, in *Reflexes of the Brain*. The Pavlovian theories of conditioned reflexes, highly controversial in their own right, added substance to the inflammatory ideas of Sechenov, who proposed that we are essentially a product of reflexes interacting with the universe around us.

Pavlov saw two kinds of reflexes. The first were inborn and constant throughout life. These he thought of as unconditioned because they were present, each ready and able to carry out a particular mission, at the onset of life. The other kind of reflexes were acquired and far less stable. These he called conditioned reflexes, for, in effect, they had to be trained. But once a conditioned reflex was established its future depended upon its treatment. It could be strengthened by use and diminished by disuse, or, in a given time, overridden by a more powerful reflex. Conditioned reflexes, said Pavlov, allowed an organism to meet the ever-changing world around it. And he felt that some could become important enough to be passed along through heredity, thereby becoming unconditioned.

The reflexes so well described by Sherrington in England were, of course, unconditioned, and, as revealed by his decerebrated animals, they were controlled along the spinal cord and brainstem. Pavlov decided that conditioned reflexes were tied to operational sites along the highest region of the brain, the cerebral cortex, which is removed by decerebration. Therefore he concluded that these reflexes, missing from brainless animals, offered a means for doing physiological research on the brain functions of whole and healthy animals. The Russian scientist saw them as a marvelous window through which the investigator standing on the outside could look into higher brain functions from a physiological point of view.

Early in the study of psychic secretion Pavlov learned how to develop and use "artificial conditioned reflexes," of which the most renowned was the classic dog-and-bell experiment. When a dog was repeatedly shown and then given food accompanied by the ringing of a bell, the creature developed a conditioned reflex that would eventually prompt salivation with no more than the sound of the bell. The bell, however, was only one of many stimuli used to condition reflexes artificially. The prick of a pin, the pat of a hand, an electric shock, odors, lights, and many different sounds became artificial stimuli for conditioned reflexes that could be activated even when omitting the food that had helped establish them. The technique allowed Pavlov to isolate conditioned reflexes and the stimuli exciting them. It became a powerful research tool for studying piece by piece the grand mosaic of the brain dealing with the environment. Through hundreds of experiments on what some of his critics called "dribbling dogs," Pavlov and many associates pushed forward the study of the nervous system.

Any attempt to cover a substantial part of Pavlov's work would be far beyond the scope of this chapter, but to illustrate the significance of his contributions to the neurological sciences, one should consider a few of the outstanding concepts that the Russian developed through his stylized look at the brain via the salivary reactions of his famous dogs.

One of the most widely discussed concepts described by Pavlov was called "irradiation and concentration of excitation." Pavlov noted that when a conditioned reflex was first established, it was remarkably undiscriminating toward the stimuli, but it soon changed and became highly selective, narrowing down until it concentrated on a single, specific stimulus.

If a dog heard a metronome used as a stimulus for a conditioned reflex, the animal at first would salivate, not only to that sound, but also to a variety of comparable sounds. This phenomenon was "irradiation of excitation." But if the beat of the metronome was continued as a stimulus, fewer and fewer sounds would excite the conditioned reflex, until only the metronome would produce the reaction. This was "concentration of excitation." Not only might the excitation prompted by the metronome concentrate on the sound in general, but eventually it would focus on a particular beat frequency. Pavlov found he could focus the excitation of a conditioned reflex within a few beats, for instance, 100 per minute, thereby eliminating reactions when the beats were under 95 or over 105 per minute.

Irradiation followed by concentration of excitation worked with other stimuli. A conditioned reflex might be formed, for example, by using the pat of a hand on the dog's left shoulder, but when it was first established, a touch to almost any point on the animal's body would elicit salivation. Then if the shoulder pats were continued as the primary stimuli, excitation of the reflex would narrow down to that particular point, leaving all the others unable to prompt the salivary reaction. With a pin prick the concentration of excitation could be narrowed down to an amazingly small radius on the dog's skin.

Pavlov did not carry his experimentation beyond the point of substantiating the existence of irradiation and concentration, so his explanation of it was mostly supposition. He believed that nervous conductors carried energy from the stimuli "to special, less numerous cells of the lower parts of the central nervous system, as well as the highly numerous special cells of the cerebral hemispheres." He continued: "From there, however, the process of nervous excitation usually irradiates to various cells over a greater or lesser area. This explains why when the conditioned reflex has been elaborated, say, to one definite tone, not only all the other tones, but even many of the other sounds produce the same conditioned reaction. . . . But afterwards the irradiation gradually becomes more and more limited; the excitatory process concentrates in the smallest nervous point of the cerebral hemisphere, probably the group of corresponding special cells. . . ."

Closely entwined with Pavlov's theory of irradiation and concentration was his concept of inhibition. He decided that this was an active rather than passive process. On a simple level he saw how one very strong reflex could inhibit a weaker one. Pain as a stimulus, for example, might inhibit a conditioned reflex excited by odor—hence the dog smells meat he is about to take, and he salivates, but then the sharp snap of a whip on his back excites a reflex conditioned by the stimulus of pain, and the salivation stops because the reflex conditioned by the odor of meat is suddenly inhibited.

On a more complicated level, Pavlov believed his theory of the concentration of excitation represented an active inhibitory process. As the nervous excitation of a conditioned reflex narrowed down to a specific stimulus, Pavlov decided that the stimuli being excluded were actually being suppressed by an inhibitory process. In the process, he concluded, the phenomenon of irradiation was at work on inhibition in a way comparable to its effect on excitation. Hence, when inhibition irradiated, it spread across the broad spectrum of excitation, slowly suppressing all but a single, specific stimulus.

The Russian physiologist supported this idea with an interesting experiment on a dog in which a conditioned reflex had been established so that it responded specifically to a note of 1,000 cycles per second. The excitation had been so finely focused that the reflex would not respond to notes only a few cycles off the thousand mark. In his experiment, Pavlov exposed the animal to a 1,000-cycle note followed promptly by one of 1,010 cycles, then immediately he went back to the 1,000-cycle note. The first sound, as expected, produced salivation, and the second stopped it, but when the 1,000-cycle note was repeated, it failed to excite the reflex for some time. Pavlov explained that the inhibitory process set up with the 1,010 cycles irradiated and temporarily extinguished the excitation caused by the 1,000 cycles.

He demonstrated the same phenomenon on a dog in which a reflex reactive to tactile stimuli on one of the forelegs had been developed. Five specific points in a line along the leg had been used in the experiment. As each of the top four points was touched, the action would excite the reflex and produce salivation. The bottom point, however, had been stimulated tactually without food, so this fifth spot would not produce salivation, having become an inhibitory point. Once it was touched, however, the inhibitory action irradiated to the point directly above, and the response of this spot to stimulation was reduced. Over a period of several minutes the inhibitory effect might spread to two or three points up the dog's leg, and then it would recede, leaving the original state of four reactive points and one inhibitory one.

From his experiments Pavlov formulated a functional picture of the brain, enlarging on that envisioned by Sechenov, who had come to see the organ as one that constantly allowed its owner to interact with his environment, internal and external, and with other organisms of the same or different species. Pavlov seemed to believe that most or all of this interaction was accomplished through reflexes. But he by no means pictured the brain as dealing with a single reflex at a time. He saw a legion of afferent signals arriving to produce a grand mixture of excitation and inhibition of reflexes, some unconditioned, having been born with the animal, and others conditioned out of thousands of experiences derived from upbringing, culture, education, social contacts, and so on. The brain envisioned by Pavlov had the power to make order, moment by moment, out of this maze of signals. He put it as follows:

"Countless stimuli, different in nature and intensity, reach the cerebral hemispheres both from the external world and the internal medium of the organism itself. Whereas some of them are merely investigated . . . , others evoke highly diverse conditioned and unconditioned effects. They all meet, come together, interact, and they must, finally, become systematized, equilibrated, and form, so to speak, a *dynamic stereotype.*"

Pavlov's idea of the brain's functioning comes close to how a modern specialist in brain waves might portray it, although the discovery of the human electroencephalogram (1929) came so near the end of Pavlov's life (1936) that he could have hardly foreseen its present-day potential. He talked about the organ as a mosaic with zones of concentrated activity—here at one moment, there the next—as billions of cells dealt in an integrated fashion with the perpetual task of interacting with an organism's internal and external environment. Pavlov's description of the dynamic process follows:

"If we could see through the cranium, and if the zone of optimum excitability was luminous, we should see, in a man who was thinking, this supposedly luminous point of optimum excitability perpetually moving about. We would watch it continuously changing in shape and size. It would be surrounded by a zone of more or less dense shadow occupying the remainder of the hemispheres."

With such thinking, Pavlov went on to develop theories for the basis of such central nervous states as sleep, hypnosis, temperament, and neurosis.

By observing how various states of drowsiness, down to a deep sleep, affected the dogs' reactions toward food, Pavlov and his colleagues drew some conclusions about the nature of sleep. They decided that sleep is brought on by the general spread of inhibition across the cortex and through cerebral regions directly below. The brain is kept in a state of wakefulness by a constant tug of war between various areas of excitation and inhibition, with neither side winning. As sleep approaches, however, the inhibitory forces gain ground until they are in control of the brain.

"Thus, the alert working state of an animal or of a human

being," explained Pavlov, "is a mobile and at the same time localized process of fragmentation of the excitatory and inhibitory states of the cortex, now in large, now in very small parts; it contrasts with the state of sleep, when inhibition at the height of its intensity and extensity is spread evenly over the whole mass of the cerebral hemispheres, as well as down to a certain level. However, even then there may remain separate excitatory points in the cortex—which are, so to speak, on guard or on duty. Consequently, in the alert state both processes are in permanent mobile equilibrium, as if struggling with each other. If the mass of external or internal stimulations falls off at once, a marked predominance of the inhibitory process takes place over the excitatory. Some dogs, in which the peripheral basic external receptors (visual, auditory and olfactory) are damaged, sleep twenty-three hours a day."

The Russian experimenter believed that the hypnotic state seen in many animals was a protective reflex closely related to sleep. He described it as "the irradiation of a weak inhibitory process . . . ," which he conceived as being able to put parts of the brain to sleep in order to lock the animal into a position for its own protection—the deer, for example, rigidly transfixed in a forest glen as hunters pass. The spread of the inhibitory process leading to the hypnotic state occurred in different degrees and encompassed different areas of the cortex depending on the stimuli.

Another product of Pavlov's extensive observations of his dogs through their alimentary reflexes was his effort to describe different types of nervous systems based on the balance or relative lack of balance between the inhibitory and excitatory processes of the brain. Pavlov concluded that the dogs' nervous systems could be fitted into four categories coinciding with the ancient classification of temperaments set forth by Hippocrates. They were (1) sanguine, (2) choleric, (3) phlegmatic, and (4) melancholic.

". . . there are strong but unequilibrated animals," wrote

Pavlov, "in which both nervous processes are strong, the excitatory process, however, predominating over the inhibitory; this is the excitable, impetuous type, or choleric, according to Hippocrates. Further, there are strong, quite equilibrated but inert animals; this is the inert, slothful type or phlegmatic, according to Hippocrates' classification. Then come the strong, quite equilibrated, but labile animals; this is the lively active type or sanguine. . . . And finally, there is the weak type, which is closest to Hippocrates' melancholic type; the predominant and common feature of this type is quick inhibitability due to internal inhibition that is always weak and easily irradiates, and especially to external inhibition under the action of various, even inconsiderable, accessory external stimuli."

With this kind of observation Pavlov was far from the kind of rigid experimental foundations that had characterized his earlier work. In that work, he remained close to what he could see and prove, but now he was projecting from his extensive knowledge of animal behavior to portray the functioning of the brain as a whole. In so doing he often seemed to be speaking as a psychologist from a sound physiological base. As a result, he was often cited by the behaviorist school of psychology established by an American, John B. Watson, who saw animals and humans as complicated machines activated by a nervous system conditioned by experience. Pavlov's new role left him badly exposed to criticism from both physiologists and psychologists. In his chosen field of physiology, scientists confined themselves to that which could be proven experimentally, which in neurology limited them to an extremely narrow view of the nervous system. They were not supposed to speculate on the workings of the system as a whole, as did Pavlov, and for this he was criticized. On the other hand, the main trend of psychology, established by Freud and Jung, was heavily committed to the concept of a mind separate from the body. Their followers were unlikely to believe that psychology was explainable from a physiological viewpoint, which is what Pavlov was attempting to do. Therefore in this quarter also he was the target of criticism.

Regardless of how his critics felt about the man, none could deny that he was faced with a formidable scientist, an internationally famous Nobel Prize winner. Right or wrong, therefore, his point of view had an impact. It invited physiologists to think more in terms of the nervous system as a whole and its relationship to total behavior. And it invited psychologists to consider that the elusive, mystical thing called "mind" was perhaps grounded in physical matter that might someday be understood through physiological experimentation.

A famous English authority on the brain, W. Grey Walter, wrote in 1953 that until Pavlov's work came along early in the century ". . . there was something like a taboo against the study of the brain." In the laboratories of England, he pointed out, workers ". . . had not permitted themselves to explore further than the top of the spinal cord. One took an anatomical glance at the brain, and turned away in despair." Walter felt that Pavlov's ability to confine his animals to a very limited number of stimuli and then to measure the responses had secured the Russian's success in breaking the taboo against studying the brain.

7

THE LAST OF THE
GALVANOMETERS

At the University of Leiden around the turn of the century a
Dutch physiologist, Willem Einthoven, was studying the
electrical activity of the heart, which had already been detected by John Scott Burdon-Sanderson and Augustus D.
Waller using a capillary electrometer, an ingenious device
for measuring small electric currents. The instrument depended on the differences created in the surface tension between two conducting liquids when a current crossed from
one to the other. But while the electrometer could detect
the tiny currents of a beating heart, it was too sluggish to
follow the organ's comparatively fast electrical variations.
By working out a mathematical method to compensate for
the sluggishness, Einthoven determined the characteristics
of the electrocardiogram with remarkable accuracy.

The method, however, was still an indirect measurement
of the heart currents, and it lacked enough precision to reveal the differences between hearts. Abandoning the capillary electrometer, Einthoven turned to another principle
to develop a more sensitive device. It was known that a varying current traveling through a wire stretched between magnetic poles would cause the wire to vibrate. The rate of
vibration was determined by the wire's tension and the frequency of the electrical variations. Applying this principle,

the Dutch physiologist rebuilt a reflecting galvanometer with a taut wire and optical system so that he could record the shadow of the vibrating wire on a moving film. After three years perfecting the idea, he published the results in 1909, and manufacturers soon built the new "string galvanometer" to Einthoven's specifications. Subsequent models were improved and so was the instrument's sensitivity. In one, the wire was of microscopic diameter, and it vibrated in a vacuum.

Meanwhile, Einthoven used the new galvanometer to record the electrical activity of the heart with considerable precision. He found that everyone's heart has certain common electrical characteristics, and he recognized that an electrocardiogram might reveal clues to heart disease. Einthoven received the Nobel Prize in 1924 for being "the discoverer of the real electrocardiogram."

The new galvanometer was also valuable in nerve physiology. Einthoven used it to study the electrical activity in the retina of the eye and the extremely small currents related to muscle tonus. Other scientists also took advantage of the sensitive device for work in nerve physiology. A Viennese psychiatrist used a string galvanometer to make one of the most remarkable discoveries in the history of brain research, one that we will cover in a later chapter.

While the instrument was a marvel and the key to a Nobel Prize, it was also the culmination of electro-mechanical measuring instruments in nerve physiology. A new age of electrical measurement was appearing, coexistent with the brand-new field of electronics that had grown out of a scientific novelty called "the Edison effect," discovered when the American inventor tried to learn why his lightbulbs were darkened by a carbon deposit on the glass. The discovery became the key to the "thermionic vacuum diode," the radio tube, invented by a British electrical engineer, John Ambrose Fleming. This invention then led the American radio pioneer Lee De Forest to the "thermionic vacuum triode," the basis of electronic amplification. With amplifiers scientists could now magnify currents and voltages of the smallest order into large quantities of electricity that could be recorded easily with a string galvanometer or other electromechanical instruments.

Alexander Forbes of the Harvard Medical School was one of the first physiologists to apply the new amplifier tube to the electrical activity of nerves. His circuit contained a single tube with the input connected to a nerve and the output to a string galvanometer recording upon a moving strip of film.

"This device," Forbes wrote in a 1920 publication, "offers great possibilities of amplifying such action currents in the nervous system as are too small to be recorded satisfactorily with the string galvanometer alone."

"As nearly as we could measure it, the amplified [nerve] current in the string galvanometer was strictly proportional to the e.m.f. [voltage] applied to the grid circuit [input]."

Eight years later an English scientist, Bryan H. C. Matthews of the Cambridge Physiological Laboratory, designed a "moving iron oscillograph" to record amplified nerve currents. It had an electromagnet with an iron tongue holding a small mirror that was vibrated by the electrical changes of amplified nerve impulses. The mirror reflected the light of an arc lamp through a lens and shutter to a whirling mirror and, in turn, onto a sheet of photographic film. When an amplified impulse vibrated the mirror, the shutter was opened for an instant, allowing the film to record the graph-like electrical characteristics of a single impulse. This instrument was an improvement over the string galvanometer.

By 1931 the amplifier with the improved recording devices was revolutionizing electrophysiology. The progress was reviewed by an English scientist and future Nobelist, Edgar D. Adrian, in a lecture at the University of Pennsylvania. "The amount of amplification which can be obtained nowadays is far greater than we are ever likely to need in physiological work," Adrian stated. "For instance, there would be no particular difficulty in demonstrating the potential change in a frog's nerve fiber as an audible signal in the course of a radio lecture. The power available in the input circuit would be of the order of 10^{-14} [.00000000000001] watts, and the transmitting station might radiate 50 kilowatts [50,000 watts] or more. . . .

"It will be seen that we have a method of detecting and recording small electrical changes which is far in advance of anything possible without amplification. We can record far smaller changes and we can record very rapid changes with far greater accuracy than before. It would be a sad confession of failure if with these new resources we had been able to learn nothing fresh about the working of the nervous system, but in fact they have already given us direct evidence on many points and the field now open is so large that it will be a long time before the method has exhausted its usefulness."

The rapid development of thermionics was closely related to another advance that was to contribute another major instrument to the neurological sciences. From the discovery of cathode rays in 1858 by a German mathematician and physicist, Julius Plücker, came the cathode-ray tube and, in the 1920's, the cathode-ray oscillograph. Instead of the sluggish mechanical parts that had impeded the investigation of high electrical frequencies, there was an unfettered electron beam shot from a cathode through a vacuumized tube to a luminescent screen. It could be made to dance in time with electricity applied to coils or plates around the side of the tube, and when their inputs were carefully designed and adjusted, the viewer was presented with a graphlike picture of the wave forms of the varying electrical activity he wished to study.

One of the earliest reports of using the new device in physiology came from Herbert S. Gasser and Joseph Erlanger in the Laboratory of Physiology at Washington University, St. Louis. They amplified currents from frog and rabbit nerves and led them to a low-voltage cathode-ray oscillograph. Gasser and Erlanger said the wave forms could be recorded from the screen photographically or simply by tracing them by hand onto paper. Actually it was some time before good photographic records could be made from the cathode-ray tube; meanwhile mechanical devices, such as Matthews' moving iron oscillograph, were the most dependable recording instruments for amplified nerve currents.

When the cathode-ray oscillograph was perfected, however, it was difficult to surpass. It allowed a scientist to: (1) detect minute voltages and currents, (2) measure both their quantities and their frequencies, and (3) look at intricate wave forms produced at high frequencies. These advantages were tremendously valuable to scientists unlocking secrets of nerve and brain held by tiny, complex electrical patterns constantly changing in form.

A third, and again a parallel, development in electronics further enlarged the neurologist's capabilities by extending his ability to see infinitely small structures at the cell level. Shortly after Santiago Ramón y Cajal did his classic work with the microscope, a German physicist, Ernst Abbe, published a diffraction theory indicating that the instrument had limitations which could not be overcome, regardless of how much its lenses might be improved. Abbe claimed that even the best conceivable microscope could not resolve the fine details of an object if they were separated by less than approximately half the wavelength of the illuminating light. This meant that visible light would prevent seeing details of less than 2,500 angstroms (the angstrom unit, Å, equals .00000010 centimeter). With a biological cell membrane approximately 150 Å thick, scientists limited to light microscopes could never visually comprehend the minute structures of the neuron. Ultraviolet light appeared to offer a solution, except that a microscope developed around it was still limited to a thousand angstroms. X rays also seemed to hold the answer, but refraction problems quickly ended that idea. However, scientists in several fields recognized the possibilities of putting electrons to good optical use. As men learned more about the basic nature of cathode rays, electrons, and light, the knowledge led to a tremendous new instrument in 1931, the electron microscope. It soon uncovered an entirely hidden world for the neurohistologist.

In 1939 a commercial electron microscope exceeded the capabilities of the best light microscope, and a year later the first was sold in the United States by RCA. By the 1960's nearly nine thousand were in use around the world. Their resolving power had steadily improved, and this in turn had forced advances in the preparation of the ultra-thin sections that are so important to viewing ultra-small structures. An electron microscope could resolve structural differences as low as two angstroms for physical materials and four or five for biological samples, which meant that magnification was on the order of hundreds of thousands of times, providing a view of the structural parts in even the smallest brain cells. Then, in the mid-1960's, a remarkable new scanning electron microscope became available commercially. It offered a three-dimensional view of specimens, which, in many cases, made visual interpretation easier and more accurate. At the University of California, Berkeley, a scanning microscope trained on nerve cells allowed investigators to make some valuable three-dimensional photographs of the synaptic junctions between nerve cells magnified twenty thousand times.

The new observational tools, which began appearing around the 1930's, helped move the neurosciences forward at an unprecedented pace. Neurophysiology, the first to profit from the electronic advances, became one of the most exciting and popular branches of the biological sciences. For a while interest in neuroanatomy slackened, and many would-be neuroanatomists were attracted to neurophysiology, but then the electron microscope re-established neuro-anatomy as a leading source of new information on the complex relationships among the warp and weft of brain and nerve tissue. In the same period new chemical understandings of the nervous system were arrived at, and neurochemistry, though off to a rather slow start, became an increasingly important branch of the neurosciences. In all branches of this science, men with different approaches were trying to unravel the same subject, and they had a great deal to gain by working together. While the scientist with electric probes could go far alone in comprehending a neurological function, he might double or triple the distance with help from someone who knew the chemistry involved. The embryologist seeking the natural plan that guides each of a million developing nerves to make exactly the right connections might profit from a histologist who could help him see what actually occurs at various embryogenic stages of the nervous system. And a computer specialist might help all these scientists compare and analyze their data. In short, the need for a multidisciplinary approach and for interdisciplinary communication became imperative as the neurosciences advanced.

Actually, the benefits of fostering such relationships were evident to scientists during the last century, and from their insights came brain research institutes in which neurological experimenters with different interests could individually and collectively enjoy the cross fertilization of ideas cultivated when scientists work close to one another. Three institutes were established late in the nineteenth century—the first in Vienna in 1882 by Heinrich Obersteiner, another about the same time at the University of Leipzig by Paul Flechsig, and a third, the Brain-Anatomical Institute, started in 1886 at Zurich when a young American zoologist, Henry Donaldson, joined Constantin von Monakow, a neurologist, to study the brain of a dog. By 1909 five more centers had been added to the list—the Instituto Cajal in Madrid, the Senckenberg

Neurological Institute of Frankfurt am Main, the Psycho-Neurological Institute at St. Petersburg, the Wistar Institute of Anatomy and Biology in Philadelphia, and the Netherlands Central Institute for Brain Research in Amsterdam.

In 1901 at a meeting in Paris of the International Association of Academies, the International Brain Research Commission was established to encourage governments to support the scientific investigation of the brain and in particular to cultivate multidisciplinary research institutes. In eight years the commission had members in sixteen countries and was associated with the existing institutes. The organization came to an end with World War I, but the international drive to form research institutes remained in force. After the war a number of new ones were founded, and the multidisciplinary approach influenced research in established schools of medicine and neurological hospitals. The most famous institutes to develop following World War I were the following.

▪ The Kaiser Wilhelm Institute for Brain Research was opened in 1931 in a Berlin suburb by two famous neurologists, man and wife, Cecile and Oskar Vogt.

▪ The Moscow Brain Institute also involved Vogt. In 1924, upon the death of Lenin, Vogt was called to Russia to arrange for the study of the leader's brain. The project, established in a former industrialist's mansion, required two and a half years and it resulted in the training of several Russian scientists. When the study was completed, the group gained independent status as the Moscow Brain Institute.

▪ The Montreal Neurological Institute was founded in 1934 under the direction of Wilder Penfield, the renowned neurosurgeon and neuroscientist.

▪ The Burden Neurological Institute was established in Bristol, England, and it became closely associated with the famous neuroscientist W. Grey Walter, a pioneer in the use of the electroencephalogram to study brain processes.

Two of the most famous hospitals connected with brain

research were the National Hospital, Queen Square, London, and the Salpêtrière, Paris. Soon after the National Hospital opened in 1860, it became associated with such famous nineteenth-century neurological scientists as Sir David Ferrier, John Hughlings Jackson, and Sir Victor Horsley. The Salpêtrière was established in 1656. Its most famous nineteenth-century practitioner was Jean-Martin Charcot, who did his classic work in neurology at the institution. Both of these hospitals, with their valuable records and hundreds of patients suffering a wide variety of neurological malfunctions, continue to play an important role in the study of the nervous system.

The development of brain research in multidisciplinary institutes was comparatively slow in the United States. One of the earliest and most famous institutes was established at Northwestern University Medical School under the direction of Stephen W. Ranson. It was founded in 1928, but the Northwestern Institute of Neurology lived only as long as its director, who died in 1942. When it was closed, another was established in Chicago, the Neuropsychiatric Institute of the University of Illinois Medical School. The research center that comes closest to being a national brain institute was established by the U.S. Public Health Service after World War II in Bethesda, Maryland, as a joint research venture between the National Institute of Mental Health and the National Institute of Neurological Diseases and Blindness. And one of the world's best examples of multidisciplinary brain research was developed at the University of California, Los Angeles, where the diverse efforts were formally drawn together as a major institute in 1961. When it opened, the UCLA Brain Research Institute was staffed by sixty-seven top scientists. The new center was representative of fourteen university departments and divisions, including anatomy, history of medicine, infectious diseases, biophysics, neurology, neurosurgery, pathology, pediatrics, pharmacology, physiological chemistry, physiology, psychiatry, psychology, and zoology. As the institute was inaugurated, its director, John D. French, illustrated the "interdepartmental attack upon problems" by describing a current research project wherein neurophysiologists were benefiting from applied mathematics, communication engineering, and computer analysis.

"This study," said Dr. French, "recognizes the current developments in these fields which render obsolete older methods of treating such data as EEG tracings or oscilloscopic recordings. Mathematicians, engineers and computer specialists join with neurophysiologists in attacking these problems collaboratively by employing skills of the physical and biological sciences which, in the recent past, would hardly have been considered complementary."

In the 1950's the multidisciplinary needs of the neurological sciences were also recognized in communication programs planned on an international scale. Symposia with participants from numerous disciplines and laboratories all over the world were held to discuss various phases of the science of the nervous system. Some of the best-known symposia were brought about by the Josiah Macy, Jr., Foundation with the American Institute of Biological Sciences. The Macy conferences gathered together world leaders in the neurological sciences for meetings centered on carefully selected topics. The participants, no more than twenty-five per conference, were chosen from the various disciplines relevant to the topics under discussion. None of the usual scientific papers were presented, for all communication came through informal talks guided by a discussion leader. Transcriptions of the discussions were edited and published. A similar series of conferences was developed under the sponsorship of the Massachusetts Institute of Technology through the Neurosciences Research Program. In the 1960's important leaders from neurologically related fields assembled at the frequently held MIT work sessions, which were covered in reports on what developed.

"At any such Work Session," explained a paper on these meetings, "twelve to twenty experts in a field important to the neurosciences try to sharpen understanding of its issues, advances, problems, and approaches, both by surveying the state of the art in that field and by reviewing its major finding and ideas . . . The fields are drawn from an extensive domain of disciplines and levels, including psychology, biology, anatomy, physiology, biochemistry, biophysics, physical chemistry, mathematics, and subspecialties of these broad disciplines."

In 1957 neurological scientists established the World Federation of Neurology, another international means for dissemination of the rapidly increasing mass of information about the nervous system. Its headquarters are in Belgium, and it has member organizations in many countries. A 1960 report on the federation stated that its central mission ". . . is to serve as an integrating force and information exchange center for neurological and other medical sciences. . . ."

From Galvani's time on, knowledge of the nervous system has increased at speeds determined largely by the rate of technological innovations. It was comparatively slow in the last century and the first decades of this century; however, the early accomplishments were stupendous when one considers the limitations imposed upon neurological scientists by primitive tools such as the early galvanometers. In recent decades, especially with the coming of electronics, the rate of innovation has increased rapidly, and with their amazing new tools, neuroscientists have moved to the most important and formidable of all scientific frontiers, that which still lies between body and mind.

8

THE MAGNIFIED MESSAGES

Neurophysiologists were fascinated in 1930 by a report in the *Journal of Experimental Psychology* from two Princeton University scientists, Ernest Glen Wever and Charles W. Bray. They had opened up the skull of an anesthetized cat and attached a copper hook to its auditory nerve. The hook was connected by a shielded cable to a powerful amplifier with a telephone receiver in a nearby soundproof room. The Wever-Bray paper claimed that a person speaking into the cat's ear could be heard in the telephone receiver with such fidelity that he was easily identified. Even a whisper in the ear was audible in the telephone. The authors concluded that their copper hook was tapping electrical messages carried by the auditory nerve from the ear to the brain.

The "Wever-Bray effect" stirred wide controversy. Was it really possible that electrical interpretations of a sound wave could be intercepted between the ear and the brain, as though the nerve were a telephone wire? Some doubting scientists suspected that currents were generated by mechanical pressures in the cochlea and were leaking off through nearby tissue to the hook. Wever and Bray felt their experiment was too well controlled for this to happen. They were supported when other laboratories duplicated their results. Then some of their most eminent critics, like two world-renowned English physiologists at Cambridge, agreed that the conclusions of the Princeton men were valid. Finally, however, Wever and Bray became their own most damaging critics. They decided the currents did originate in the cochlea and leak off to the hook—which was later proven to be correct. It was not until 1954 that a Japanese scientist first succeeded in tapping the real currents that bear messages along the auditory nerve.

Although Wever and Bray were wrong, scientists of the day wouldn't have been too surprised to find they were right. In the two decades between World Wars I and II many remarkable advances were made in understanding the nerve impulse as a message carrier. The most important contributions came from physiologists who recorded the intricate variety of patterns in nerve currents magnified by the radio amplifier. The best known included Alexander Forbes at the Harvard Medical School, Edgar Adrian of Cambridge University, and Joseph Erlanger and Herbert Gasser at Washington University Medical School, St. Louis. All four lifted nerve physiology off a plateau where it had settled down for lack of instruments of sufficient sensitivity to probe the unknown.

One of the most significant advances came from understanding the "all-or-none" principle of nervous conduction. Since du Bois-Reymond had described the electrical activity of nerves, scientists had assumed that the impulses carried the nervous system's messages, but how they did it was a mystery. It was recognized, however, that an active nerve transmitted a series of impulses, with each impulse followed by a brief refractory period in which no electrical activity could occur. The combined time of a single impulse and refractory period was only a few thousandths of a second, so in a full second a long train of impulses might move along a nerve. The impulses reminded observers of the dots and dashes of Morse Code, with its short and long impressions, but as improvements of the last century's comparatively primitive instruments came along, scientists recognized that nerve impulses were not dots and dashes, but dots of equal length.

This phenomenon was seen by Francis Gotch, one of England's foremost authorities on nerve physiology. He was trying to determine if a relationship existed between the time duration of a nerve impulse and the intensity of an electric shock stimulating it to act. He learned that regardless of the size of the stimuli each of the resulting impulses lasted the same time as all other impulses. However, Gotch noticed that larger stimuli prompted larger impulses, even though their time durations were constant. The explanation, he suggested, might be found in the structure of a nerve, which is like a trunkline with a bundle of fibers, each being an axon of a nerve cell. Gotch proposed that a weak stimulus sent fewer fibers into action than a strong stimulus, and as the strength of the stimuli increased, more and more fibers came into action, one adding to another to form one large, single impulse.

He was close to the idea of the all-or-none principle. His proposal suggested that, regardless of the stimulus, a single cell (i.e. fiber) always reacted in the same way. Upon stimulation it gave its all or nothing—no minimum or medium activity, only a maximum effort if anything happened at all.

The idea was not new. It had already been described for the heart by America's first full-time professor of physiology, Henry Pickering Bowditch of Harvard. He had found that when the heart was subjected to electric shocks in varying strengths it responded with the same force regardless of the stimulus. Both an English and an American scientist also had evidence that the all-or-none principle applied to skeletal muscle fibers, which have much in common with nerve fibers.

At Harvard early in World War I Forbes and a medical student, Alan Gregg, conducted experiments that indicated the all-or-none principle applied to nerves. It had been assumed that electrical activity prompted in peripheral nerves by signals from the brain and spinal cord would differ from activity stimulated electrically in an isolated preparation of nerves in the laboratory. But Forbes and Gregg showed that it made no difference. What happened in a nerve, whether stimulated naturally or artificially, was always the same. This finding again indicated that nerve fibers gave all or nothing regardless of the stimuli.

But the principle could not really be proven in a nerve until someone could measure the electrical activity of a single fiber, which meant dealing with a few millivolts (thousandths of a volt) persisting for only a few thousandths of a second. In the days before the amplifier this electrical activity was far too small and much too fast for existing measuring devices. Unable to reach definitive proof, scientists held a number of conflicting views about the nature of nerve activity among the fibers of a nerve trunk. There was, for example, controversy about how the impulses were spaced as they proceeded along a nerve fiber. Some authorities felt they came fast upon one another; others were convinced that the frequency was comparatively low. And while there was evidence to favor the all-or-none principle for nerves, the proof of measurement still lay in the future with men like Adrian.

In the English physiologist's classic work, he and his co-workers experimented on the peripheral nerve trunks of small animals, like frogs and cats. They used two experimental preparations designed to get at the electrical activity in single nerve fibers in the trunklines, one for motor nerves carrying impulses from the central nervous system out to the muscles, the second for sensory nerves transmitting impulses into the central system. In the motor nerves the experimenters had no way of stimulating a single fiber from within the animal; they had to depend on natural stimuli and then somehow isolate a single fiber to analyze the impulses it carried. Adrian and a colleague, Detlev W. Bronk, accomplished this by gingerly slicing down across nerve after nerve until in one they would succeed in severing all but a single fiber. The impulses picked up from such a nerve preparation could then be analyzed, since they were the electrical activity of the only one of the trunkline's many fibers with a closed circuit. Adrian spoke of spending "many hours in this tedious pursuit, for it is the only way of dealing with the motor fibers.

"With the sensory nerve fibers," he explained, "it is usually much better to leave the nerve alone and try to arrange matters so that only one end organ [a receptor of the senses] will be thrown into action by the stimulus."

To accomplish this, the scientists sought out simple nervous systems where single fibers led away from single sensory end organs. Such was available in a toe muscle of the frog. In other animals, single endings were found in the skin. In any instance, the stimulus was a tiny pinch of the skin, the stretch of a muscle, or the tweak of a single hair—all done at points known to connect with only one sensory fiber. In both the motor and sensory preparations an intact section of the nerve was connected to the input of an amplifier that picked up impulses from the single fiber and recorded them with a special oscillograph on a moving strip of photographic film.

These intricate experiments led Adrian and his co-workers to a number of conclusions about the messages borne by the impulses coursing through millions of fibers forming the trunklines of the nervous system. The findings had something to say about the way the sending stations function in the sensory endings of peripheral nerves. And the work added to the fundamental knowledge of how the nerve cell functions.

First the English scientist clearly established the all-or-none principle of the nerve fiber. "When a nerve is stimulated electrically," explained Adrian, "the potential [voltage] change in each fibre is of fixed magnitude and duration; it depends only on the state of the fibre and not on the strength of the stimulus which set it in motion."

This was evident to anyone who studied Adrian's oscillograph recordings. Each looked like the blade of a saw with sharp, spike-like teeth representing the impulses moving through the nerve fiber. The vertical dimensions of the spikes, which indicated the strength of the impulses, were all equal, and the shapes were alike, revealing that one pulse was characteristic of the next. The similarities in size and shape remained throughout a recording, even though the experimenter changed the strength of the stimulus. In one test, stimulation was varied by stretching the muscle of a frog's toe at different rates, yet the sizes and shapes of the recorded spikes remained the same. Such results provided the long-awaited experimental proof of the nerve cell's all-or-none characteristic.

The changing amounts of stimulation, however, did have one important effect on the impulses. Larger amounts of stimulation increased the numbers of spikes per second. In one experiment on a sensory fiber from a frog's toe, seven impulses were recorded in 0.1 second when the toe was stretched just a little, but as tension was increased, the number of spikes nearly doubled for the same split second. The impulse frequency was also affected by the rate at which a stimulus increased, i.e., the more rapid the increase, the higher the frequency of recorded spikes. In these phenomena, Adrian and his associates uncovered what could be part of a message-carrying code for the nervous system.

"The nerve fibre is clearly a signalling mechanism of limited scope," explained Adrian. "It can only transmit a succession of brief explosive waves, and the message can only be varied by changes in frequency and in the total number of these waves. Moreover, the frequency depends on the rate of development of the stimulus, as well as on the intensity; also the briefer the discharge the less opportunity will there be for signalling by change of frequency. But this limitation is really a small matter, for in the body the nervous units do not act in isolation as they do in our experiments. A sensory stimulus will usually affect a number of receptor organs, and its result will depend on the composite message in many nerve fibres. A good example of this is to be found in the discharge which passes up the nerve from the carotid sinus at each heart beat. Bronk and Stella [who were associated with Adrian] have shown that as the blood pressure rises, the impulses in each nerve fibre increase in frequency and more and more fibres come into action."

This principle was also evident when Adrian and his associates analyzed the efferent signals of motor nerves. As a motor nerve signaled for a muscular contraction, it began with a low impulse frequency in each fiber, five or ten per second, and increased to forty or fifty per second. When the frequency approached the maximum in one fiber, another fiber came into action, and its impulses started ascending the frequency range. And so it would go, bringing fiber upon fiber into action and, in turn, innervating more and more muscle cells until the contraction was accomplished.

As other scientists experimented on other nerve fibers, they found essentially the same message system at work. In 1934, for example, Haldan K. Hartline (a Nobel Prize winner of 1967) recorded impulses that came from an optic-nerve fiber of a horseshoe crab. For stimulation he exposed the crab's eye to one-second flashes of light with different intensities. At a relatively high level of light the recordings revealed some twelve nerve impulses per fifth of a second. As the intensity was reduced, the number of impulses per fifth of a second dropped until the level was too low to fire the nerve cell at all. Regardless of the frequency of the impulses, they remained the same size and shape, in keeping with the all-or-none principle.

One of the most important scientific accomplishments to come from Adrian's laboratory was the description of a phenomenon that his amplifiers helped perceive in the peripheral sensory endings, at such receptors as those sensing pressure, heat, cold, pain, and muscular movement. Observing signals from these endings, Adrian and his collaborators formulated the concept of "adaptation."

The phenomenon had actually been recognized for a long time, since physiologists had realized that if a constant flow of electric current were applied as a nerve stimulus, it would produce only a single impulse regardless of how long the stimulus lasted. To produce a train of impulses, a stimulus had to be constantly changing. Furthermore, the rate of change had to be within a certain critical range if the train were to continue. Therefore, it was said that a nerve "adapts" to a stimulus by first responding, but then ceasing, although the stimulus persists. The phenomenon was scientifically explained with a series of remarkable recordings made by Adrian and his co-workers during the 1920's. Using experimental animals, they recorded signals from deep-seated receptors within the limb muscles related to posture. When an animal's posture changed, the recordings revealed that afferent impulses were transmitted, but they quickly stopped once a new posture was established. Thus the muscle sensors adapted to each new position and remained inactive until the posture changed again. Other sensory endings showed the same kind of response. Tension applied to a hair by pulling it caused a related sensory ending to transmit a burst of impulses, which quickly ended even though the tension remained. Adrian predicted that adaptation was a general phenomenon to be found with sensory receptors all over the nervous system, and he was later proved correct.

With this work the English physiologist scientifically described one of the great marvels of the nervous system. It is crucial to our sensing the world around us without being inundated by the millions of signals streaming in upon us every split second of a lifetime. Adaptation allows us to sense change in our environment, but once the notification has been made, the signals fade. The warm bath upon immersion seems unbearable, but if the bather waits awhile, the skin's sensory receptors adapt and the temperature feels normal. Let the bath burn, however, and the process doesn't work. Pain is a phenomenon for which adaptation doesn't and shouldn't apply. Here the signals are obviously calling for action against the cause of the discomfort; therefore, adaptation would overrule the very purpose of pain. In fact, we now know that adaptation has many variations, which range from some receptors that don't adapt at all to others that adapt with great rapidity. Those in between reveal a wide variety of adaptation needs—each according to the demands placed on it by the function it serves.

Adrian shared the Nobel Prize for Physiology or Medicine in 1932 with Sir Charles Sherrington. In the presentation speech, Professor G. Liljestrand of the Royal Caroline Institute said: "Adrian's investigations have given us a highly important insight into the question of the nerve principle and the adaptability of the sense organs. In reality they open new paths within important fields which have only to a slight extent been accessible for research hitherto."

Twelve years later another Nobel Prize went to the two American physiologists Erlanger and Gasser, and the presentation speaker, Ragnar Granit, said that theirs was the third of three "milestones in the development of our knowledge of nerve physiology." The first was established by du Bois-Reymond and Helmholtz, the second by Adrian.

The Washington University scientists were pioneers in the use of both the amplifier and cathode-ray oscillograph. In 1922 they were the first to photograph the electrical response of a nerve from a cathode-ray tube, which was remarkably faithful in tracing the wave form of a nerve impulse. With their new-found measurement techniques Erlanger and Gasser experimented with the nerves of small animals and made some of the most fundamental discoveries in nerve physiology.

For some time scientists had been aware that the composite impulse recorded from the many impulses running simultaneously through a nerve trunkline was not a single, simple spike. Instead, the wave form consisted of a spike trailing off into a series of different elevations. This indicated that the spike did not represent a single, smooth increase in electrical potentials followed by a comparable decrease. This was unexplainable until the two St. Louis scientists made a fundamental discovery about the conduction of nerve impulses along the axons of nerve cells.

Erlanger and Gasser recognized from their recordings that impulses did not always travel at the same velocity over different nerve fibers, and that the speed was determined by the diameter of a fiber. Essentially they found that large fibers allow impulses to move faster than smaller ones. The scientists assigned all nerve fibers to one of three categories, which they labeled A, B, and C. They described A fibers, the largest, as those that conduct impulses at velocities from five to one hundred meters per second. B fibers, the medium sizes, carry impulses from three to fourteen meters per second. And C fibers, the finest, work at speeds of two meters per second and below. The three categories covered fiber diameters as high as twenty-two microns for the A group to as low as 0.3 micron for C fibers (one micron is a millionth of a meter).

This discovery said a great deal about the wave form of a nerve's composite impulse. While scientists had thought of it as the sum of many fibers firing together, Erlanger and Gasser revealed that at most points along a nerve trunk the fibers do not fire together. The scientists found that when a nerve was electrically stimulated at one end, it set off impulses that momentarily traveled together, but soon some gained on others, because of the differences in velocity determined by different fiber sizes in a single trunkline. Thus at a point out along the trunk, the wave form of the composite impulse broadened out from the relatively sharp spike created when impulses were traveling together near the starting point. At the distant point the rear of the spike flattened out into a series of different elevations dropping off to zero. This after-part of the wave form was named the "after potential."

The investigations by the Washington University scientists revealed that different-size fibers had different functions in the message-carrying duties of the nervous system. For example, the messages of pain are comparatively slow, since they travel on fibers of small diameter, but motor transmissions prompting muscular movements travel at relatively high velocities over larger fibers. Think of these differences in terms of a person stepping on a sharp object. The sensory signals arriving at the spinal cord from the foot quickly lead to the return of motor signals that force a reflexive contraction of muscles to withdraw the foot. Meanwhile, the original sensory impulses proceed on up the spinal cord to the brain to inform the individual of the accident and permit him to take evasive action or to do anything else necessary beyond the reflexive act. Last of all, the person feels the pain, relayed by the slowest impulses from the injury. Gasser described the injured foot incident as follows:

"The first report would come to the spinal cord in about 13 milliseconds; two milliseconds later impulses would be on their way out over the motor nerves, and only 10 milliseconds later (on the basis of data obtained in animal experiments) would the first impulses arrive at the brain at the level of the medulla. In the meantime, impulses would be approaching the cord over some of the more slowly conducting lines. The first of the impulses capable of arousing a sensation of pain would require 40 milliseconds to reach the cord, and the sensation itself would be felt only after a half a second. . . . Even at that time, however, the first impulses over the slowest fibres would not yet have reached the cord. The fastest impulses in the slow pain system would require three-quarters of a second, and the slowest about a second and a half."

The time ratios discovered by Erlanger and Gasser were of great importance for understanding the nervous system. Consider that signals from a combination of several cells working in unison may act upon another single cell via synapses, and they either cause it to react or they inhibit it, thereby reducing the possibility of a reaction. The single cell in turn may be part of another network of many neurons directing impulses at still another single neuron. And when one remembers that these arrangements are repeated billions of times in the central nervous system, one may begin to sense why the varying velocities of nerve fibers become a crucial factor. The differences in millionths of a second in the times that impulses take to reach the synapses between many transmitting neurons and a single receiving cell become crucial as to whether the latter cell shall act, remain inactive, or be inhibited toward electrical activity. So the diameter of fibers plays a key role in the message-carrying system of the nerves. In a sense a fiber could even be an involved part of the message itself because it may determine how far and where a signal shall travel.

In Professor Granit's presentation speech awarding the Nobel Prize of 1944 to Erlanger and Gasser "for their discoveries concerning the highly differentiated properties of single nerve fibers," he pointed out that "their achievement was not born, fixed and armoured, in the manner of the birth of Pallas Athene. But no sooner had their first result given them the key word than discovery followed hard upon discovery until their colleagues everywhere in the world came to realize that a great new synthesis had been born to nerve physiology. This synthesis is based on new facts, well-hardened by a masterly technique cementing them into a groundwork on which will be erected whatever structure the future has in store for the physiology of the central and peripheral nervous system."

In the 1930's new discoveries led to another important principle of nervous conduction. They were made in Tokyo, chiefly through work on isolated single fibers of the Japanese toad. The scientists responsible were M. Kubo, S. Ono, and I. Tasaki. Their results provided a basis for understanding "saltatory conduction" in what had long been known as "myelinated" fibers.

The fibers had been recognized in the nineteenth century after the German zoologist Theodor Schwann found and described a special cell that now bears his name. The "Schwann cell" wraps itself around a portion of an axon of a nerve cell to form a covering called the "myelin sheath." Over the length of a fiber, several Schwann cells each provide a segment of the total sheath. Between the segments there are distinct breaks, first described in 1878 by the French histologist Louis Antoine Ranvier, and subsequently named the "nodes of Ranvier." The myelin sheath is found in most peripheral nerves, while myelination in the central nervous system is less well known. It appears, however, that such coverings do exist centrally, but as products of cells other than Schwann cells. Finally, myelinated fibers are unique to vertebrates, but not all vertebrate fibers are so covered. Incidentally, the experiments described in the past several pages were conducted on unmyelinated fibers.

For many years the functions of the myelin sheath were not understood and, for that matter, are not fully comprehended even today. But one essential function was found just before and during World War II. In 1925 an American scientist, Ralph S. Lillie, suggested that when a myelinated nerve conducted an impulse, the electrical activity occurred only at the nodes of Ranvier and the impulse proceeding along a fiber skipped from one node to the next. The word "saltatory," which means to move in leaps, was adopted to describe the action. Lillie's idea that the discontinuous action occurred only at the nodes of Ranvier contrasted with the theory of continuous action of an unmyelinated fiber, which maintained that an impulse at any part of an axon prompted activity in the region immediately adjacent and thus spread over the length of the fiber.

Evidence in support of Lillie's theory came from experiments performed in the 1930's, first by Kubo and Ono, and then by Tasaki. Kubo and Ono used a variable electrical stimulus applied with an electrode so fine that its point affected only a tiny segment along the surface of an isolated myelinated nerve fiber. Depending on where their electrode contacted the fiber, the Japanese scientists discovered that a varying amount of stimulus was required to excite the nerve. The least was required when an electrode was over a node of Ranvier, and the most when it was on the myelin sheath between two nodes. Tasaki improved upon the experiment and definitely verified that an electrical stimulus was most effective if applied at a node. Obviously the sheath between two nodes acted as a partial insulator, at least to the direct current of the stimulus.

The importance of the nodes compared to the sheathed areas between them (internodes) was further demonstrated by another kind of experiment conducted by Tasaki and co-workers. In previous tests on unmyelinated fibers it had been established that when certain "blocking agents," such as cocaine and urethane, were applied to a nerve, they interfered with the conduction of impulses. The Japanese experimenters applied these agents to myelinated fibers and found that electrical activity was reduced only when a blocking substance was applied to the nodes of Ranvier. It made no difference when applied to internodes. In subsequent years many blocking agents, including ultraviolet light, were found to affect nodes but not internodes.

While these experiments revealed that the nodes of Ranvier were the electrically sensitive parts of a myelinated fiber, they did not directly prove that impulses leaped from one node to the next. However, the direct evidence soon came from some complex experiments conducted on a motor fiber of the Japanese toad by Tasaki and another Japanese scientist, T. Takeuchi. They arranged about five millimeters of a single fiber so that it extended through three pools of Ringer solution (a nutrient preparation capable of keeping

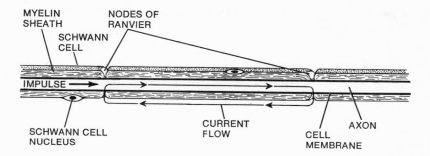

Diagram of a nerve cell's myelinated axon to illustrate saltatory conduction. Electrical activity across membrane occurs only at nodes of Ranvier so that current flows around myelin sheath between nodes. A length of axon can have many nodes, so, in effect, impulse jumps from node to node.

the fiber alive). Each pool was electrically insulated from the other two. The dimensions of the setup were such that a fiber, with slight adjustments, could be placed in either of two ways: (1) with a node of Ranvier in each of the three pools, or (2) with a node in the two outer pools and an internode in the center one. With three electrodes, one touching the fiber in each of the three pools, the scientists recorded the electrical characteristics of the double combination of isolated nerve sections. From their results they were able to prove that an impulse generated in a myelinated fiber traveled by means of the saltatory conduction suggested by Lillie some seventeen years previously. But the proof was arrived at in Japan and published in Germany during World War II (1941 and 1942), so it was several years before the findings were generally known to the world's scientists.

Saltatory conduction is essential to vertebrate nervous systems because it provides small nerve fibers with the capability of conducting impulses at relatively high speeds—which is essential where large numbers of fibers must extend long distances. This demands that nerves be both small and capable of high conduction velocities, so the myelinated fiber with saltatory conduction is the answer. It has the speed of a large fiber but the economy of space of a small fiber. We now know that the myelinated nerve conducts impulses twenty to twenty-five times faster than the unmyelinated one of comparable size. In a mammal the conduction speed of a myelinated fiber is about 225 miles per hour, which means that an impulse can travel from a man's head to his toe in about one fiftieth of a second.

In the decade and a half following World War II numerous studies of the myelin sheath were made with the electron microscope, and the investigators added considerably to the knowledge of the nerve cell covering. In peripheral nerves, it turned out that the sheath of an axon is a series of membranes extending from the Schwann cell and wrapping themselves spirally around the fiber, layer upon layer, so that the completed sheath is laminated. The electron microscopists found that a myelinated axon may be wrapped with more than one hundred spiral laminations, one tightly squeezed against the next. In the 1950's and the early 60's electron microscope studies on the central nervous systems of cats, mice, and rats revealed that myelin sheaths are formed by "glial cells," which surround and support the neurons. It was observed that flattened extensions of these cells, which outnumber nerve cells ten to one, surround adjacent axons.

As scientists continue their studies of the myelin sheath, one of the more important benefits is likely to be realized in clinical medicine. Among the most serious malfunctions of the nervous system are the "demyelinating diseases." The best known, multiple sclerosis, affects a quarter million or more Americans, most of whom are afflicted between twenty and forty years of age. With multiple sclerosis the myelin sheaths on nerve fibers of the brain and spinal cord disappear in scattered patches and are replaced by hard fibrous tissue. This damages the basic cable qualities of the fibers, the nerve messages go wrong, and the victim suffers from symptoms such as shaking or tremor, general weakness, and progressive paralysis. Several theories on the cause of multiple sclerosis exist, but none have been verified. Some interesting studies have revealed that the person whose childhood was spent in colder climates has a greater chance of suffering multiple sclerosis than one who grew up in a warm climate. No one knows why. Many treatments—from medicines to diets—have been tried, but none has been consistently successful. The only solution is to help the victim live as normally as possible. Physical therapy may be useful. Rehabilitation helps some victims regain lost skills through special training. Meanwhile a worldwide research effort is attempting to find the true cause in hopes the knowledge will lead to prevention or a cure.

Men like Adrian, Erlanger, Gasser, and their fellow scientists in Japan mined fundamental knowledge of the most crucial functions of nerves. In a system laid out by natural design to be the most complex communication network likely to be known, these men dealt with the messages, and they discovered some of the system's basic procedural rules for the electrical transmission of information. While they were at work, other researchers were dealing with much the same problem from a chemical point of view. Their efforts were to be equally important.

9

FROM ELECTRICAL TO CHEMICAL

One afternoon in April 1943 in Basel, Switzerland, Albert Hofmann, an organic chemist, suddenly and unexplainably went berserk in his laboratory and had to be carried home. Until he was put to sleep with the help of a sedative, the chemist was the victim of strange hallucinations, illusions, and other psychotic symptoms. The next morning, his sanity restored, Hofmann returned to his laboratory to seek the cause of this weird spell. He had decided it must have had something to do with a new compound he had been using. It was d-lysergic acid diethylamide, better known as LSD, and the chemist suspected he might have accidentally swallowed some. To test his theory he placed a quarter milligram of LSD in a glass of water and drank it. Again he went out of his mind and had to be taken home.

Hofmann's accidental "trip," the first known pharmacological effects of LSD on a normal human being, led to nearly fifteen hundred investigations over the next fifteen years as scientists sought the pharmacological facts about the drug. At the same time the chemist's experience initiated a revolution in psychiatric thought. Controversies arose on two major fronts, one around the LSD experience as a model of schizophrenia, and the second around the use of the drug as a tool for exploring the mind, and for altering personality and behavior.

142

The strange incident in Basel came at a time of great scientific interest in the chemical activity of the nervous system, a subject that had received worldwide attention over the preceding twenty years. The two leading figures in the events that opened up this field were Otto Loewi, an Austrian physiologist, and Henry Hallett Dale, an English biologist. In the 1920's and 30's Loewi and Dale began settling the question of how electrical activity is transmitted from one nerve cell to another or from a cell to a muscle fiber. Their work was of such fundamental importance that they were jointly awarded the 1936 Nobel Prize for Physiology or Medicine.

For three quarters of a century, from the time when du Bois-Reymond characterized the nerve impulse, most scientists had assumed that an impulse proceeded from cell to cell, or cell to muscle by electrical transmission. The assumption, however, had been seriously questioned almost as soon as it was made. About 1850 the French physiologist Claude Bernard made an observation that undermined the electrical transmission idea.

Bernard was experimenting with curare, the South American Indian arrow poison, to learn if a muscle might be excited independently of its nerve supply. He paralyzed a frog with the poison and then isolated a muscle along with a connecting nerve. Bernard found that electrical stimulation applied directly to the muscle caused a contraction, but when applied to the nerve, it failed to produce a muscle contraction. From this result he deduced that the poison blocked the electrical transmission from the nerve to the muscle. Further experiments showed the French scientist that curare did not affect a nerve's ability to conduct an impulse along its own fibers, which supported his feeling that the transmission-blocking phenomenon occurred at the nerve-muscle junction.

Bernard's work stirred interest in the influence of drugs on nerves, and other experimenters sought other drugs that might affect nervous action. One that caught attention was nicotine. A small amount applied to a nerve-muscle preparation caused a muscular contraction. However, if curare was then added, it stopped the muscular response. Curare produced the same results if the muscular contraction was being elicited by electrical stimulation of the nerve instead of an application of nicotine. About 1910 an investigator found that when nicotine droplets were applied at various points on a muscle fiber, their contraction-producing capabilities varied with the size of the drops, or with the distance at which they were placed from the nerve-muscle junction—the larger the drop the larger the contraction, or the nearer the junction the larger the contraction. But when the experimenter mixed curare with the drops, the poison had little of its usual adverse effect on contractions if the drops were applied at a distance from the junction; the muscle reacted to the nicotine as always. Near the junction, however, the nicotine mixed with the arrow poison reduced or stopped the muscular response. From these results it was decided that either electrical or nicotine action produced some kind of chemical activity at the nerve-muscle junction, an action that could be blocked by curare.

All these experiments raised doubts about nervous transmission being totally electrical. Two of the doubters were du Bois-Reymond and his foremost student, Julius Bernstein, who became one of Europe's leading neurophysiologists. But despite these doubts, the electrical theory remained strong for decades, as illustrated by the Croonian lecturer of 1888, Wilhelm Kühne, who flatly stated: "A nerve only throws a muscle into contraction by means of its currents of action."

Indeed, the assumption stood up until 1921, when in the middle of one night an interesting thought occurred to Otto Loewi, the Austrian physiologist, as he suffered from insomnia. According to his own account, the idea for an intricate physiological experiment came to his restless mind at three a.m. Loewi wrote down his thoughts and went back to sleep, only to find the next day that he couldn't read the handwriting. At the same hour the following night the idea returned to the sleepless physiologist, and this time he went directly to his laboratory to perform an experiment that was to become a classic in nerve physiology.

It involved a preparation with two frogs' hearts. In one, the cardiac branch of the parasympathetic vagus nerve, which acts to inhibit the heart muscle and reduces the amplitude and frequency of the beat, was severed. In the other it was left intact. A portion of Ringer's solution, the nutrient fluid, was introduced into the chambers of both hearts. First Loewi electrically stimulated the vagus fibers of the heart in which the nerve was intact, and then he transferred some of the Ringer's solution from that heart to the second heart. As he suspected, the fluid, upon transferral, caused the same inhibitory action in the denervated (nerves cut away) heart as the electrical stimulation of the vagus had caused in the first heart. Loewi repeated the experiment with other frogs, but this time he worked with the sympathetic nerve, which causes the heart to accelerate. He found that this nerve action, once prompted by electricity, could also be transferred to the denervated heart along with a little of the nutrient fluid. This ingenious experiment made it substantially clear that upon stimulation the nerves had secreted substances into the hearts that were directly responsible for the muscular action producing the changes in their beats. Loewi's classic work undercut the electrical transmission theory, and the chemical theory was on the way to acceptance.

What substance was released by the stimulated nerves? Loewi couldn't say. Direct analysis was next to impossible because the chemicals were ejected in such minute quantities. He believed that the sympathetic and parasympathetic substances were not the same, because of the different reactions they elicited. Soon he decided that the chemical secreted from the sympathetic nerve was adrenalin, or at least something comparable to it. He was much less sure of the substance secreted from the vagus nerve so he simply called it "Vagusstoff" (vagus material). Somewhat later, as we shall learn below, Loewi decided that Vagusstoff was a compound called acetylcholine, but positive proof did not come until the 1930's and the persistent efforts of the English biologist Henry H. Dale.

When Dale learned of Loewi's experiments, he had reason to be particularly interested. In 1914 he had isolated acetylcholine in the natural state, although it had been produced artificially as early as 1867. Dale had found it while working with extracts from the fungus ergot. Subsequently he had discovered that acetylcholine applied to a muscle at certain nerve endings produced a response in the muscle. In reporting these discoveries, the English biologist speculated that the chemical might be found in animals. Naturally, then, Leowi's work was of immediate interest to him, as he later related:

"When, therefore, some seven years later, Loewi described his beautiful experiments, showing that stimulation of the vagus nerve produced its . . . effects on the frog's heart by the liberation of a chemical substance; and when his successive papers provided cumulative evidence of the similarity of this substance to acetylcholine . . . ; I believe that I was more ready than most of my contemporaries for immediate acceptance of the evidence for this 'Vagusstoff,' and more eager, almost, than Professor Loewi himself, to assume its identity with acetylcholine. There was wanting, it seemed to me, only one item of evidence to justify certainty as to the nature of this substance, namely, a proof that acetylcholine itself, and not merely some choline ester of closely similar properties, was an actual constituent of the animal body."

In 1929 Dale and a colleague, H. W. Dudley, reported a laborious experiment that they claimed was "the first occasion on which the substance [acetylcholine] has been found to occur naturally in the animal body." The work began at a slaughterhouse, where the scientists collected the spleens of twenty-four horses killed between 7:00 in the morning and 8:15 in the evening. In the laboratory the spleens were minced after they had been soaked in alcohol. The resulting extract, weighing over seventy-one pounds, was then filtered and reduced in several ways to a volume of 1,120 cubic centimeters. An examination of this solution indicated that it held the equivalent of 334 milligrams of acetylcholine.

Knowing that the substance was present in animals, Dale and his laboratory colleagues conducted further experiments to see if acetylcholine was actually involved with the action of peripheral nerves. In January 1936 he and two of his co-workers presented a paper to the *Journal of Physiology* with proof of what had been suspected. They had worked with motor nerve endings and muscles in a cat's tongue, and in the legs of cats, dogs, and frogs. In each case the scientists stimulated a connecting nerve with an electrical device that delivered fifteen shocks per second, producing repeated twitches in the muscle. Meanwhile the throbbing muscle was perfused with a liquid called "Locke's solution"—i.e., the substance was forced through the tissue with a special pump. The Locke's solution was then tested by applying it to a leech muscle while investigators watched for a response that acetylcholine was known to cause in the worm's tissue. The 1936 paper reported that Dale and his co-workers finally had evidence substantial enough to say that acetylcholine was secreted following the electrical stimulation of motor nerve fibers. They also stated that the substance appeared when a muscle was directly stimulated by electrical means. However, when the muscle's connecting nerves were cut away, stimulation of the same muscle failed to produce acetylcholine, which added to the proof that the compound was secreted by the nerves. And they revealed that when a nerve, stimulated to the point of exhaustion, failed to conduct any longer, it also failed to secrete acetylcholine. Subsequent experiments in Dale's laboratory further substantiated the fact that acetylcholine was the chemical agent by which nerves worked upon muscles. Using both a muscle preparation complete with nerves and another that was denervated, the scientists found that small doses of acetylcholine injected into the empty blood vessels could by themselves cause contractions comparable to those produced by nerve stimulation. The trying nature of the search in nerves for acetylcholine is clear when it is realized that the scientists were seeking an amount of the compound close to being nonexistent. A single nerve impulse, according to a later statement from Dale, released only .000000000000001 gram of acetylcholine.

The English biologists had finally pinpointed the first, and still the best known, of the chemical transmitters of nervous action. Through their pioneer experiments, the English biologist and his co-workers had given the neurological sciences an extremely important insight into the events that occur when a nerve impulse travels from one cell to another and to a muscle.

If nervous transmission was chemical, a fundamental question about the process had to be answered. For decades scientists had recognized in the twitch of muscles under stimulation that a nerve impulse was, as the name implied, brief and transitory. But if impulses were chemically transmitted, their transitory nature was hard to explain. It seemed that a chemical applied by one cell to another would remain at the point of contact and continue producing nervous activity. The resulting muscular response would, in turn, be continuous rather than impulsive. In 1926 Loewi and a co-worker, E. Navratil, found the answer as they were trying to identify the transmitter substance at work in the original heart experiment.

As noted earlier, Loewi suspected the substance was acetylcholine. He had arrived at this idea by a circuitous route. First he had discovered that the substance, whatever it might be, was blocked by atropine, an alkaloid extracted from belladonna and other plants. He then looked for chemicals that could be destroyed by the alkaloid, and the research led him to Dale's 1914 report in which the English biologist had postulated that his newly isolated acetylcholine might be broken down by the hydrolyzing action of an enzyme. Loewi decided acetylcholine could be the chemical transmitter, and then he wondered if an enzyme might not play a key part in nervous transmission. If it was secreted by nerves, this might explain the impulse's transitory nature.

Then in 1926 Loewi and Navratil discovered such an enzyme, a "cholinesterase," in the heart of a frog, and it destroyed acetylcholine. But proof that it was the key to the impulsive character of nerve transmission was not complete until the two scientists found that the cholinesterase could be inhibited by an alkaloid of the calabar bean, physostigmine. When this substance was applied to a frog's heart, it became evident that the scientists had discovered an anticholinesterase, which, in effect, protected acetylcholine from cholinesterase. With the anticholinesterase present the action of the frog heart, following stimulation of the vagus nerve, indicated that the nervous transmission was being prolonged and intensified. It was pretty clear now that the enzyme, cholinesterase, was responsible for the impulsive chemical transmission.

Loewi felt that this work was as important as his first major finding with the two frogs' hearts, for he believed it was strong support for the chemical transmission theory, and for his belief that the transmitter was acetylcholine. Definitive proof, as we have already seen, was subsequently provided by Dale and his colleagues.

While the English scientists were at work on acetylcholine, a well-known Harvard scientist, Walter Bradford Cannon, was experimenting with sympathetic nerve fibers, in which, Loewi had proposed, adrenalin was the transmitter substance. Cannon was trying to prove it with an intricate experiment on a cat. First he removed the animal's liver and suprarenal glands to eliminate two known sources of adrenalin in the animal. He then carefully severed all the nerves to the heart, and he cut the animal's spinal cord apart at a point that ensured the termination of all nervous connections between the cat's forward and hind quarters. With the animal still alive, Cannon stimulated the sympathetic nerves leading from the severed part of the spinal cord to the smooth muscle of the tail hairs, which rise when the animal is emotionally excited. As he did so, the creature's heart rate and blood pressure increased. The changes in the heart could not be attributed to the disrupted nervous communication, so the flow of blood from the tail forward to the heart had to be the mode of communication, and Cannon proved it. By shutting off the blood supply to and from the tail area, he found that the nerve stimulation no longer speeded up the heartbeat. It was pretty good evidence that the stimulated nerve was secreting a chemical that got into the bloodstream and acted upon the heart. He couldn't identify the chemical, but called it "sympathin." His results were subsequently supported by the findings of other scientists. Most of them agreed with Loewi's proposal that the substance was adrenalin.

The correct identification finally came from Sweden in the 1940's, when Ulf von Euler, a scientist at the Caroline Institute in Stockholm, analyzed the substance extracted from sympathetic nerves of cattle and horses. Von Euler discovered that sympathin was actually noradrenaline, "the nearest relative to adrenalin." He did not determine how the effect of noradrenaline is quickly terminated after its release in order to maintain the impulsive character of the nervous action. The question has not been fully settled yet, but it is well accepted that the transmitter substance is taken up through a chemical process of the cell that releases the transmitter. For his discovery of noradrenaline and for other contributions to knowledge of the sympathetic nervous system, von Euler was chosen as one of three scientists to receive the Nobel Prize for Medicine or Physiology in 1970. A second recipient, Julius Axelrod of the National Heart Institute, Bethesda, Maryland, also made important contributions to the understanding of sympathetic nerves. The third recipient was Bernard Katz of University College, London, who was honored for his research on the role of acetylcholine in the nervous system (to be discussed below).

As the transmitter substances were identified, nerves were categorized as (1) "cholinergic," and (2) "adrenergic." Cholinergic nerves, which secrete acetylcholine, include: (1) all peripheral nerves outside the autonomic nervous system, and (2) all the parasympathetic nerves of the autonomic system. Among the sympathetic nerves of the autonomic system, only some are cholinergic, those called "preganglionic," for they lead from the central nervous system to a collection of nerve cell bodies called ganglia. Axons extending on out from the ganglionic cells, "postganglionic" fibers, are adrenergic. The postganglionic nerves, secreting noradrenaline, can send the living organism into hyperactivity comparable to what its companion chemical, adrenalin, can do in the body's hormonal system. These adrenergic nerves can step up the beat of the heart, prepare the lungs for greater oxygen intake, open up the blood vessels for the increased flow of blood, stimulate mental activity, and take several other measures to prepare the entire organism for action. They counterbalance the autonomic system's cholinergic nerves, which tend to slow the organism down.

While pioneers like Dale, Loewi, Cannon, and von Euler came up with fundamental information on chemical transmission in the peripheral nervous system, comparatively little direct evidence of transmitter substances was found in the central nervous system. Here the research problems were formidable because the smallest nerve cells of all are packed together by the billions, and to obtain and analyze chemicals released by specific cells or groups of cells appears next to impossible. Evidence generally came from indirect methods. For example, once a possible transmitter substance was isolated or synthesized it could be tested by applying it to nerve tissue and observing the reaction, if there was any. Or if a scientist suspected that a certain chemical was a transmitter, he might check it out by treating pertinent nerve tissue with a second chemical known to modify the one in question. If the treatment affected the normal nervous action, the investigator might conclude that he had discovered a new transmitter substance.

The clearest case for a central nervous system transmitter was made for acetylcholine. The first evidence appeared in 1941 from two Oxford University scientists, Edith Bülbring and J. H. Burn. They worked with the spinal cord of a dog that was perfused with a Ringer's solution (the liquid was forced into the spinal tissue via the blood vessels). Bülbring and Burn then stimulated the sciatic nerve so as to send impulses into the perfused cord. Subsequent analysis of the Ringer's solution taken from the tissue revealed that the solution had picked up acetylcholine in the amount of one part in fifty million. In 1956 at the University of Edinburgh, L. Angelucci, a pharmacologist conducting a similar experiment on a frog, found acetylcholine in the spinal cord after the skin of one foot had been electrically stimulated once a minute for six to eight hours. And in the early 1960's J. F. Mitchell in Cambridge, England, reported that acetylcholine was found in the cerebral cortex of sheep and cats after the brain had received messages from sensory stimulation. For any given test, Mitchell opened an animal's skull and placed a special cup upside down on the exposed cortex. The cup, which was filled with a certain solution, was located over a sensory area of the brain related to the contralateral forepaw. After the paw was stimulated and the solution was tested, Mitchell found that it had acquired a small amount of acetylcholine. His continued experimentation revealed that the amount of the chemical picked up by the solution was proportional to the amount of stimulation applied to the paw.

During the 1950's scientists in America and Europe found evidence of several related chemicals in the central nervous system; classified as monoamines, they were assumed to be transmitters, although direct evidence is still difficult to attain. They include noradrenaline with its precursor, dopamine, and a complicated but fascinating chemical, 5-hydroxytryptamine, or serotonin. The discovery of all these substances in the brain had the widespread effect of bringing more attention to brain chemistry, brain pharmacology, and drugs for mental diseases.

In 1954 a University of Edinburgh pharmacologist, Marthe Vogt, provided the first convincing evidence that noradrenaline has a part to play in the central nervous system. She stimulated the sympathetic nerve trunks of dogs and cats to produce nervous activity in their brains. The animals were then quickly killed, and their brains were dissected and tested for noradrenaline. She found the substance in all cases, although it was unevenly distributed, with "some parts containing at least twenty times as much as others."

In the previous year, two scientists in Cleveland, Ohio, Betty M. Twarog and Irvine H. Page, investigated serotonin, which had been previously isolated from several sources, including beef serum and the salivary glands of the octopus. In their studies Twarog and Page found they could obtain relatively large quantities of serotonin from rat and rabbit brains. Their work was confirmed by three Edinburgh scientists in 1954, and subsequently in other laboratories.

While acetylcholine and the monoamines have received the greatest share of attention as transmitter substances in the central nervous system, others have also been identified as possible candidates, and scientists believe that still more will be found. In 1950 seven American scientists, in three different papers published in the *Journal of Biological Chemistry*, reported isolating gamma-aminobutyric acid (GABA) in the brain. Four of the scientists found the chemical in beef brain, while the others identified it in the brains of mice. Four years later scientists in Montreal isolated a brain substance that could affect the stretch-receptor neuron of a cray-fish when it was used in a test. Not knowing what the chemical was, they called it Factor I, but in 1957 it was identified as GABA. Its effect on the neuron led to the supposition that GABA was a transmitter. Since then much has been learned about the substance, and the case for it being a transmitter is fairly strong. A much weaker case has been developed for another substance, glutamate, which was cited in the 1960's as a possible neuro-transmitter because of studies on the nervous systems of crustaceans, such as the lobster. Other chemical transmitters will undoubtedly be discovered, since there are nerve cells, alive and active in their natural state, that fail to react to any of the known or suspected transmitters when the chemicals are applied to the cells artificially.

The fresh view of nervous transmission that grew out of Otto Loewi's nocturnal thoughts led to many new under-standings of how the nervous system functions and malfunc-tions, and of how it is chemically modifiable. It had an impact in many diverse fields of science and medicine. The most dramatic undoubtedly came with new drugs capable of affecting mental states and behavior.

Once the monoamines were discovered in the brain, they were soon the subject of a voluminous literature that largely reflected pharmacological investigations of brain chemistry, especially involving noradrenaline and serotonin. The reports were often startling, for these substances appeared to be deeply tied to patterns of the mind and behavior, both in human beings and animals. On the one hand a drug acting on the brain's monoamines produced sedation, or even de-pression comparable to that associated with mental illness. On the other hand a drug might stimulate the subject, lift-ing him to high levels of emotional excitement. The expla-nations at times seemed to follow simple lines of chemical action, but as more drugs became involved in the experi-ments, the simplicity quickly faded.

Early in the pharmacological quest for understanding,

an American and an English scientist, working independently, found that the action of serotonin could be blocked in a certain kind of muscle by a small quantity of LSD. It was then easy to speculate that the wild mental effects of LSD resulted from its blocking of serotonin in the brain. Assuming that serotonin was a nerve transmitter, a scientist could further assume that its blockage literally throws the brain's complex circuitry out of kilter. Subsequently it was learned that the drug not only blocked serotonin, but also noradrenaline and adrenalin. The idea of a simple explanation for LSD was soon upset, and by the mid-1960's scientists were not at all sure how the exotic drug acted on the fabulous fabric of the brain. In 1967 two authorities on such drugs, A. Hoffer of University Hospital, Saskatoon, Canada, and H. Osmond of the Princeton Neuropsychiatric Institute, co-authored a book, *The Hallucinogens*, wherein they proposed that "LSD could block transmission of stimuli in the brain by any one" of six mechanisms that involved noradrenaline, serotonin, and other chemicals associated with the brain.

Back in the 1950's, soon after the monoamines were discovered in the central nervous system, a tranquillizer, reserpine, also became the subject of extensive literature. When applied to animals, reserpine created a marked sedation, and in human beings it generally toned down an overexcited mental state, except that it lowered some individuals into a depression which persisted until the effects wore off. In 1962 scientists at the National Heart Institute, Bethesda, Maryland, found that the drug released serotonin until the cells were depleted of the substance. Again it was surmised that such interference with the possible neuro-transmitter upset the normal electrical patterns of the brain. Then, as in the case of LSD, it was found that the action of reserpine was not limited to serotonin; it also affected noradrenaline and its precursor, dopamine, to the point of depletion in the brain. Again the view of what was really happening became murky.

However, in the course of studying the monoamines, pharmacologists increased our knowledge of how many drugs work on the brain. In general, those that lift mood and increase activity seem somehow to make noradrenaline more available at the synapses of the central nervous system. An example is benzedrine (amphetamine), which inhibits sleep despite considerable fatigue. Those drugs that depress mood and lower activity somehow impair the storage and release of noradrenaline, making it less available at the synapses. The tranquillizer chlorpromazine is an example.

While knowledge of chemical transmission produced new pharmacological insights into the nervous system, it also increased our understanding of the system's malfunctions. For example, it soon helped find the basic cause of the dreaded disease botulism, a type of food poisoning associated with canned or sealed foods. It was long understood that such foods fostered the growth of a bacterial toxin capable of attacking the nervous system. The main symptom was muscular paralysis that particularly caused problems in swallowing and speaking. The mortality rate of the disease was high, some sixty-six percent of the cases, with death usually resulting from respiratory failure. In 1949 at the Middlesex Hospital in London, Arnold S. V. Burgen and his co-workers found that botulinus toxin does its lethal work at the neuromuscular junction, where it prevents the release of acetylcholine. The blockage causes muscles to become limp and flaccid so that the victim is unable to move his limbs. Tetanus is closely allied to botulism. It also attacks the nervous system, but the victim of this affliction, which often results from deep, dirty lacerations, suffers from muscles becoming locked in a state of spastic paralysis, leaving the person unable to move. The jaw muscles are often affected first, whence comes the name "lockjaw." In 1898, European scientists found that tetanus toxin was taken up by nerve tissue, but the meaning was not evident until investigators began understanding the mechanisms of chemical transmis-

sion. Evidence developed at the Oxford University laboratory of W. E. van Heyningen now indicates that tetanus
toxin is taken up by the membranes of nerve cells in the area
of their synapses. It occurs specifically in the spinal cord
with nerves whose impulses lead to inhibitory action on the
part of certain reflex systems. Muscular contractions normally
countered by the inhibitory action are no longer opposed,
and the muscles are locked into the state of paralysis long
associated with tetanus. The tetanus toxin in the spinal cord
apparently affects a chemical transmitter, which has yet to
be identified. Before these basic causes were known, medical
scientists curbed botulism and tetanus by the development
of antitoxins.

Parkinson's disease, a far more baffling, long-lasting illness, has been the subject of intensive research in the decades
following World War II, and its cause, though still unknown,
is suspected to be related to chemical transmission in the
nervous system. In the 1960's scientists developed a new
theory for Parkinsonism that may explain why the disease
leads to serious disorders of movement control. The theory
postulated that normal movement depends on a continuing
balance maintained by two pathways of motor-control nerves,
one set being cholinergic, the other adrenergic. Parkinson's
disease, said the theory, occurred when this balance was lost
by a reduction in activity of the adrenergic side of the two
pathways. It was found that symptoms of the disease could
sometimes be reduced by lowering activity in the cholinergic side through drugs or surgery. The other approach
would be to restore activity in the adrenergic side, and in
the latter half of the 1960's scientists discovered a way. They
found that large doses of a drug called L-DOPA (levo-
dihydroxyphenylalanine) apparently restored the lost balance. L-DOPA raises the level of dopamine in the central
nervous system. Dopamine, as stated earlier, is the precursor for noradrenaline, which is thought to be the transmitter
substance in adrenergic nerves. For many victims of Parkin-

son's disease, L-DOPA brought help, especially those sufferers known as "postencephalitics," whose affliction was apparently related to the encephalitis pandemic that occurred between 1916 and 1927. In tests conducted with L-DOPA at Beth Abraham Hospital in the Bronx, New York, severely disabled postencephalitics responded favorably to the new treatment. In 1969, Dr. Oliver Sacks, a Beth Abraham neurologist supervising treatment with L-DOPA, stated: "Close to 90 percent have benefited. It's been spectacular in about 30 percent, of very substantial help in about 30 percent, and of modest help in about 30 percent. A minority appear either refractory to the medicine, or have adverse reactions." In the most dramatic cases the new drug returned Parkinson victims from a mummified state to a relatively normal existence. When L-DOPA was first manufactured, it cost five thousand dollars a kilogram. Several years later (1969) it was down to five hundred dollars, and the cost of treating a patient for a year was about one thousand dollars.

In another area of medical research the growing appreciation of chemical transmission led to a fascinating research tool. As noted in an earlier chapter, the neurophysiologists of the nineteenth century began exploring the brain by electrical stimulation, and as this century produced its electronic technology, advances led the electrical stimulators to remarkable discoveries (a subject to be discussed in a forthcoming chapter). However, these scientists, despite their fine probes and tiny electrical stimuli, were forced to stimulate comparatively gross areas of brain tissue, for their currents were bound to spread through thousands of cells with many different functions. They often wished their stimuli could be much more specific in selecting only cells with certain functions. With the understanding of chemical transmission and realization that different cells respond to different transmitters and drugs, a possible answer to the specificity problem appeared. Instead of using electric probes, neuroscientists began to consider using probes capable of depositing tiny drops of chemicals in minute areas of the brain. With this technique an experimenter might employ carefully selected chemicals to stimulate only certain cells of the many cells encountered in even the smallest corner of the vastly complicated organ.

The first attempts to put this idea to work failed, but in 1953 a Swedish scientist, Bengt Andersson, succeeded when he guided a chemical probe into a goat's brain and deposited a five-percent salt solution at a precisely chosen spot of the hypothalamus, which governs the autonomic nervous system. The goat responded by becoming extremely thirsty and drinking huge quantities of water. By the 1960's chemical stimulation of the brain was being practiced in many laboratories, and the equipment for carrying it out was greatly refined. Tiny hollow shafts were being permanently implanted in the brains of experimental animals. The shafts were put in place with stereotactic instruments designed to guide them precisely through holes in the skulls to points selected from three-dimensional brain maps of the animal subjects. Once in place, a shaft would be fastened to the skull with jeweler's screws and adhesive. Four or five such shafts might be inserted into the brain of a rat, while a monkey might receive as many as one hundred. When the anesthesia wore off, an experimental animal would be free to move around its cage and resume a relatively normal existence. The experimenter then repeatedly used the implanted shafts to deliver test chemicals and observe the animal's reactions.

Some of the most fascinating experiments with chemical stimulation were performed by Alan E. Fisher, first at McGill University and then at the University of Pittsburgh. In 1954 he injected the male sex hormone, testosterone, into the hypothalamus of a male rat, fully expecting it would cause the animal to mount a female rat even though she was not in the receptive state. To his surprise Fisher found that the male acquired maternal instincts and treated the fully grown female as a baby, even to the point of building a nest. The same tests in females led to the same results: they acted out their normal parts. Puzzling over the outcome, the scientist continued stimulation and found that testosterone delivered at a point in front of and to one side of the male rat's hypothalamus produced the results he had expected originally. But when the same spot was stimulated with testosterone in a female rat, she acted like a male, trying to mount any likely partner.

To explain the incongruous results Fisher hypothesized that the male hormone applied to areas particularly sensitive to the female hormone, progesterone, acted like the latter. It was already known that the male hormone under certain circumstances could become a weak substitute for the female hormone. This idea led to two possible conclusions: (1) that brain cells are selectively responsive to chemicals, and (2) that the male and female brains are essentially alike, the differences in the animals being caused by the kinds of hormones arriving at the brain via the circulatory system. Other scientists confirmed Fisher's work and added to it.

Subsequently a Yale University graduate student, Sebastian Grossman, produced some interesting responses in rats by injecting acetylcholine and noradrenaline in a brain site just above the hypothalamus. He showed that noradrenaline caused a satiated rat to become hungry and eat again. Acetylcholine applied at exactly the same point caused the rat's thirst to increase, although the animal had just drunk his fill. When these results came to Fisher's attention at the University of Pittsburgh, he and a collaborator set out to map the brain circuits of the thirst drive through carefully placed injections of acetylcholine and muscarine, which mimics the former's action as a transmitter substance. During their experiments the Pittsburgh scientists found that in an hour a stimulated rat would drink twice his normal daily water intake of twenty-five to thirty-five milliliters. The initial map of the thirst circuits turned out to be amazingly like one prepared in 1937 at Cornell University by James W. Papez, who had traced them with anatomical methods. However, Fisher found that nerve pathways supporting this basic drive to drink in the rat were not anatomically the same in the cat. When acetylcholine was injected into the cat's brain in spots comparable to those that caused thirst in the rat, the result was anger, fear, or a sleep-like trance. Meanwhile an experimenter in Mexico City, Raúl Hernández-Peón, independently found he could trace a sleep circuit in the cat that practically followed the anatomical course of the rat's thirst circuit. He, too, relied on acetylcholine as the chemical stimulator. The explanation for these chemical differences between the animals was not evident.

Such experiments firmly established chemical stimulation as an important tool for studying the brain. Fisher, writing in *Scientific American*, said ". . . chemical explorations of the brain have established at least two significant facts: first, that certain brain cells are stimulated selectively by specific chemicals and, second, that drive-oriented behavior can be triggered and sustained by chemical means. It seems safe to predict that chemical stimulation of the brain will become an increasingly important tool in the investigation of the neurophysiological bases of behavior."

While the knowledge of chemical transmission that grew from Loewi's discovery was beginning to serve the life sciences, it also played a less laudatory role in what have been called the "death sciences." The story goes back to Germany and World War II, when two compounds, Tabun (ethyl phosphorodimethyl amidocyanidate) and Sarin (isopropyl methyl phosphonofluoridate), were manufactured in industrial lots. They came from the work of synthetic chemists, led by Gerhard Schrader, who were developing insecticides that turned out to be compounds with an amazing toxicity to human beings. Tabun and Sarin were considered for use as new forms of war gas that would be far more lethal than anything employed in World War I. They were not used, fortunately, but became known as nerve gases for reasons found in their mechanism of action. The compounds are inhibitors of the enzyme cholinesterase, which, as we learned earlier, hydrolyzes acetylcholine to preserve the impulsive nature of nervous transmission. The nerve gases, it was found, prevent the destruction of the nerve transmitter at the synapse, thereby causing its action to persist. In experiments with animals the nerve gases were found to be the most toxic substances ever known. A few millionths of a gram of Sarin injected into the bloodstream of a dog or cat caused respiratory distress in 15 to 30 seconds, and death in less than five minutes. The gases can do their deadly work if inhaled, or if the liquid, from which come the vapors, is swallowed or even dropped on the skin. The symptoms of nerve gases before death are terrifying to contemplate, including increased nasal secretions, constriction of the pupils of the eyes, tightening of the chest with wheezing during expiration, nausea, vomiting, diarrhea, increased urination, pallor, general convulsions, and depressed respiration. Sarin presented its makers and handlers with a tremendous storage problem, for it rapidly ate away most anything it contacted. Silver-lined equipment had to be used to deal with it. At the end of World War II a plant was found in Germany producing Tabun at the rate of a thousand metric tons per month. The United States Army Chemical Corps began producing nerve gas at its Rocky Mountain Arsenal near Denver and loading it into munitions. In 1970 the disposal of these munitions became an immensely difficult and controversial problem.

But in the future the great contributions of those who opened up the secrets of chemical transmission will not be found in the death sciences; they have the most to offer in revealing the basic functions of the nervous system, which means opening up the mysteries of life and thought.

10

THE GIANT AXON

At the Cold Springs Harbor Symposium on Quantitative Biology in 1936 a British biologist, J. Z. Young, unceremoniously reported a discovery that was to become the key to some of this century's most significant work in nerve physiology.

"The nerves of the Decapod Cephalopods such as the squid, *Loligo,* or the cuttlefish, *Sepia,* are particularly interesting," said Young, "because they contain enormous axons, the largest of them in a large Atlantic squid *(Loligo pealeii)* being as much as one millimeter in diameter. In spite of their great size these axons seem to have been referred to previously only by Williams (1909), who described them very briefly." He was referring to Leonard W. Williams, who had written about the nerve fibers in a privately published thesis.

The squid "giant axon," as it became known, is anything but giant with its diameter of .03937 inch—unless compared to the largest nerve fiber in a human being, which is around .0003937 inch in diameter. The thread-like giant axon is an unmyelinated cylindrical rod filled with clear protoplasm, or "axoplasm," with the consistency of stiff jelly. In the squid's body it is surrounded by a fluid very much like sea water. The large fiber is part of the mechanism that allows the creature to swim (or jet propel itself) backwards at a relatively high speed by taking water into a large cavity, then squirting it out under pressure through a funnel in front. When a few centimeters of the axon are cut off from the rest of the cell and placed in sea water, the fiber will continue to conduct impulses for many hours. The animals are plentiful in the waters near two laboratories where experiments with the giant axon led to important scientific advances: the Marine Biological Laboratory, Woods Hole, Massachusetts, and the Laboratory of the Marine Biological Association, Plymouth, England.

To realize the significance of Young's 1936 report, one should know about a theory that had been extant, but unverifiable, for over thirty years. It was proposed in 1902 by a University of Halle physiologist, Julius Bernstein, who had been du Bois-Reymond's foremost student and an assistant to the famous Helmholtz. Bernstein had emerged from the nineteenth century as a leading pioneer in nerve physiology, and his proposition, the "membrane theory," commanded attention, for it offered a possible explanation for the basic mechanisms behind the electrical activity of the nerve cell.

Bernstein envisioned the living nerve cell in its resting state as holding a potential for producing a flow of electricity, as does a battery before its terminals are connected. Such a "resting potential" would show up as a small voltage that could be detected between the inside and outside of the surface membrane. The internal fluid, Bernstein explained, contained a high concentration of potassium ions compared to the outside, while the external fluid held a high concentration of sodium ions compared to the inside. These ionic differences, said the physiologist, produce a negative charge inside the cell and a positive charge outside. The result is an ionic attraction, with potassium ions inclined to move outward and sodium ions inward, except that the cell membrane prevents the migration. This was the same as saying that a potential (a voltage) exists across, or "polarizes," the membrane. The potential remains there, ready to move the ions and equalize their internal and external differences should the membrane stop blocking the effort. In that case the resulting ionic movement would result in a flow of electrical current, continuing until the membrane was "depolarized."

Evidence to support Bernstein's membrane theory was available from a past discovery made by the Italian Carlo Matteucci, when he recognized the "current of injury" in muscle tissue. He found that when the living tissue is injured, electricity flows from the damaged area. The phenomenon, which could also be produced in nerve tissue, could be explained by the membrane theory: the injury breaks the membrane barrier of the nerve cells involved in the injury, and they are depolarized—which, as discussed above, is indicated by a flow of electric current.

In his theory, Bernstein went on to postulate that in the normal neuron the thin living cell wall does not always remain a barrier to the ionic flow. He decided that a temporary breakdown occurs when a nerve impulse is relayed from the cell body along the thread-like axon. He believed that during the split second of the passing impulse the cell membrane becomes "selectively permeable" to the internal potassium ions (but not the external sodium) and some of them move out. At this moment, according to the theory, electricity flows across the membrane out of the cell until it is depolarized. Thus the impulse could also be characterized as a wave of depolarization moving along a nerve fiber. As it passes any given point, Bernstein concluded, the resting potential, becoming an "acting potential," falls to zero. This part of his theory was not entirely correct, as explained below.

Bernstein's idea of a wave of depolarization could undoubtedly explain why the nerve impulse travels, not at the speed of light, but at a far slower rate, as determined by Helmholtz in the mid-nineteenth century. According to the membrane theory, nerve electricity does not move in a smooth uninterrupted flow parallel to the fibrous physical length of the cell, as it does through a wire. Instead it flows in an infinite number of small, local circuits more or less at right angles to the cell fiber. This form of electrical action, with one circuit exciting the next, would, of course, have an indirect and much slower forward movement than would an uninterrupted flow of current parallel to the physical length of the cell.

The process was described in 1918 by the American scientist Ralph S. Lillie, who was trying to develop a model for nervous transmission with a specially treated iron wire. "The state of activity aroused in the irritable living system [like nerve] by a localized stimulus," said Lillie, "does not itself remain localized, but tends to spread; the region immediately stimulated imparts a similar state of activity to adjoining regions, these then activate the next adjoining, and in this manner a wave of activation or excitation is propagated over the entire irritable element, often to a long distance from its point of origin. In many cases, as in nerve, there is no decrease in the intensity of the local process as it passes along the element; its characteristics are reduplicated both qualitatively and quantitatively at each point which it reaches in its course; the local excitation is temporary and quickly dies out, each successive region of the tissue becoming active and then returning automatically to its original state of rest. Transmission of this type is know to physiologists as 'conduction,' and is exhibited in its most highly developed form in the nerves of higher animals."

Lillie attempted to demonstrate this kind of conduction with his iron wire model, which became famous among neurophysiologists. In an experiment reported in 1918, the scientist dipped a piece of No. 20 piano wire into a strong solution of nitric acid for a few seconds to produce a coating of oxide. He then immersed the oxidized wire in a dilute solution of nitric acid in a flat dish and was ready for the experiment.

"The wire if left undisturbed remains bright and unaltered

for an indefinite time," explained Lillie. "If then it is touched at one end with a piece of ordinary iron, or with zinc or another baser metal, the bright metallic surface is at once darkened (through formation of oxide) and active effervescence begins; this change is transmitted rapidly, though not instantaneously, over the entire length of the wire; the velocity of transmission varies with the conditions, and is of the order of 100 or more centimeters per second in this experiment. The wave of excitation may also be initiated *mechanically*, *e.g.*, by bending the wire or tapping it sharply with a glass rod; or *chemically*, *e.g.*, by contact with a reducing substance such as sugar; or *electrically*, *e.g.*, by making the wire . . . the cathode in any battery circuit (of two or more volts potential). . . . Activation with the electric current is thus typically a polar phenomenon, just as is the excitation of a living irritable element like a nerve."

The change that Lillie witnessed moving along the surface of his iron wire was attributed to electro-chemical activity between the wire and the thin surface film acquired when the metal was dipped into the nitric acid. He felt that this surface action might be comparable to the excitation process of a nerve as it carried an impulse along its length. The idea was discussed for many years and offered as one of several possible explanations on how a nerve impulse is conducted. But as scientists learned more about the nerve cell, Lillie's model was recognized as inadequate to explain the complex process of nervous transmission.

Actually Bernstein's membrane theory had to remain unproven, because it could not be tested with the comparatively gross measuring instruments of the time. They could not deal with the minute amounts of electricity involved, but more than that, investigators could not even reach the proper points of physical contact to make the decisive measurements, i.e., the inside as well as the outside of a cell wall. They had neither the microscopes that would allow them to see what they were doing, nor probes small enough to pick up the sources of electrical differences along the membrane of a single cell. The discovery of the squid's giant axon was, therefore, a major accomplishment for those interested in testing Bernstein's theory.

In the summer of 1939 scientists at Woods Hole and Plymouth successfully conducted an experiment on the squid axon that became a landmark in the neurosciences. The work at Plymouth was conducted by A. L. Hodgkin and A. F. Huxley. The same experiment, except for minor differences, was carried out at Woods Hole by Kenneth S. Cole and Howard J. Curtis. In each instance the experimenters inserted an extremely fine electrode into the axoplasm of a giant axon resting in a solution of sea water and still capable of conducting impulses when stimulated. At Woods Hole the tiny electrode was made of a fine platinum wire. The scientists at Plymouth used a silver wire electrode. In both cases a second electrode was placed outside the cell so that its tip was opposite that of the internal electrode just across the membrane. At both Plymouth and Woods Hole the four scientists found they could measure a relatively large electrical potential between the tips when the cell was at rest (meaning that no impulse was passing). This "resting potential" was measured in England at forty-five millivolts and in the United States at fifty-one millivolts. The results meant that the axon's internal fluid was minus forty-five or fifty-one millivolts compared to the outside fluid.

Measurement of the resting potential was strong evidence in favor of Bernstein's membrane theory. The difference in electrical potential between the inside and outside of the cell made it clear that the electrical activity of the neuron took place across the membrane. Cole and Curtis provided additional evidence in favor of what Bernstein had proposed. As part of their experimentation, they increased the potassium concentration of the external solution of a giant axon while measuring the resting potential. When the added potassium made the solution approach the concentration of that on the inside, the resting potential dropped until the membrane was depolarized, and the voltage-measuring device read "zero." This finding supported Bernstein's contention that polarization depended upon the internal potassium concentration remaining higher than the external concentration.

But measurement of the resting potential was only part of what was accomplished on both sides of the Atlantic in 1939. When the giant axon was stimulated and an impulse passed by the opposing electrode tips, a surprise was in store for the investigators in both laboratories. The wave form of the fleeting impulse recorded by their oscilloscopes revealed that the action potential was not, as supposed, equal to the resting potential. It was considerably larger. Hodgkin and Huxley measured it as 86 millivolts. Cole and Curtis recorded 108 millivolts.

The results didn't jibe with what the Bernstein theory would lead one to believe, and the oscilloscope revealed the difference. It showed that during the passage of a nerve impulse the action potential goes through a much greater change than the theory would predict. There is an "overshoot," said the investigators, and it happens in the following way: On a vertical scale, with zero in the middle, the electrical action begins at the negative value of the resting potential, rises up through zero (where it becomes a positive potential), and continues upward to a relatively high plus value. It then reverses itself, dropping back down through zero to the minus value of the resting potential. Hodgkin and Huxley noted that the potential shifted from minus forty-five to plus forty-one millivolts—making the total change of eighty-six. Put in terms of electric current flow, the scientists' instruments indicated that the following occurred: As the impulse passed the electrode tips arranged across the membrane, current first flowed into the cell until the internal fluid became positively charged with a potential of forty-one millivolts. It then reversed direction and flowed out of the cell until the interior was again negatively charged at the

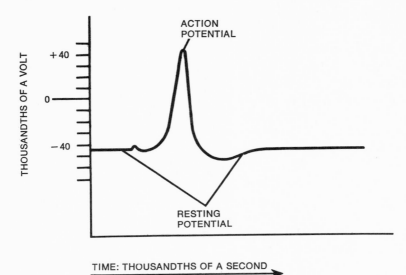

Curve of action potential of squid axon measured between inside and outside of cell membrane. Voltage differences across the membrane are plotted against time during passage of nerve impulse.

resting potential of minus forty-five millivolts. Curtis and Cole also found that during the activity the electrical resistance of the cell membrane dropped tremendously, from a thousand to twenty-five ohms per square centimeter, allowing for the sudden current flow associated with the nerve impulse.

As the summer of 1939 ended, the scientists at Plymouth and Woods Hole were pretty sure that Bernstein's proposition was partly right and partly wrong. His basic idea that the electrical action of a nerve cell takes place across the surface membrane was still intact. But his construction of what happened to the ionic exchange through the membrane could no longer be supported. It was apparently not enough to say that the impulse was a wave of depolarization resulting only from the exit of potassium through a membrane that momentarily became permeable to the ions. Had this been the case, the oscilloscope would have indicated a change in potential only from the negative resting value up to zero and return. The "overshoot" to the plus side of the scale would not have occurred. Henceforth Bernstein's idea of the nerve impulse as a wave of depolarization had to be abandoned in favor of it being a transient reversal of the resting potential, from negative to positive and back to negative.

For several years scientists were unable to prove what happened across the cell membrane during passage of the nerve impulse, although, oddly enough, a good clue was available in the same journal and volume carrying Bernstein's 1902 presentation of the membrane theory. It was part of a lengthy paper from a Würzburg University scientist, E. Overton, published in *Pflügers Archives of Physiology*, Volume 92. Overton noted that the excitation of muscle depended on the presence of sodium in the immediate environment, and he went so far as to propose that the electrical activity of nerve might involve the exchange of potassium and sodium across the cell membrane. In the late 1940's his proposition was shown to be correct. A number of scientists, including Hodgkin and Huxley, altered the sodium content in the environment of nerve cells and revealed that it was the key to the unexpected results obtained by the 1939 experiments at Plymouth and Woods Hole.

On the one hand, they found that lowering the sodium content in the external fluid of squid and other axons reduces the over-all action potential and that eliminating it renders the fiber unexcitable. On the other hand, they discovered that raising the sodium concentration increases the action potential. This was a good indication that sodium ions were entering the cell via the membrane. And the electrical flow associated with an impulse makes it likely that the entry of sodium occurs in the initial phase of the activity, when current rushes into the cell and the potential changes from a minus to plus value.

Around 1950 more direct evidence favoring this idea came from experiments in England and America, where scientists employed sodium labeled with the newly developed radio isotopes to prove that the ions definitely enter the cell during passage of an impulse. Indeed, the new labeling tool provided for such precise measurement that one of the English experimenters, R. D. Keynes, was able to show that with one impulse twenty thousand sodium ions entered each square micron of a particular axon's surface.

While such results were strong support for Overton's idea of a sodium-potassium exchange, they still did not provide scientific evidence of precisely how it happened. However, scientists were now fairly certain that while the influx of sodium occurs during the first phase of the action potential, when current rushes inward, the efflux of potassium coincides with the second phase and the outward flow of electricity. If this was the case, the cell would have to shift its permeability characteristics during an impulse so that first the membrane's tiny gates would open to sodium but not potassium, and then quickly reverse their selectivity to favor potassium but reject sodium.

In 1947 the technical equipment that would substantiate the facts of this ionic flow was devised in the United States by Kenneth Cole and an associate, G. Marmont. The equipment, which was to be improved and used in England by Hodgkin and Huxley, was called the "voltage clamp." It involved a complex electronic feedback system that, in effect, allowed an investigator to stop a nerve fiber's action potential at any point of the activity and look at it. This is impossible under normal circumstances because the electrical event occurs so rapidly. In the squid giant axon, the impulse moves over the fiber at nearly fifty feet per second, so at any given location along the membrane the full sweep of the action potential occurs in about a thousandth of a second.

To analyze the ionic basis of the wave, therefore, required a split-millisecond-by-split-millisecond inspection of the explosive burst of electrical activity. The voltage clamp was the answer. It allowed an investigator to change the potential across a membrane in controlled steps without triggering the all-or-none firing action characteristic of nerve. For example, he could take the potential from its forty-five millivolt resting level a few steps at a time up the scale to zero and on to a maximum action potential of forty-one millivolts. Along the way the experimenter could then analyze what was happening in relation to the membrane's permeability.

From 1948 to 1951 Hodgkin, Huxley, and Bernard Katz, working at Plymouth in the summer and Cambridge in the winter, compiled a large amount of experimental data that greatly clarified what occurs along the cell membrane during the passage of a nerve impulse. Through tests using the voltage clamp and a variety of ionic concentrations around nerve fibers, the scientists were able to describe what happens to the action potential during its two main electrical phases, and thus offering proof that: (1) the inward current flow is created by the influx of sodium ions, and (2) the outward flow results from the efflux of potassium ions. Hodgkin and Huxley then developed mathematical equations with which they could predict the electrical behavior of the giant axon with considerable accuracy. The equations, for example, could help predict such factors as the form, duration, and amplitude of the action potential, the conduction velocity of the axon, and the ionic movements involved in the electrical activity.

For their brilliant work on the physiology of the nerve cell, Hodgkin and Huxley were awarded the Nobel Prize for Physiology or Medicine in 1963. They shared the award with another English scientist, John Eccles, who also made an outstanding contribution in the same field with his work on synapses, which will be discussed in the following chapter.

Around 1960 Hodgkin and two other scientists at Plymouth, P. F. Baker and T. I. Shaw, developed an interesting technique that made it possible to provide added proof about the role of potassium in the nerve cell. Since 1937 it had been recognized that with the gentle strokes of a glass rod or pressure applied by a small roller, the axoplasm of the giant axon could be extruded from a cut end of the fiber. No one assumed, however, that the cell membrane could survive the pressure so that the fiber could function again, but Baker and Shaw proved it could. They developed a method for re-inflating a flattened axon with an isotonic solution of potassium so that it functioned again in about seventy percent of the cases. A re-inflated, or "perfused," axon, which could conduct impulses for several hours, allowed the scientists to control the ionic concentrations on both sides of the cell membrane and to make further tests of the membrane theory. An experimenter, for example, could now take a perfused giant axon through the electrical phases of its action potential simply by altering the internal and external concentrations of potassium and sodium, thereby altering the electrical potentials across the membrane. Such tests added to the already substantial proof that the nerve cell's activity is largely a matter of ionic transfer across the cell membrane.

Experimentation in the 1960's at Duke University and other institutions added an interesting dimension to the study of membrane permeability. The work involved a powerful poison found in the delicious (but infamous if improperly cleaned) puffer fish and in the California newt. After ingestion, the poison, tetrodotoxin, strikes at the nervous system, and the victim usually suffers its effects within ten minutes. He experiences numbness of the lips, tongue, and inner surfaces of the mouth, and then he grows weak, and his limb and chest muscles become paralyzed. Vomiting may occur. Blood pressure drops, and the pulse rises. Death often comes within a half hour. The experimentation of the 1960's indicated that the poison damages the specific mechanism which allows the influx of sodium ions in the beginning phase of the nerve impulse. This fact was learned from voltage-clamp experiments on squid and lobster axons when a solution with tetrodotoxin was bathing the fibers. The poison, the investigators discovered, reduced and then abolished the part of the impulse carried by the flow of sodium ions.

The membrane theory now has a firm basis in the idea of an interchange between the internal potassium and external sodium of a nerve cell. It can be applied not only to unmyelinated axons, like that of the squid, but also to myelinated fibers. Here, however, the electrical action takes place mainly at the nodes of Ranvier.

Two important questions about the membrane theory remain unanswered. First, what is the mechanism that can selectively open the cell membrane gates during the passage of an impulse so that in one split millisecond it is permeable to sodium ions and the next to potassium ions? Second, how are the internal-external differences between potassium and sodium maintained after thousands of impulses have forced a continual exchange of the two ions across the cell membrane?

Scientists trying to answer the first question generally agree that the change in the membrane's permeability is triggered electrically. As we have already learned, an impulse, once started, propagates itself like a chain reaction, with each active point exciting the next. This idea, which has been current since the nineteenth century, was supported by the experimentation of Hodgkin and Huxley, with the former publishing on the subject as early as 1937. It is now well accepted that small local currents flowing out from an active point on an axon depolarize the adjacent area until it reaches a critical electrical value called the "threshold." At this point the permeability of the membrane to sodium ions suddenly increases, and the action potential occurs explosively. And thus the impulse proceeds down the axon, with each minute segment giving its all or nothing, then passing the action along to the next segment. The nerve cell, therefore, doesn't depend on any outside source for energy. With each impulse it derives its own power from the ionic differences waiting for the tiny membrane gates to open and release the energy.

But what opens and closes the membrane gates? It is not enough simply to say that the electrical action spills over from an adjacent active area of an axon. Some scientists think that a chemical mediator is involved. This possibility was indicated by some delicate measurements made in 1932 by Archibald Vivian Hill, who had already won a Nobel Prize for discoveries related to the production of heat in muscle. The English scientist used some extremely sensitive equipment to measure "nerve heat," which he found was in the order of .000001 calorie per gram of nerve per single nerve impulse and .0004 calorie per gram per second when impulses were sustained. The infinitely small measurements indicated that a chemical reaction occurs in a nerve cell when it fires. In 1953, a Columbia University scientist, David Nachmansohn, offered an explanation for this action. He suggested that while local electric currents are responsible for impulse transmission along an axon, they depend on a chemical mediator, namely acetylcholine, to open the membrane gates. He further postulated that subsequent closing of the gates is accomplished by the swift destruction of acetylcholine by cholinesterase. This enzyme, he pointed out, is found in the surface membrane of the squid axon, but not in other parts of the fiber, such as the axoplasm. Nachmansohn also explained that inhibiting cholinesterase in such a membrane blocked the passage of an impulse. Nachmansohn's "new conceptual scheme," as he called it, was not readily accepted by all scientists, for they felt he had failed to offer sufficient proof to warrant his contentions. Nearly two decades after the scheme was proposed, the possible role of acetylcholine in the membrane processes is not discounted, although the subject remains controversial.

The second question remaining about the membrane theory—how are the external-internal ionic differences maintained around the axon?—has not been answered. Overton's paper of 1902 pointed out that in seventy years of life the muscle of the human heart contracts tens of billions of times, but the distribution of sodium and potassium remains the same. If, with every impulse, sodium enters and potassium leaves via the nerve cell membrane, why are not the all-important internal-external differences in concentration eventually spoiled? The answer is that sodium gets back out of the cell and potassium gets back in. How this happens is still a puzzle. In either case, the ionic movement would appear to be a difficult "uphill" flow. Sodium ions, having arrived inside a cell, must move outward against the external sodium ions trying to enter—and vice versa for potassium ions. The action, regardless of how it happens, takes energy. Where does it come from? Authorities on the subject talk about sodium and potassium pumps with metabolic drives capable of forcing sodium back out of the cell and potassium back in. The workings of these theoretical pumps are yet to be explained. Whatever they may be, they are essential to maintaining the ionic differences that are in turn the basis for the electrical activity of the nervous system. In life these differences are everything; in death they disappear and the electricity goes off. Scientists trying to explain these metabolic processes are reckoning with life itself.

11

SECRETS IN A SEA OF DETAIL

Shortly before Santiago Ramón y Cajal died in 1934, he was visited by a famous neurosurgeon from Montreal, Wilder Penfield. "He was confined to bed with a cold, dressed in a gray sweater and cap, when I last saw Don Santiago Ramón y Cajal," said Penfield when he later wrote an appreciation for the Spanish histologist's final book. "The manuscript of this book—'Neuronismo o Reticularismo. The Objective Proofs of the Unity of Nerve Cells'—lay in his lap. As we came into the room . . ., he put down the goose quill with which he had been writing and smiled a courteous welcome. The wall adjacent to his impatient right hand was spattered with ink.

"The master was then in his eightieth year, alone in his home in Madrid, for Señora Cajal had passed on. He was feeble, and deafness was closing doors to the world around him. But within him there burned the boundless enthusiasm of the born explorer and his eyes blazed at us through shaggy brows as he talked."

The manuscript on the aged Spaniard's lap was a detailed monograph defending his neuron theory for one final time against the reticular theory that had been held religiously by Camillo Golgi until the Italian's death in 1926. Now it was still being pressed by Hans Held, a reticularist prominent since the last days of the nineteenth century.

"Despite the wealth of objective evidence favoring the doctrine of individuality of the constituent elements of the gray substance," Cajal began, "now and then we observe new interest in the reticular theory."

The theory, as we learned in an earlier chapter, proposed that the nervous system consists of a continuous network of cells with each connected to the other. This idea was opposed by the neuron theory, for which Cajal had provided substantial proof. His theory claimed that each cell is a separate entity with processes reaching out and touching other cells at the synapses. Now, a half century later, Cajal was still defending the proposition.

"I propose to describe briefly *what I have seen* during fifty years of work and what any investigator can verify for himself. It is not based on this or that nerve cell (which may be of abnormal type or very badly fixed) but rather on millions of neurons strongly stained by different methods of impregnation." And Cajal went on through nearly 150 pages of print and sketches to provide detailed support for his theory.

In those fifty years Cajal and other microscopists, like David Bodian and George W. Bartelmez at the University of Chicago, had used the conventional light microscope, the polarized light microscope, and X-ray diffraction studies to expand anatomical knowledge of the nerve cell. They had been able to describe the contours of nerve endings well enough to say that tips of axons expand into bulbous endings that contain mitochondria close to the synaptic interface (mitochondria, intracellular particles known to cluster close to areas of intense activity, are considered the "powerhouses of cells"). But there at the interface the investigators were stopped, because the best microscopes lacked the resolution to provide a clear picture of what structures, if any, exist between connecting neurons. At best the instruments revealed only a thin line, and, as Cajal conceded, there were enough variations—among different kinds of nerve cells and different qualities of preparations—for the reticularists to question that the line was really a separation between cells.

While most scientists had accepted Cajal's proposal over the fifty years of its life, the textbook writers of the 1930's and 40's still felt obliged to present the reticular theory. A standard textbook of histology revised in the early 40's carried a section on the neuron by a well-known scientist, Stephen Polyak, who explained: "In the light of this [reticular] doctrine, the nervous system in all animal forms at all stages of their development forms a cellular and fibrous syncytium in which the 'cells' are little more than local condensations in an otherwise uniform and continuous mass." He continued, saying that the doctrine remained "in its primitive state" and that "no successful attempt has ever been made to give a functional interpretation of the structure of the nervous system by means of it." Polyak felt the controversy persisted only because of "the assumption that crude histological methods can give evidence regarding the most delicate of cytological structures, viz. the synapses in the central nervous system and relations of peripheral nerves to end organs."

In the next decade, the 1950's, the old argument was settled when scientists first trained the electron microscope upon synapses. Some of the earliest work was done by George E. Palade of the Rockefeller Institute of Medical Research, Sanford L. Palay of Yale University, and Eduardo D. P. de Robertis and H. Stanley Bennett at the University of Washington, Seattle. With their new, powerful microscopes these men were soon describing what the synapse was really like, and it was bad news for anyone still promoting the reticular doctrine. It was even revealed that Sherrington's designation, synapse (from the Greek word meaning "to clasp"), was not entirely accurate.

The early electron micrographs showed that two cells at the synapse did not clasp, but were separated by an ultrafine gap, about two hundred angstroms wide. It was named the "synaptic cleft." The cleft was apparently the site for chemical action when one cell (on the "pre-synaptic" side of the gap) acted upon another cell (on the post-synaptic side). Hence this submicroscopic canyon might be considered among the most important, if not *the* most important structure in the nervous system, for apparently it is in this gap that the system's communication signals are mediated.

On the pre-synaptic side of the cleft the electron microscope revealed some important structures for understanding chemical transmission. Within the knob-like ending of the pre-synaptic axon the electron microscopists could observe many tiny vesicles along with the mitochondria that light microscopists had seen earlier. In the cells of frogs and earthworms that were used by the modern experimenters the vesicles were only two hundred to five hundred ang-

TERMINALS

(PRE-SYNAPTIC)   (POST-SYNAPTIC)

AXON

IMPULSE ⟶

IMPULSE ⟶

MITOCHONDRIA

SYNAPTIC VESICLES
WITH TRANSMITTER
SUBSTANCE

SYNAPTIC
CLEFT

DENDRITE

Synapse in diagrammatical form. When impulse arrives at pre-synaptic terminal, transmitter is released into cleft, and impulse is reactivated in post-synaptic terminal, on dendrite of second cell.

stroms in diameter. Their circumferences were darker than their centers.

"The synaptic vesicles immediately adjacent to the pre-synaptic membrane," explained de Robertis and Bennett, "show a special arrangement and relationship, being elongated or drawn out in a direction normal to the membrane, and coming in contact with the membrane in many cases. Some of these vesicles seem to perforate the pre-synaptic membrane, so that portions of the vesicle lie in the intermembranal space [the synaptic cleft] and come into direct contact with the post-synaptic membrane."

These observations gave the impression that vesicles serve as repositories for the transmitter substances that are released into the synaptic cleft when impulses move down the axon. The presence of mitochondria reinforced the idea that here in the pre-synaptic ending was a small generating plant for restoring the chemical supplies used up in the process of nervous transmission. But evidence on the storage and release of transmitter substances remained mostly circumstantial, and by the 1970's scientists still couldn't give a definite explanation of the chemical processes involved.

In the meantime the electron microscope was used to study the synapses in various regions of the mammalian central nervous system, and the results largely supported the earlier observations of vesicles and mitochondria near the pre-synaptic membrane. But details were added of what the synapses looked like in different cells. One scientist, E. G. Gray at University College, London, decided that synapses could be placed in two categories, determined by where on the post-synaptic cells their junctions were located and by the membrane shapes on the opposing sides of synaptic clefts.

However, to go much beyond these descriptions of synaptic structures in the central nervous system, scientists using electron microscopes faced the formidable problem of trying to discern fine detail among a great number of cells and their processes twisting and turning around one another to form an unimaginably complicated thicket of fibers, even in the smallest possible sample of tissue. Often a viewer simply couldn't make out what parts went with what cells in tiny areas laced with many different kinds of neurons. The histologist naturally wanted a look at the synaptic endings of single cells in the central nervous system.

In the early 1960's this was made possible through techniques developed largely by de Robertis and an English scientist at Cambridge, V. P. Whittaker. They found that by gently homogenizing brain tissue in a special preparation and then treating the resulting substance in a centrifuge, they could break apart (fractionate) the tissue into some interesting particles that were high in acetylcholine content. It seemed that they had isolated synaptic vesicles containing the chemical, but upon observation with the electron microscope it was discovered that the fractionation actually delivered pinched-off nerve endings. But more than that, it produced entire synapses, including a part of the post-synaptic membrane. Whittaker named the fractions "synaptosomes." While they gave the investigators a good chance to look at isolated synapses, the very fact of their existence also revealed how strong the attraction is between the pre- and post-synaptic membranes across the synaptic cleft.

In 1964 Whittaker reported on having broken down the pinched-off nerve endings into seven subfractions, including synaptic vesicles, mitochondria, post-synaptic membrane, and soluble cytoplasm (the liquid substance of the cell). He further reported that his results clearly indicated "the separate localization within the synaptic region of the three components . . . of the acetylcholine system." These three were acetylcholine itself and two enzymes, choline acetyltransferase and cholinesterase, the latter being the enzyme that destroys acetylcholine.

This capability of separating nerve cell endings from the rest of the neuron and of then breaking it down into the cell components was regarded by Whittaker as one of the most

important technical advances in the study of synaptic functions. In turn he felt that this study was central to the
entire science because, "The processing of information by
the central nervous system is largely determined by the number, arrangement and properties of synapses." Whittaker
envisioned that in the future the fractionation process could
become important in two ways. First, it could be used in
the identification of new transmitter substances throughout the nervous system. Thus when fractionation turned up
an unknown substance, it could be extracted from the fractionate and applied in a functioning nervous system to see if
it would act as a transmitter. Second, Whittaker could see
where properly prepared synaptosomes could be used to
observe the action of drugs upon synapses.

In 1965 Whittaker fractionated cerebral cortex from
guinea pigs and coypus (beaver-like rodents) and obtained a
pure preparation of synaptic vesicles from which he cal-
culated the acetylcholine content of a single vesicle. It
amounted to the unimaginably small quantity of about three
hundred molecules.

While fractionation methods were being developed, a
group of scientists at the Caroline Institute in Stockholm
devised a technique that allowed microscopists to map the
monoamines in the brain. By specially treating brain tissue
with a layer of dried protein exposed to gaseous formal-
dehyde, the Swedish investigators found that cells with
noradrenaline and dopamine fluoresced with a green or
yellow-green color, while those with serotonin fluoresced
with yellow. This development revolutionized the knowledge
of where these chemicals are located in the central nervous
system. It even led to the mapping of certain pathways in
the nervous system that are delineated by the presence of
the monoamines.

Such sophisticated techniques allowed neuroscientists to
become better and better acquainted with synaptic structures, so that in 1967 Palay could write: "Synaptic vesicles,

like chocolates, come in a variety of shapes and sizes and are stuffed with different kinds of fillings." Indeed, electron microscopists, like those sweet-toothed people who have learned to pick their candy fillings by the shapes of chocolates, learned that they could often do the same with synaptic vesicles. In the mid-1960's scientists found that they could separate synaptic bulbs with excitatory functions from those with inhibitory functions by the differences in shapes and sizes of synaptic vesicles. In some cases they could also name the transmitter substance in a synaptic ending by the characteristics of the vesicles. This developing capability was considered one of the most important modern advances to come from the electron miscroscopist.

At times, however, the increasing knowledge of the intricate details of nerve cells made the forest of the nervous system seem more confusing than ever because the explorer occasionally found a tree that spoiled the chance to generalize about the forest. Just as everyone was accepting the idea that communication between all nerve cells depends on chemical transmission, a series of experiments indicated that the contention was not always supportable. In fact, the findings even seemed to offer an ounce or two of support for the discredited reticular theory. For example, in the late 1950's readers of *Nature* and the *Journal of Physiology* encountered papers from the Biophysics Department of University College, London, where two experimenters, E. J. Furshpan and D. D. Potter, explained how they had worked with the "giant motor synapses" of the crayfish and found evidence to indicate that electrical activity spread from one cell to the next by electrotonus (direct electrical transmission). Furshpan and Potter also decided that this unusual synapse acted as a rectifier that allowed the current to flow only from the pre- to the post-synaptic fibers. Later, other such synapses were found in other organisms, although some were nonrectifying, meaning that they allowed current to flow in either direction. The electron microscope showed that the opposing surfaces of these various synapses were very close to each other and even fused.

In the mid-1960's scientists recognized another variation on the synapse as they looked at some special central nervous system cells, Mauthner cells in the brains of goldfish, and Purkinje cells in the cerebral cortex of such animals as the rat. Here they found the axons of the pre-synaptic cell ending in a maze of branching twigs filled with small vesicles. But instead of meeting the post-synaptic cell, the branches formed a field that enclosed, but did not touch, the axon of the post-synaptic cell. These cells, known to inhibit the action of their post-synaptic neurons, were thought to work by changing the ionic environment around the post-synaptic membranes, rather than by a specific injection of a chemical transmitter.

The discovery of such a synapse caused Palay to ask: "Is this kind of junction a synapse? It lacks the important characteristic of contact or apposition between cells, but it is certainly a place where the activity of one cell specifically and critically affects the activity of another. Physiologically it must be called a synapse, and the morphological definition must be expanded to include it. But it must be recognized, in so doing, that morphological criteria for identifying a synapse become less compelling, less useful. They turn out to be characteristics of certain *kinds* of synapse, chemical or electrotonic. These are, fortunately for the investigator, the most common kinds, but they do not restrict our imagination."

While microscopists were focusing their ever more powerful instruments upon the synapse to study its form, physiologists were applying sophisticated new techniques and equipment to study the function. A giant step forward was taken in 1951, when John C. Eccles and his associates at the University of Otago in New Zealand employed an ingenious technique for electrically recording the internal activity of nerve cells. They used an extremely fine glass "micropipette" with a tip diameter of about 0.5 micron. The infinitely thin glass tube was filled with a salt solution that acted as a conducting core for electricity. The scientists at Otago found that by carefully probing with the micropipette they could impale a nerve cell so that the fine glass tip projected into the internal fluid. Fortunately the cell membrane sealed itself around the glass intruder, and the impaled neuron continued to behave normally for many hours. The experimenters were unable to use a microscope to guide the micropipette visually (the tip being smaller than the wavelength of light), but they did so with the help of electrical observations. The tiny probe was connected to an oscilloscope, and as it was forced into the tissue, the scientists could tell from the wave forms on the screen when the tip broke through a cell membrane. This was a major accomplishment, for it now gave the neurophysiologist an electrical avenue right down to the inside of neurons functioning normally in their natural environment. Eccles used the new technique to study the physiology of the synapse. His subjects were mostly anesthetized cats in which the necessary nerves were dissected free so that the desired cells could be impaled by the glass pipettes.

The work, which began at the University of Otago and continued at the John Curtin School of Medical Research in Canberra, Australia, first dealt with certain large nerve cells, "motoneurons." The cell bodies with their synaptic connections lie in the spinal cord, and the axons lead out to muscles. Each motoneuron has several synaptic inputs that derive from sensory fibers bundled into a nerve and enter the cord from stretch receptors that lie within muscles to sense when the muscles stretch. This combination was valuable to Eccles and his colleagues because it allowed them to vary the amount of stimulus applied to the motoneuron via the synapses. This work was accomplished by electrically stimulating the sensory nerve trunk in different amounts so that the resulting "volley" of impulses involved different numbers of fibers leading to the synapses. Hence a low stimulus activated only some of the fibers, but as its strength increased, it forced more and more fibers to come into play in the transmission. Thus able to control the synaptic inputs, the experimenters proceeded to record the results in the single receiving motoneuron. In this way they could observe the actual electrical communication across the synaptic junctions between the nerve and the motoneuron. The results can be summarized as follows:

A low stimulus involving few synaptic inputs failed to fire the motoneuron. However, the cell's internal potential became more positive—say, from the minus seventy millivolts of the resting potential to minus sixty. Such a change is referred to as an "excitatory post-synaptic potential" (EPSP). As stimuli of added strength brought more synapses into action, the EPSP became increasingly positive until suddenly the motoneuron reached its threshold voltage and fired. Then the spike-like wave of an action potential replaced that of the EPSP on the oscilloscope screen. Eccles and his collaborators now had experimental proof that multiple synapses excite a neuron according to the algebraic sum of their activity, i.e., the more the synapses that are activated, the higher the EPSP, until it reaches the threshold value, and the cell fires with an all-or-none impulse. They found an EPSP of ten to eighteen millivolts was necessary to force the cell's internal potential over the threshold.

In similar fashion the scientists Down Under experimented with synapses that inhibit rather than excite a motoneuron. They found that a volley arriving at the cell via multiple inhibitory synapses caused the internal potential to become more negative rather than positive in relation to the resting potential. This voltage change, called an "inhibitory post-synaptic potential" (IPSP), appeared on the oscilloscope in what the scientists referred to as a "mirror image" of the EPSP. It moved the cell's internal potential down the scale away from the threshold, from the minus seventy millivolts of the resting potential to minus seventy-five or eighty millivolts. The IPSP, therefore, meant that excitatory synapses trying to make the neuron fire would need to add up to an extra five or ten millivolts to overcome the threshold value.

As Eccles and his associates studied these changing potentials with their oscilloscopes, they could actually observe why the action of inhibitory synapses reduces the chances for a receiving cell to fire an impulse, and it helped explain one of the fundamental features of nerve cells at work in the vastly intricate nervous system. Any given cell may be reached by synapses with many other cells, both inhibitory and excitatory (a given neuron is either one or the other, not both). Whether the receiving cell fires or not depends upon the algebraic sum of the EPSP and IPSP that may be prompted at a given moment. The IPSP's negative force pulls the cell away from the threshold and the positive EPSP pushes it toward that critical value. The winner of this electrical tug of war determines whether or not the receiving neuron shall fire and add one more tiny impulse to the billions and billions that continually race around the nervous system.

Eccles and his colleagues were also interested in the chemistry of synapses, especially with regard to two questions: How do chemical transmitters affect the post-synaptic membrane? How do they make one cell inhibitory and the other excitatory? Eccles chose to research these problems through experiments with the ionic concentrations in the post-synaptic cells.

In innumerable experiments he and his collaborators altered the ionic contents of nerve cells by injecting them with solutions containing various ions. Again the scientists used the micropipettes, but this time the tiny tubes served to transport the ionic solutions into the cells. In each case the membrane was impaled by a pipette filled with a solution, and a small, brief electric current was sent down the tube to carry the ions into the cell. As this altered the cell and caused synaptic action, electrical records were made and analyzed. The scientists thereby learned a good deal about the functions of chemical transmitters, even though they didn't necessarily know their identity.

Essentially they found that transmitters from excitatory cells affect the permeability of the post-synaptic membrane so as to permit the influx of sodium ions and the efflux of potassium ions. The incoming sodium develops the more positive EPSP, and then, when the cell's threshold is reached, there occurs a more rapid influx of sodium. From that point on through the ensuing action potential, the post-synaptic membrane experiences the sodium-potassium exchange associated with passage of an impulse (as discussed in the previous chapter).

On the other hand the scientists in Eccles's laboratory found that transmitters from inhibitory cells produce a different change in permeability in the post-synaptic membrane. Somehow they open only gates allowing potassium ions to flow outward, while preventing sodium ions from entering the cell. This increases the potential difference between the internal and external ions, thereby driving the inside potential in a negative direction, accounting for the IPSP.

While these findings would clearly seem to say that the transmitter substance determines whether a cell is to be inhibitory or excitatory, scientists still aren't entirely sure. In fact, a 1966 review of considerable evidence indicated that acetylcholine, noradrenaline, dopamine, and serotonin work for both excitatory and inhibitory cells at various areas of the central nervous system. GABA, on the other hand, seems to be predominantly associated with inhibition, while glutamate is predominantly associated with excitation. The explanation of why one cell excites while another inhibits may yet be found in some other nerve cell mechanism besides the chemical transmitter.

Eccles, who moved to the United States in the 1960's,

continued his studies of these fundamental secrets of the nervous system. Meanwhile he received the highest of honors for his important contributions to the neurosciences. He was knighted by Queen Elizabeth in 1958 and five years later received the Nobel Prize for Physiology or Medicine with Hodgkin and Huxley.

In 1970 a share of the Nobel Prize went to one of Eccles's early colleagues, Bernard Katz, who had joined him in 1939 to study neuromuscular transmission at the Kanematsu Memorial Institute of Pathology in Sydney, Australia. After World War II Katz returned to England, where for a time he collaborated with Hodgkin and Huxley at Plymouth as they were beginning their classic work on the action potential. He then joined another neuroscientist, Paul Fatt, and they used the new micropipettes to study what is known as the "end-plate potential," which occurs in a motor nerve axon at the neuromuscular junction.

As Fatt and Katz were studying these tiny potentials, their oscilloscope frequently indicated extremely small, spurious voltages at random intervals. Apparently the two scientists first assumed these odd potentials were only undesirable electrical activity in their instruments, technically known as "noise." But then they recognized that the voltages were not present all the time, only when a micropipette was in a muscle fiber near the area of a nerve end-plate (terminal of a motor fiber). Wondering if these small potentials might not be occurring at the neuromuscular junction, the scientists applied curare (which, it will be recalled, blocks the action of acetylcholine), and the noise stopped. From this accidental discovery came an important theory about nervous transmission.

Fatt and Katz proposed that their pipettes were actually picking up "miniature end-plate potentials" caused by the occasional, spontaneous release of small packages, or "quanta," of acetylcholine. They further postulated that when stimulation of the nerve caused the normal transmission of an impulse, acetylcholine was released in a large number of these quanta. After some careful experimentation by Fatt and Katz and then by Katz and another colleague, José Delcastillo, it was shown that the transmitter substance was definitely released in small, fixed amounts—as if the chemical had been care.ully packaged so a user could obtain various amounts by ordering different numbers of packages.

Delcastillo and Katz subsequently formulated the "quantum hypothesis" on the release of transmitter substances. It proposed that each terminal of a nerve axon is the store-house for large numbers of packages of the nerve's chemical transmitter, and the inventory awaits the arrival of an action potential to prompt the release of a certain number of the quanta. Tests by the two proponents of the theory and by others showed it was valid, not only at the neuromuscular junction, but also at a wide number of synapses involving different transmitter substances in both the peripheral and the central nervous systems of many different creatures.

This was extremely important information for anyone try-ing to comprehend the exact workings of the synapse as the key point of communication in the enormous and intricate system of communication formed by nerve and brain. In a sense it offered a statistical hook that helped in studying the entire process of chemical transmission. Subsequent investi-gation of the process could not ignore that what happens at the synapse is directly related to the quanta release of the transmitter substance.

For this and other important contributions to our under-standing of the synapse, Katz was awarded the Nobel Prize of 1970 with Ulf von Euler and Julius Axelrod, whose work was described earlier.

Thus far this chapter has been limited to the synapse in discussing the form and function of the nerve cell. But while the synapse was the subject of major advances, other areas of the cell were also being explored. The scientists' new microscopes and generally improved technological capability were leading to a large body of knowledge about the entire structure and function of the neuron.

Experimenters found that nerve cells fit no one description, but mature in a wide variety of complex geometric patterns and dimensions. However, there are common features. Each cell has a central body, the "perikaryon." Therein lies the metabolic center to provide for the cell's own maintenance and to supply its functional needs. Many of the internal elements, the "organelles," which carry on the work, are structures found in other types of living cells: the mitochondria and Golgi complex are two examples. One of the perikaryon's main jobs is the synthesis of carbohydrates, lipids, and, most important, proteins. "The biological significance of proteins cannot be overemphasized," explains a standard textbook of biochemistry. "If carbohydrates and lipids, generally speaking, can be considered the fuels of the metabolic furnace, proteins may be regarded as forming not only the structural framework, but also the gears and levers of the operating machinery. Indeed, at the risk of pushing the analogy to extremes, we may regard the protein hormones (which act as regulators of metabolism) as the policy-forming top management of the enterprise."

Another significant task of the nerve cell body is the synthesis of deoxyribonucleic acid (DNA) and ribonucleic acid (RNA), the genetic materials of cells. In animals DNA is the chemical repository for genetic information central to the development of cells (neurons in our case) with the same characteristics as their predecessors. The most powerful support for this contention came from the model for DNA structure proposed by James D. Watson and Francis H. C. Crick, who shared the 1962 Nobel Prize in Physiology or Medicine with Maurice H. F. Wilkins.

In short, the nerve cell perikaryon has been identified as the main chemical plant of the neuron, and, as indicated by some ingenious work at the University of Chicago in 1948, many of the products flow out to the cell's extremities. This conclusion came from over three hundred experiments conducted by Paul Weiss and Helen B. Hiscoe, mostly on the nerves of rats. The Chicagoans developed a method for constricting a tiny segment of an axon by slipping a short, tight-fitting piece of artery over the cut end of the nerve containing the fiber. The artery soon contracted and squeezed the axons forming the bundle. Microscopic observation of a single fiber then revealed that the constriction caused a damming up of material on the side of the fiber near the cell body, while the opposite side decreased in diameter. When the constriction was suddenly removed, the dammed-up substances proceeded slowly down the axon at about one millimeter per day. Subsequent studies indicated that some specific materials may move along nerve cell axons at higher rates of speed.

Following World War II neuroscientists with their new investigative tools made rapid advances toward settling an old controversy over some thin, delicate strands within the neuron. These "neurofibrils" were first characterized microscopically in 1871, although they were so fine that they barely came within the purview of the light microscope's resolving power. They were used by the reticularists in support of their doomed theory, for the long, thin filaments seemed to stretch endlessly from one cell to another across synaptic junctions. Eventually this assumption was shown to be false; neurofibrils do not extend outside the surface membranes. The electron microscope and other modern techniques available by the 1950's allowed scientists to identify such tiny filaments as fibrous protein. The strands could be seen in all areas of the liquid cytoplasm that fills the internal space of nerve cells, including their axons, and the numerous dendrites, which stretch out from cell bodies like limbs of trees to make synaptic connections with the axons of other cells. A few years later the nature of some comparable structures was cleared up. They had been noted in 1948 at the MIT Department of Biology by Francis O. Schmitt and Eduardo de Robertis, who referred to them as "dense-edged fibrils" and tentatively named them "neurotubules." Later they, too, were identified as protein structures. As the name neurotubules implies, they are like microscopic pipes, and as is true with the delicate neurofilaments, they are also seen throughout the cytoplasm of neurons.

Scientists are still speculating on the roles of both these fibrous protein organelles, although it is pretty much agreed that whatever their function, they are vital elements in all nerve cells. They are often found in abundance throughout axons and dendrites, which has led investigators to believe that they may provide a transportation avenue for substances moving to and from the peripheries of neurons. Neurotubules are also thought to play an important structural role in helping nerve cells maintain their forms.

Optical and electron microscopes in the hands of twentieth-century neuroscientists have also revealed much from the clear view they afford of the neuron's external structure. A great deal has been learned of the cell's receiving-transmitting functions over and above that which has come from detailed inspection of the synaptic junction. While numerous synapses may form on the surface membrane of a cell's perikaryon, more are likely to occur on the fibrous processes that are part of the neuron's receiving facilities, the dendrites. These projections are largely responsible for the diverse physical patterns of nerve cells. Functionally they provide added surface space to allow for large numbers of synaptic connections with many other cells. At a given moment it is possible for a particular cell to receive multiple transmissions from hundreds or even thousands of synapses. Around ten thousand synaptic knobs have been seen on certain individual nerve cells of the brain, namely Deiters's cells. The multiple transmissions feeding into a given cell can, as we have seen, be both excitatory and inhibitory in nature, and the receiving neuron is either excited or inhibited according to the momentary sum of the transmissions arriving via the many synaptic junctions.

While the perikaryon receives from multiple synapses, its outgoing impulses travel over a single process, the axon that we have considered so often. However, the single outgoing fiber does not necessarily deliver impulses only to a single synapse. In most cases the axon branches near its outer end to form several junctions with other cells. Recently scientists have also discovered that the branches sometimes extend from the nodes of Ranvier on myelinated fibers. In any case, the single impulse from one cell may fan out for transmission to many cells.

In sum total, the receiving-transmitting mission of a nerve cell can be a baffling affair. As we just discovered in discussing cell inputs, hundreds or thousands, with either inhibitory or excitatory messages, may impinge upon a single cell whose mission in turn is either inhibitory or excitatory. If an impulse is activated in the receiving cell, the electrical activity proceeds out along the axon and is distributed through its branches. Each of these then reaches a synapse among many other synapses (both inhibitory and excitatory) forming the inputs of still another cell, which again is either inhibitory or excitatory. Such complexity defies comprehension when it is recalled that the central nervous system of man involves enough synaptic connections to tie together ten or twelve billion nerve cells. Even the separate functional parts such as the eye challenge any attempt to imagine the intricate circuitry. The retina depends on around 130 million receptor cells, and the fibers leading back into the brain number over a million.

In recent times microscopists studying almost unfathomable arrays of tens of billions of synaptic junctions concluded that the patterns of connections in themselves may be fundamental to the functioning of nervous systems. From highly magnified observations they have recognized some interesting associations between the input-output connections of cells and nervous functions. Wherever gross actions are required, there are comparatively few neurons, with large numbers of branches leaving their axons. Where precise, refined action is called for, there are more neurons, with less branching. The latter is evident in the peripheral nervous system, where different kinds of muscular movements are on order. Nerve fibers leading to finger muscles, which need refined, precise control, have comparatively few branchings, but for leg muscles involving massive contractions and less control, a single motoneuron may branch out to innervate over a thousand muscle fibers. These principles of neural connections are also visible to microscopists looking at central nervous systems. Many cells with fewer branchings appear where scientists are aware of well-defined channels of communication.

The more neuroscientists learn about the complexities of nerve cells, the more they wonder if perhaps much of their knowledge to date may not be a gross oversimplification of nervous functions. The questioning is understandable after a look at modern research in which investigators have studied the functions of single neurons or comparatively small groups of them. From here one can come away with the impression that thought is at work even down to the single cell level, and that individual neurons or small systems of them have specific problems to work at.

This conception of specialized activity was beautifully illustrated in a classic paper published in 1959 by four scientists at the Research Laboratory of Electronics of MIT: J. Y. Lettvin, H. R. Maturna, W. S. McCullouch, and W. H. Pitts. Their paper, entitled "What the Frog's Eye Tells the Frog's Brain" appeared in the *Proceedings of the Institute of Radio Engineers*. The simple purpose of the frog's vision, explained the scientists, "is to get him food and allow him to evade predators no matter how bright or dim it is about him . . ." And, they continued, "he will starve to death surrounded by food if it is not moving." With this in mind they began a meticulous exploration of the fibers of the optic nerve, which are axons of "ganglion" cells connecting with nerve tissue directly behind the retina. One of the team (Maturna) had already discovered with an electron microscope that the optic nerve's fibers numbered about five hundred thousand. The team's research was accomplished with a fine platinum-tipped electrode probing the fibers to pick up nerve impulses while the creature's eye was trained on carefully selected and controlled images. Through this technique the experimenters found that four separate kinds of information processing are performed by the ganglion cells in relation to the image in the frog's eye. This was evident from the electrical activity of the fibers bundled into the optic nerve, which were categorized as follows:

1. *Sustained Contrast Detectors.* These fibers remain unexcited unless the sharp edge of an object, either lighter or darker than the background, moves into the frog's field of vision, in which event the cells fire as long as the object remains in view. The excitation ceases or is greatly reduced if the lights are turned off, leaving the frog in the dark, but if the illumination is restored and the object is still in sight, the nerve cells resume firing.

2. *Net Convexity Detectors.* This group of cells remains quiet when a sharp edge comes into the frog's visual field, but if a small dot arrives on the scene, the fibers commence firing. If the dot stops within view, the fibers continue reacting, but if it passes out of sight the cells quit. If a dotted pattern goes by, it will not cause the fibers to act, but if one of the dots follows a course inconsistent with the others, the net convexity fibers fire. The experimenters exposed their frog's eye to a color photograph of his habitat and found that it did not affect these fibers whether the picture was moved or held still. When they put a fly-sized speck on the photograph and moved it across the stationary picture, the fibers fired, but when the speck and photograph were moved together, the cells remained quiet. "We have been tempted

. . ." said the MIT scientists, "to call the convexity detectors 'bug perceivers.' Such a fibre . . . responds best when
a dark object, smaller than a receptive field, enters that field,
stops, and moves about intermittently thereafter. The response is not affected if the lighting changes or if the background . . . is moving, and is not there if only the background,
moving or still, is in the field. Could one better describe
a system for detecting an accessible bug?"

3. *Moving Edge Detectors.* These fibers are like the first
in that they respond to an edge, but it can be any distin-
guishable edge rather than one that is sharply outlined
against the background. Also in this case the edge must remain moving for the fibers to continue firing. If it stops,
even though in view, the impulses stop.

4. *Net Dimming Detectors.* When the frog's eye perceives
a reduction of the light level, as though a shadow were cast
in front of him, these fibers fire. The degree of activity
among the fibers is dependent upon the nature of the darkness and the speed with which it occurs. A large dark object
moving directly into the field of vision produces a prolonged
response from the fibers, but if the object is small and off
to the side, the activity is less.

The main point of the scientists' findings at MIT is that
interpretation of what the frog sees is not a function of the
brain alone, but of the nerve cells between the eye and
brain. In brief, the ganglion cells with their fibers forming
the optic nerve are more than simple transmitters of information. They also seem to be able to think about and act
on the messages that are en route to the brain.

Other provocative examples of the nerve cell's sophistica-
tion are found in the work of Cornelius A. G. Wiersma, a biologist at the California Institute of Technology. From 1928,
when he was a graduate student in Holland, Wiersma
studied the nervous system of the crayfish, whose nerve
cells are relatively large but comparatively few in number
(below a hundred thousand). In these crustaceans he recog-

nized that certain fibers are in charge of entire behavioral patterns, and they were named "command fibers." A most dramatic instance of such a fiber is found in the crayfish. When this kind of cell is stimulated with a fine needle electrode in a particular way, the creature suddenly assumes a defensive position. In more recent years of his career Wiersma concentrated largely on the crayfish's optic nerves, each of which consists of some seventeen thousand separate fibers. By 1966 the California biologist had decided that about seven thousand were sensory fibers leading to the eye from fine hairs at the front of the crayfish. Of the other ten thousand Wiersma had gathered data on about a hundred and fifty. Among them, for example, were "space-constant" fibers that send impulses back to the brain only in response to light seen from the sky. Even if the whole creature is revolved, the space-constant fibers respond only to light that enters the turning eye from the direction opposed to the pull of gravity. Wiersma also found what he calls "sustaining-fibers," which fire continually when light enters the eye, but shut off with darkness. Conversely, "dimming fibers" fire only when light entering the eye is reduced. "Jittery movement fibers" described by Wiersma react whenever a moving object enters the crayfish's visual field, but they soon cease firing and remain quiet unless the object changes speed or direction, at which point the fibers fire again. One such fiber was nicknamed after the scientist's black pet dog, a constant laboratory companion. The "happy dog fiber" momentarily responds to any black object entering the crayfish's field of vision, but then it ceases and remains off until the object does something unusual. "If my black dog enters the field," Wiersma once explained to a visitor in his laboratory, "the fiber responds, but then stops. But if the dog wags his tail, it will cause the fiber to respond again." Wiersma speculated that the happy dog fiber serves as an attention-getter to alert the creature for a possible attack.

One of the most dramatic of all reports illustrating the

individuality of nerve cells came from another Cal. Tech. scientist, Felix Strumwasser. Working with a mollusk, the sea hare *Aplysia,* he found that a certain cell fired on a twenty-four-hour rhythmical basis, its most active period occurring a few hours before sunset. In an attempt to disrupt the scheduled firing, Strumwasser controlled the temperature and light, but found that the cell refused to abandon its circadian rhythm.

Such results make scientists believe that down in the fantastically minuscle electrical-chemical works of the neuron they may find the most important but most difficult secrets of the nervous system.

12

THE PSYCHOPHYSIOLOGICAL
WAVES

In 1940, a year before committing suicide, Hans Berger, a German psychiatrist, published his last paper, and in it related a story revealing why he had turned to the study of the brain. At the age of nineteen during service in the German army he barely escaped serious injury, or death, one spring day when he and his mount accidentally fell down an embankment into the path of a horse-drawn artillery unit. That evening Berger was surprised to receive a telegram from his father inquiring if he were safe and well. As it turned out, the father had sent the wire because his daughter had had a premonition of her brother being in great danger. In his 1940 paper Berger explained: "This is a case of spontaneous telepathy in which at a time of mortal danger, and as I contemplated certain death, I transmitted my thoughts, while my sister, who was particularly close to me, acted as the receiver."

The event altered the course of the young man's life. Back in school after serving in the army, he changed his astronomy major to medicine. While this subsequently led into psychiatry, his real interest was the investigation of the relationships between physical and psychical life, which he felt must have played a role in his sister's premonition. Berger referred to this interest as his "psychophysiological attitude," and it remained a major personal force throughout his life. As this attitude matured, it became rooted in at least three fundamental scientific concepts developed in the nineteenth century. One biographer, Pierre Gloor of McGill University, described them as follows: "(i) the law of conservation of energy, (ii) the total dependence of biological processes upon physiochemical mechanisms which fully obeyed the law of conservation of energy and thermodynamics, and (iii) the knowledge gained from clinical observations that mental processes were completely dependent upon brain functions." Such concepts led Berger to question the long-held notion that mind is separate from matter, that mental processes are totally apart from physical processes. "The persistent search," says Gloor, "for this elusive connection between the material and the psychical world, which he firmly believed could ultimately be described in terms of observable and measurable physical or physiochemical phenomena, was the underlying motive for all his scientific studies. . . ." The most important result of these studies was Berger's discovery of the electroencephalogram of man.

In 1897 Berger received his doctorate at the University of Jena, where he remained with the institution's psychiatric clinic until his retirement in 1938. His first published research—"On the Circulation of the Blood of the Cranial Cavity of Man"—described his earliest attempt to explore the relationships between the brain's material processes and mental functions. He continued the exploration through a line of study that involved temperature measurements with small thermometers introduced into the brains of patients whose skulls had been punctured for medical purposes. Meanwhile he became familiar with the work of Richard Caton and other early investigators of the electroencephalogram of animals. Berger tried comparable experiments with animals, but by 1910 he was discouraged for lack of meaningful results. After World War I, however, his interest in the electroencephalogram returned, and in the 1920's he decided to see if it could be found in the human brain.

Berger was poorly equipped for the research he attempted. He had little experience as an electrophysiologist, and his electrical-mechanical knowledge was limited. Although radio amplifiers and cathode-ray oscilloscopes were becoming available, the psychiatrist relied upon relatively primitive string galvanometers designed to record the much higher potentials of the electrocardiogram. Because of an unusual penchant for secrecy—which perhaps reflected his shyness— Berger did not seek advice, although he could have asked for and received help from some well-qualified scientists. While his university lectures alluded to his psychophysiological interests, he did not discuss the related experiments he was conducting a few hours every evening in a secluded laboratory next to the psychiatric clinic.

Berger failed in his first attempt to detect the electroencephalogram of man, which he described as follows: "As early as 1920, in a medical student who had lost almost all his hair and who, upon my request put himself most obligingly at my disposal, I had attempted to obtain current oscillations from various places on his scalp, especially from the corresponding areas on the right and left half of the head. I used *Piper's* funnel electrodes and subcutaneously inserted needle electrodes, which were connected to the small *Edelmann* string galvanometer which was then available to me in addition to the *Lippmann* capillary electrometer. However, I was completely unsuccessful."

In the next few years Berger worked with people whose defective skulls had left openings in the bone between the scalp and the brain. Also he obtained an improved, more sensitive model of the string galvanometer, and for the first time he began to enjoy some positive results. One evening Berger finally saw the galvanometer string vibrate slightly as an electrode was placed over a defect in the skull of a seventeen-year-old subject. The psychiatrist's diary for that day, July 6, 1924, included the following remark: "A type of work which agrees well with me and my whole— psychophysiological—attitude." He found more such subjects and in a short time was regularly recording feeble potential changes from defective areas of their skulls. His recordings, made by a dancing spot of light on a moving strip of photographic paper, came out as a wavy line which indicated that the tiny cerebral voltages were changing with a regular rhythm of about ten beats per second. It was amazing that Berger's equipment, designed to pick up the comparatively large potential changes associated with the heart, ever found what he was seeking. The potentials of the human brain are around fifty millionths of a volt, while those of the heart are roughly ten times higher.

In 1924 the psychiatrist decided he was well enough equipped in instruments and knowledge to try again to record through an intact skull. His foremost subject was now his son, Klaus, who was used for seventy-three recordings between the ages of fifteen and seventeen. From the boy came the first published electroencephalograms of man. They were made with many different kinds of electrodes—needles of zinc, platinum, lead, and others—placed on or in the scalp in many different ways. The best results were obtained when they were fixed to the forehead and occiput (lower rear of the skull). The tracings clearly showed the ten-cycle oscillating potentials picked up earlier from the defective skulls.

Here was a major discovery, but Berger waited five years before reporting it. Apparently unsure of his results, he continued making test after test on many subjects, and even upon himself. He was concerned that his electrodes were picking up extraneous currents, "artifacts," that could deceive him. He particularly feared that the waves might be an electrical reflection of the blood circulating through the head. Many of his tracings were therefore made with an electrocardiogram recorded simultaneously for comparative purposes on the same paper from the same subject. He also employed a "pulse telephone" to record the changing blood pressure in the head to compare it with simultaneously recorded tracings supposedly coming from the brain.

Berger was also concerned that the potential changes might be the result of muscle currents. He found that muscular movements in a subject's jaws and eyelids caused changes in his tracings, but he felt they were completely apart from the regular waves, which he believed were coming from the brain. Perhaps the waves were developed in the skin, said Berger at one point, and he set out to test his question with specially insulated needles that could be inserted so as to pick up the electrical variations just below the skin. The results were the same as before, and they reinforced the experimenter's belief that his tracings were truly coming from the brain.

Finally, in 1929, Berger published his findings for the first time and after a lengthy review of his work he said: "I therefore, indeed, believe that I have discovered the electroencephalogram of man and that I have published it here for the first time.

"The electroencephalogram represents a continuous curve with continuous oscillations in which . . . one can distinguish larger first order waves with an average duration of 90σ [thousandths of a second] and smaller second order waves of an average duration of 35σ. The larger deflections measure at the most 0.00015—0.0002 Volts."

"We see in the electroencephalogram," he continued, "a concomitant phenomenon of the continuous nerve processes which take place in the brain, exactly as the electrocardiogram represents a concomitant phenomenon of the contractions of the individual segments of the heart."

Berger concluded that ". . . these studies as well as those of the problems indicated above will be continued as far as time will allow me, and I hope to be able to report on them later. In the pursuit of these questions and investigations it would of course be desirable if one could use still more sensitive instruments of the type which technology is in fact able to provide."

His 1929 report, entitled "On the Electroencephalogram

of Man," was the first of fourteen that Berger published with the same title, one or more a year until his retirement in 1938.

By February 1930 he had made 1,133 recordings on seventy-six persons and was ready with a second report. In it he first assigned names to the two orders of waves that he had seen from the beginning of his electroencephalograms in human subjects. The larger ones of longer duration were called alpha waves, and the smaller ones of shorter duration were named beta waves. Berger also decided henceforth to use the initials EEG rather than the word electroencephalogram.

The bulk of the report then took up one of the most fascinating parts of his discovery. In his earlier paper he had noted that the largest deflections of the string galvanometer came when the experimental subjects were lying down with their eyes closed with "complete bodily and also, if at all possible, mental rest." Now he discussed what happened to the recordings if this state of bodily and mental rest was disturbed.

"I had been struck early by the fact that in many experimental subjects opening of the eyes while recording the curve from the skull surface, caused an immediate change in the EEG and that during mental tasks, e.g. when solving a problem of arithmetic, the mere naming of the task sometimes caused the same change of the EEG."

But the change that Berger observed in his tracings came with a surprise. He assumed that sensory stimulation leading to increased mental activity would cause a larger deflection of the EEG waves, whereas the opposite was true. When the subject's eyes were opened, or when he made a mental effort, the large alpha waves often disappeared, leaving only the smaller beta waves. The experimenter found this result hard to believe, but it was supported by further tests. Pricking a subject's hand or even stroking it with a glass rod caused alterations of the EEG. Berger anesthetized a small spot on a subject's hand and found that jabbing it with a sharp point had no effect on the EEG, but if the point was moved to an unanesthetized area, it caused a reduction in the alpha waves. When a subject was startled by the shot of a cap pistol, his reaction was revealed by the EEG. When he was ordered to do something, the command eliminated the alpha waves.

What were these waves? Berger was not sure. He only knew that they arose from the central nervous system, most likely the cerebral cortex, the top layer of the brain. He also felt his experiments had indicated that alpha waves were associated with consciousness. When a subject was physically and mentally at rest, but still conscious, the waves developed from the entire brain. But the second he concentrated upon an external stimulus a single region of the brain went to work and the over-all waves ceased for the moment. ". . . we know from our psychic life," said Berger, "that there exists a narrowness of consciousness. When our attention is fully directed toward a sensory impression, all other mental processes are simultaneously shut off for a brief period of time. We can see something similar here in the EEG. Directing attention to a sensory stimulus, *e.g.* towards a touch, causes an immediate extinction of the alpha wave of the EEG. . . ." Further study, he believed, would either extend, improve, or completely eliminate this hypothesis.

The next year Berger conducted EEG experiments with subjects asleep and under the influence of drugs. His record of a thirty-five-year-old fellow physician, who had been asleep for ninety minutes, showed the alpha waves diminished from what they were with the man awake. When another subject was put to sleep with scopolamine, his EEG flattened out until it was practically a straight line. The opposite effect was produced on the EEG by the drug cocaine, which stimulates psychic processes. Finally, in testing patients while they were being anesthetized with chloroform, Berger saw that the amplitude of the alpha waves decreased as narcosis deepened until it was recorded as nearly a flat line. Such tests strengthened the psychiatrist's belief that alpha waves are physiological evidence of the psychological phenomenon known as consciousness.

This experimentation was discussed in Berger's third report, in which he also began talking about the possibilities of the EEG in clinical neurology. He said that if drugs acting upon the central nervous system produced significant changes in a person's brain waves ". . . then one also ought to expect that those diseases of the brain which are associated with disturbances of psychophysical processes should produce similar changes." His tests indicated that he was right. The EEG of a woman suffering from severe intracranial pressure resulting from a head injury revealed that the duration of her alpha waves had become abnormally long. Some of Berger's most significant findings came from fourteen patients suffering from epilepsy. In eleven of the cases he found waves of surprisingly large amplitude. Berger also noted that there were "clear pathological alterations" in the EEG's of patients suffering from multiple sclerosis and Alzheiner's disease, both of which strike at the central nervous system.

Berger, however, professed disappointment over the normal EEG's indicated for a number of patients suffering central nervous system malfunctions. In manic-depressives, "whenever a satisfactory examination was possible," he could find no signs of pathological alterations in the brain waves. The same was true with cases of severe melancholia and schizophrenia. Advanced cases of arteriosclerosis, with such symptoms as loss of speech (aphasia), left Berger puzzled as to why the EEG's appeared normal. And he expressed great disappointment over finding normal EEG's in patients classified as imbeciles.

Regardless of these disappointments, he had obtained enough evidence of the EEG's capabilities with abnormal functions to say that his discovery had great potential as a

diagnostic tool. Future investigations with improved technology, Berger concluded, would reveal the possibilities—
and he was correct.

In 1931 the Carl Zeiss Foundation presented the psychiatrist with a technical assistant and an amplifier and oscillograph especially constructed for his work. Berger was
amazed by the sensitivity of his new equipment. It was so
sensitive, in fact, that X-ray machines and other electrical
devices, including the university laundry, had to be shut
down or else they interfered with the recording of brain
waves. Even the electric light wires around his laboratory
had to be shielded to prevent them from influencing the
experiments. Berger also was forced to select subjects who
could remain absolutely still during their tests; otherwise
sudden movements could produce muscular currents that
would send the tracings completely off the moving strip
of record paper. But he was willing to grapple with these
problems to take advantage of the "far-reaching improvement" that the Zeiss Foundation had provided.

He immediately repeated and substantiated a number of
earlier experiments. For example he found that when his son
Klaus (now nineteen) solved the arithmetic problem, 22
× 43, the youth's EEG clearly indicated the moments when
the mental task began and ended. The EEG of Berger's
fourteen-year-old daughter revealed the same as she divided 196 by 7. One day as Berger was connecting his new
equipment to an epileptic patient, she experienced a violent
seizure before the electrodes could be attached to her head,
but then she fell into a state of unconsciousness, giving
Berger a chance to complete the test, which resulted in
practically a straight-line recording instead of the usual
curves. As consciousness slowly returned, so did the woman's
alpha waves. In other instances, the sensitivity of his amplifier and oscillograph indicated that, contrary to former tests,
a difference did exist between the brain waves of severely
retarded and normal subjects. Those of mentally deficient

patients represented abnormally low voltage measurements. Berger used one subject, described as an "idiot," who had to be soaked in a warm bath for several hours to quiet him down enough to take the tests.

Around this time the discoverer of brain waves in man made the first EEG's of very young children. "Many of the small children and smallest infants," he said, "quietly tolerated the application of the electrodes, especially when they had been nursed immediately before. A few children, however, screamed incessantly and became so restless that it was impossible to obtain the kind of continuous records necessary for interpretation." In six children, eight to thirteen days old, Berger found no EEG. He then discovered that the waves showed up at two months and over, all of which, he concluded, was a demonstration of the fact that the brain is still incomplete during the earliest weeks of life, when areas of the cerebral cortex contain cells that still have not acquired their myelin.

A friend suggested that Berger compare the EEG's of infants with one that he might make on a dying man, but the psychiatrist ruled out such an experiment as "inadmissible on moral grounds." He did, however, make such recordings on a dying dog along with its electrocardiogram. As respiration ceased and the heart beat less and less frequently, the dog's brain waves increased in duration, and then their amplitude slowly diminished until, in death, only a flat line was traced by the oscillograph.

One might assume that Berger's unusual reports about these spontaneous electrical rhythms of the brain would have caught widespread attention, but for nearly five years he was practically ignored. For one thing the results must have seemed preposterous. Alexander Forbes of Harvard later explained: "We supposed that to record the electrical activity of the cerebrum [the top part of the brain] would be like trying to tap all the telephone wires in the world at once; you would get just a confused roar and would learn nothing from it. But Berger had the audacity to try it. . . ." A famous electroencephalographer of the Burden Neurological Institute, Bristol, England, W. Grey Walter, had other ideas as to why Berger's work was ignored for a half decade.

"First," said Walter, "it was not considered really respectable to study the activity of the brain with measuring tools. Classical scientific methods depend on measuring one thing at a time as exactly as possible, and it was plainly impossible to isolate the individual functions of the complex human brain. Second, the 'brain waves' Berger published were altogether dull—merely a tiny electrical oscillation at about ten waves per second. It was inconceivable that these simple, regular lines could disclose anything significant about so mysterious an organ as the human brain. Third, Berger had rather unwisely admitted that he was looking for what he claimed to have found; psychiatrists, rightly or wrongly, have a reputation for being able to find proof of their wildest ideas when it suits their beliefs."

The general disregard of Berger's work abruptly stopped in 1934, when two of the world's best-known physiologists, one a Nobelist, confirmed the German psychiatrist's original findings. They were Edgar Adrian and B. H. C. Matthews of the Cambridge Physiological Laboratory. Their paper in the journal *Brain* noted that in the previous five years Berger had "published a series of papers dealing with a remarkable electric effect which can be detected in the human subject by electrodes applied to the head." Adrian and Matthews described the spontaneous, regular waves that Berger had found and decided they should be called the "Berger rhythm," a name the German soon rejected.

"We found it difficult," said the Cambridge scientists, "to accept the view that such uniform activity could occur throughout the brain in a conscious subject, and as this seemed to us to be Berger's conclusion we decided to repeat his experiments. The result has been to satisfy us, after an initial period of hesitation, that potential waves which he describes do arise in the cortex, and to show that they can be explained in a way which does not conflict with the results from animals."

Adrian and Matthews used an amplifier and oscillograph connected to electrodes consisting of copper gauze covered with lint and soaked in a warm saline solution. With subjects including themselves, the famous physiologists were able to duplicate Berger's alpha rhythm. They reported that: "There are . . . considerable variations between one subject and another in regard to the persistence of the rhythm and the fluctuation in the size of the waves. One of us (E.D.A.) gives the rhythm as soon as the eyes are closed, and maintains it with rare and brief intermissions as long as they remain closed. The other (B.H.C.M.) is better in the role of observer than of subject, for in him the rhythm may not appear at all at the beginning of an examination, and seldom persists for long without intermission. In another subject an extremely uniform series of waves appear suddenly ten seconds or more after the eyes are closed, the record giving the impression that the beat is harder to achieve but more perfectly synchronized when once it has developed."

But while the English scientists had found Berger's alpha waves, they could not agree that the electrical activity occurred over the entire cerebral cortex; they felt it was present only in a region associated with vision.

"We believe," said Adrian and Matthews, "that the potential waves are due to the spontaneous beat of an area in the occipital cortex which is normally occupied by activities connected with pattern vision. When the area is unoccupied the neurons discharge spontaneously at a fixed rate (as in other parts of the central nervous system) and tend to beat in unison. . . . In man a large area is normally occupied with visual activities; thus when the area has nothing to do and is free to develop a synchronous beat the potential changes are large enough to be detected outside the skull."

The two scientists claimed to have proven their point by exposing a subject's eyes to a uniform field of light that could be made to flicker at varying rates. The alpha waves, which would appear as soon as the eyes were settled upon the field, could then be varied in frequency by changing the rate of the flicker. The Englishmen also pointed out that in tests of blind subjects they were unable to record alpha waves, which they claimed as support for their theory about the origins of the electrical activity.

Berger, after a half decade of being all but totally ignored, welcomed this attention from the two illustrious scientists of Cambridge, although he was not ready to abandon his theory in favor of theirs about the origin of alpha waves.

The Adrian–Matthews paper on the "Berger rhythm" suddenly made the electroencephalogram of man acceptable fare to the neurological scientists of the 1930's, and a rapidly growing number soon became involved with the fascinating spontaneous waves issuing from the human head. The German discoverer of the EEG became world-famous, except in Germany, where he had fallen into disfavor with the Nazis, whose oppression hung heavily over the University of Jena. Not only did Berger remain unknown in his homeland, but also his fame elsewhere remained unknown to him. In 1937, when he attended an international congress in Paris, he was surprised to find himself a world celebrity. But back home a year later he was subjected to the most humiliating experience of his life. On September 30, 1938, while making his rounds of the psychiatric clinic, he was called to the telephone, where the voice of a Nazi official peremptorily announced that Berger was to retire the following day. The remainder of his life was marked by tragedy that ended in suicide. According to one of Berger's associates, Rudolf Lemke, the discoverer of brain waves in man was twice considered for the Nobel Prize, once before and once after his death, but in both cases the Hitler regime prevented its acceptance.

As worldwide interest in the EEG flourished, it was seen primarily as a clinical tool for diagnosing impaired functions of the human brain. Exactly a year after publication of the Adrian-Matthews paper, three doctors at the Harvard Medical School, Frederic A. Gibbs, H. Davis, and William G. Lennox, reported on their work with abnormal EEG's. For an oscillograph they modified a Western Union "undulator," which worked with an ink-filled pen that wrote upon a moving strip of paper. Their most important recordings agreed with tracings that Berger had eventually been able to make on epileptics during seizures. The Harvard scientists found that in certain seizures a patient's alpha waves slowed down to as low as three per second while the amplitude increased many times. In other words, the voltage represented by the patient's brain waves increased greatly, but the shocks, in effect, came less than a third as often. The process was described a few years later by W. Grey Walter: "In Petit Mal [epilepsy] . . ., when the patient suddenly becomes unconscious for a short time, the whole brain generates enormous regular slow waves a hundred times bigger than any normal rhythm, each one with a short spike indenting its crest. One may consider a patient generating these 'wave and spike' rhythms . . . as being electrocuted by his own brain."

Medical scientists of the 1930's, however, were not easily convinced that the EEG was a dependable tool. Some felt it was exceedingly complicated, and because of the tremendous chance for error, it hardly offered a safe approach to the diagnosis of serious problems of the brain. At a 1936 conference, Herbert H. Jasper, a well-known neurologist, warned that the EEG could be easily confused with electrical artifacts from sources having nothing to do with the brain's electrical activity. He claimed that by wiggling his ears, and moving his eyes and scalp, he had learned to produce electrical waves around the head that imitated those which Berger and Gibbs had claimed were characteristic of petit mal epilepsy. "First, it must be kept in mind," said Jasper, "that the electrical potentials under consideration are extremely small electrostatic potentials from 0.000010 to 0.000200 volt in magnitude. The same sort of potentials of magnitudes up to many volts, or one million times as great, may be produced merely by drawing a comb through the hair. With as sensitive a recording instrument as this and with the recording electrodes separated from the cortex by several layers of poorly conducting materials, it is surprising, at first, that it is at all possible to obtain records of brain activity which are not grossly distorted or masked completely by potentials of extracranial origin. The eyes, for example, act like small batteries in the head since the retina is positively charged with respect to the cornea. The movement of the eyes may produce potential disturbances in electrodes placed over the frontal portion of the head especially, which are much greater than normal brain potentials and the same form as some pathologic brain potentials. Slight movements of the scalp beneath the recording electrodes may also produce changes of potentials which resemble closely some of brain origin."

But these problems were overcome, and the EEG soon became a respected, widely used medical tool. Its clinical development was pushed during World War II because of the new instrument's capabilities for helping to diagnose brain damage caused by head injuries. At the same time technological spinoff from such wartime marvels as radar led to the improvement of brain-wave machines. By the end of the war England had fifty EEG laboratories compared to two at the beginning of the conflict.

In the pioneering years the practitioners of the new science soon realized that the human brain is a sea of electrical waves that cannot be portrayed by drawing potentials from only two points on the head. For a more comprehensive picture electroencephalographers began working with many electrodes spotted over the skull—six, eight, and, as time went on, many more electrodes. Each point of contact with the head was led through its own amplifier channel and, in turn, to its own moving oscillograph pen. During a single recording such a complex of electrodes, amplifiers, and oscillograph units produced a battery of wavy lines, each representing the EEG from a point on the skull.

The earliest electroencephalographers were primarily interested in the wobbly lines for what they might reveal concerning malfunctions of the brain, especially in epilepsy. First, however, they had to identify and describe the normal EEG in order to say what was abnormal. It was an engrossing search, which engaged leading scientists on both sides of the Atlantic. Walter in England thought of it as a detective job with the sleuths hunting for "brainprints" left in EEG records by brain diseases. They are as distinctive as a criminal's fingerprints, said the English scientist, and they are useful in medical practice "for precisely the same purpose—to identify the culprits."

On the most basic level these studies revealed that Berger's alpha and beta rhythms had company, for other notable frequencies were evident in brain waves. In most cases the newly discovered waves were also labeled with letters of the Greek alphabet.

One was the "theta" rhythm. It was very evident in such animals as the cat and rabbit, but traces were found to remain in humans and monkeys. In humans it was strongest in children. The waves, recorded at frequencies between four and seven cycles per second, emanated from the brain's temporal and adjacent parietal regions, roughly midway between the front and rear of the head. They were strongest on the left side of the skull. In subjects of ages two to five, theta rhythms were found to dominate the EEG, but at ages five and six theta and alpha waves appeared about equal. At subsequent ages theta waves became smaller than alpha waves. They somehow seemed to be a function of emotions, especially frustration. In children, electroencephalographers found that the theta rhythm increased with laughter, crying, and signs of hunger. Any unpleasant stimuli increased the waves in a youngster. And in adults the termination of pleasant stimuli heightened the theta rhythm. Like alpha, theta rhythms were also increased in all subjects when they closed their eyes.

Brain waves with the slowest oscillations per second were named "delta." Delta waves, with frequencies as low as a half to three and a half cycles per second, included the large, slow potentials recorded with epileptic seizures. Thus their name became associated with "destruction" and the abnormal EEG. But they couldn't always be characterized as bad, because such slow waves were found in the normal brains of the young and in sleeping adults. Indeed, delta rhythms were recognized in infants up to age one as dominant waves which then continue, but to a lesser degree, over the next few years of maturation. But in adulthood, scientists generally agreed, a person is unlikely to exhibit delta waves while he is awake unless something is wrong. Despite their destructive side, delta rhythms were thought of by some scientists as a protective feature of the brain. Walter once compared them to the "dead man's handle" of a machine. When, for some reason, the neurons of the brain are in trouble, the English scientist surmised, the large, slow waves are called upon—probably by some genetically controlled mechanism—to shut down the organ until order can be restored, or until fatigue is overcome, in the case of sleep.

"During delta activity," he explained, "no useful work can be done by the neurones concerned. Sometimes the delta waves are so large that we may suspect them of paralyzing the cortex by electrocution, as it were, and we may speculate as to whether this may not be their special function in certain conditions, just as the function of pain is sometimes to immobilize an injured part."

Scientists exploring the EEG's various frequencies also

recognized and named gamma, kappa, lambda, and mu rhythms. Gamma waves, having very small amplitudes, were found in the 35-to-50-cycle-per-second range, but they never played much of a part in electroencephalography. The kappa rhythm, oscillating about ten cycles per second, was thought to be related to thinking processes, but it was also largely ignored. Lambda waves were identified as single waves occurring at random times from the back of the head. Associated with vision, they were conspicuous in a few subjects while their presence in the remainder of the population was much more difficult to detect. Mu rhythms were found in about seven percent of all subjects under the age of thirty. These waves, oscillating around nine cycles per second, were picked up from the central regions of either side of the head. They disappeared when the subject moved or thought about moving the limbs on the opposite side of his body.

Making good use of all these different frequencies drawn simultaneously from a dozen or more points on the human scalp was an immensely formidable undertaking. The waves were a continuum, an endless river of electrical potentials with infinite mixtures of forms and frequencies. Spatial differences added complications. What was happening to the EEG at one point on the head was not occurring anywhere else at any given moment. The electroencephalographer could not say precisely where his recorded waves were originating or what they represented, because at any single electrode he was always receiving a summation of potentials drawn from a three-dimensional cerebral region of which he knew very little. Finally he was forever in danger of being buried by his own work. While he was trying to figure out the tracings accumulating in one minute, yard upon yard of tracings would be pouring from the same machine attached to the same head. Precise visual analysis was impossible. It was an art at best—with the persistent danger of the investigator suffering mental strangulation by his own raw material.

From the earliest days of their science, brain-wave authorities recognized the need for automatic analytical assistance —mechanical, electrical, or both. Mainly it had to come in two ways: (1) in dissecting the frequencies of the EEG to tell which frequencies were the more prominent in the ever-changing spectrum of frequencies, and (2) in understanding the spatial relationships of waves issuing simultaneously from different regions of the brain.

The first frequency analyzer was developed in 1938 at Harvard and the Boston City Hospital by Albert M. Grass and Frederic A. Gibbs, whose machine was modeled on a mathematical tool, the Fourier Transform, based on the principle that any complex, periodic wave form (like the EEG) can be broken down into its sine-wave (simple, periodic) components. The device, which contained a rapidly whirling belt of thirty-five mm. film with a photographic record of a thirty-second EEG sample, was capable of dissecting the sample's different frequencies and presenting them on a graph-like chart indicating their relative voltages. The process was greatly improved in England during the war, when Walter developed a fully electronic analyzer that accomplished the same results and even transcribed the results directly on the record of the EEG being analyzed. This model became the basis of frequency analyzers for the next several years.

However, the rapid development of computers and sophisticated tape recording methods eventually provided the best answers of all to the problem of automatic frequency analysis. In 1964 a well-known neuroscientist at the University of California, Los Angeles, W. Ross Adey, said that the recent use of computers with magnetic tape recording equipment was "perhaps the most significant change in the last 150 years of physiological data acquisition." At the time Adey was particularly excited about the development of a single magnetic tape capable of simultaneously recording many more channels of information than previously possible. While earlier tapes had been limited to accepting fourteen to sixteen tracks of data, neuroscientists had frequently needed to record as many as twenty to thirty EEG channels along with data being recorded from the heartbeat, eye movements, and other sources. Meanwhile scientists in the military field of missile telemetry developed a special tape capable of handling as many as twenty-eight channels of data with conventional recording machines. This advance took the recording of brain waves many giant steps away from the scribbling pens tracing waves on a wide, endless paper belt that literally buried the observer physically and mentally. Now the human EEG gathered by a scalp full of electrodes could all be recorded on a narrow band of magnetic tape that was easily stored, readily retrieved, in full or part, and definitely the raw material for analysis by large, modern computers. With this elaborate equipment neuroscientists finally had an analytical tool that offered both the speed and capabilities necessary to deal with the fantastic rivers of human brain waves and to compare their infinite forms and frequencies with the subject's actions and responses to various stimuli.

The new analytical tools that came with the computer helped solve a problem that had blocked an important avenue of research related to the EEG. The work was aimed at mapping out the areas of the cerebral cortex where sensory signals arrive. It had been known for a long time that stimulation of the senses—a flash of light in an eye, a tap on the hand, a sound in the ear—produced electrical activity at appropriate sites in the brain, and it appeared superimposed on the endless river of brain waves. The location of these "evoked potentials" or "evoked responses" on the cortex when the various senses were stimulated offered a good clue to how sensory systems are connected into the brain.

Originally the sensory mapping work was conducted on anesthetized animals with electrodes drawing electrical potentials directly from the cortex. In the late 1930's and early 1940's a number of scientists reported on such investigations with various animals. In 1937, for example, three scientists at Johns Hopkins Medical School used a camelhair brush to stimulate the skin of a monkey tactually while fine wires on the creature's exposed cortex picked up the evoked responses to be recorded on a cathode-ray oscillograph. In 1943 Edgar Adrian, the Nobelist at Cambridge, conducted one of the more unusual sensory mapping experiments with a Shetland pony. The lightly anesthetized animal was supported by a frame in an upright position, and the brain was exposed. A fine silver wire carried the evoked potentials from the cortex to an amplifier with a loudspeaker. When sensory stimulation produced brain activity, Adrian, listening to the loudspeaker, could hear "the characteristic sound of a volley of impulses in the afferent fibres of the cortex." He moved the wire electrode from point to point around the surface of the pony's brain, and at each point he located the corresponding area on the animal's skin where tactile stimulation evoked brain potentials at the electrode site. In this way Adrian mapped the somatic receiving areas of the animal's cortex.

The method worked fairly well in anesthetized animals where the experimenter picked up electrical potentials directly from the brain, and the anesthesia reduced the natural brain waves so the evoked potentials stood out. But with unanesthetized humans, where the scientist is ordinarily limited to drawing from the scalp, the procedure didn't work as well because evoked potentials were simply lost in the mass of EEG potentials. In 1951 G. D. Dawson, a scientist at the National Hospital, Queen Square, London, proposed a "summation [or 'averaging'] technique for detecting small signals in a large irregular background [such as the EEG]." By repeating a stimulus and then averaging all the electrical activity from simultaneously recorded EEG's, the evoked potential would stand out in the confusing mass of brain waves. Dawson's technique was based on one proposed in the eighteenth century (and later verified) for recognizing a lunar tide in the atmosphere; it depended upon averaging great amounts of data on atmospheric pressure. To demonstrate his technique, Dawson painstakingly measured and averaged many complex EEG curves by hand, but it was the kind of work suitable for the relatively new computer. At any rate, the technique was the answer to studying evoked potentials in humans in order to map the sensory receiving areas of the brain.

A few years later the averaging method was immensely improved by W. A. Clark, Jr., at the Lincoln Laboratory of MIT. He designed an "average response computer" that not only did the averaging of EEG's to unmask evoked potentials, but did it almost immediately. This machine allowed a scientist to apply sensory stimuli and simultaneously observe the averaged results on a cathode-ray screen or a special plotting device.

With this kind of capability available to neurology, evoked response, otherwise hidden in the EEG, could be carefully studied, so that experimenters were soon able to make a fascinating generalization about them. Besides helping to unravel the intricate wiring system of the brain, the work revealed that the evoked potentials themselves vary according to the brain involved. The potentials, in general, were found to grow more and more complicated in wave form as the experimenters moved up the evolutionary scale through various animals to man. A flash of light in the human eye, for example, not only evoked a sharp, single response in the visual area of the brain at the rear of the head, but also prompted a train of electrical waves immediately following the main response. Such results led scientists to wonder if this kind of response might not be an indication of how the brain in higher animals processes a sensory message for storage as a memory. The idea was supported by evoked-response experiments on human subjects under anesthesia, or with hypnotically induced blindness.

Here a flash of light still evoked the main response in the brain, but not the subsequent train of waves—and, of course, the person tested did not remember the flash.

While electroencephalographers were pioneering with such sophisticated problems of frequency analysis, they were also working at the problems of spatial analysis of brain waves. The difficulties in this area were once explained by W. Grey Walter through the analogy of a phonograph recording (representing the EEG) and an orchestra (representing the brain). "When you listen to the complex air vibrations from a phonograph disc or a tape record of an orchestral composition," he said, "you cannot assert scientifically that you are hearing an orchestra. For all you know, the complex wave-forms may have been generated by a single instrument. How can you be sure it was really an orchestra with many individual instruments identifiable by their position as well as their *timbre?* A stereophonic reproduction would indicate this of course, but there are two other possible explanations of your impression that the instruments are spatially separated. The imaginary complex instrument may have been dashing about the recording studio, or the recording company may merely have put some frequencies on one tape and some on the other. . . . In the case of the brain we have to suppose that this last explanation, deliberate deception, is unlikely, though we sometimes sadly suspect it may be true. But we cannot be so sure whether a single complex EEG is due to an intricate mobile process or to an instrumental synthesis of many simple relatively stationary processes arising in different regions. Actually both effects are present most of the time and only a combination of frequency analysis with spatial analysis will resolve the ambiguity."

Walter was a leader in spatial analysis, and from 1947 into the 50's he worked with an elaborate analyzer called a "toposcope." In one advanced model, twenty-two cathode-ray tubes with circular faces like small TV screens were arranged in an elliptical pattern to represent the shape of a subject's head as viewed from above. Each tube was connected by an electrode to one area of the head to pick up brain waves from there. But more than that, an electron beam excited by the EEG was made to sweep around the face of each screen like the hand of a clock, and whenever it was made to do so by the EEG the electronic hand left a brief luminous trail of light. By controlling the speed of the sweep the observer could compare the brain's natural timing of waves from different areas. The toposcope could also deliver carefully controlled stimuli to a subject—such as flashing lights for visual stimulation—and the operator could observe their direct, immediate effect on the EEG in different cerebral regions. The toposcopic results were often recorded with a high-speed movie camera or a series of still photographs.

The machine with its twenty-two screens and whirling beams of flashing lights was a startling creation to behold. It emphasized to any viewer the power and complexity of the brain's machinery silently at work in the human skull. Many a beholder recalled a poetic description of the brain set down by Sir Charles Sherrington when he pictured the organ as "an enchanted loom where flashing shuttles weave a dissolving pattern: always a meaningful pattern but never an abiding one."

In 1954 Walter reported: "When we began to use this machine, we found the time maps hard to understand. But gradually the new code has begun to penetrate our thick heads, and much of what was quite bewildering in the ordinary brain-prints now seems to be taking on a new form and luster." A few years later, after much more experience with both spatial and frequency analysis of brain waves, the English scientist said: "We know that within the brain, a great many electric processes can be identified, each with its own limited domain, some apparently independent, others interacting with one another. We must accept that in the EEG we are dealing essentially with a symphonic orchestral composition, but one in which the performers may move about a little, and may follow the conductor or indulge in improvisation—more like a jazz combination than a solemn philharmonic assembly. Only rarely can we sit in on this session—in ordinary EEG recording we hear only the rhythm section and an occasional break from far off."

While Walter was deeply involved with his complex machinery, a French scientist, Antoine Rémond, was working in Paris at the famous neurological hospital, La Salpêtrière, on another fascinating method of analyzing brain waves. Rémond's EEG records, displayed on the usual long sheets of paper, looked more like contour maps than representations of brain waves. The conventional wriggly EEG lines scribbled out in parallel were now contour lines like those that indicate the lay of the land on topographical maps, or like the isobars showing high- and low-pressure areas on a weather map. Rémond's lines, however, represented the rise and fall of electrical potentials over a thin, straight section of the brain, as plotted against the passage of time. His electrodes, eight in number, were arranged in a straight line that he laid out on the subject's scalp according to the regions of the brain he wished to map. A special computer translated the changing EEG to the contour lines on Rémond's record paper. In such a display of brain waves, the swirling lines made interesting, ever-shifting patterns revealing the rise and fall of potentials coming from the slice of brain under the electrodes. At a glance the experienced eye could recognize the changing frequencies and voltage within the span of the brain covered by the line of electrodes. While the French scientist had made a contribution to both frequency and spatial analysis, he saw his topographical method as essentially a new way of looking at the EEG, one that could be most fruitful in making better use of brain waves.

By the mid-1960's Rémond's Paris laboratory was an

elaborate complex of equipment for preparing topographical EEG records. At one side of the laboratory there was a small room with a subject's chair, like a dentist's chair, where a person connected with EEG electrodes could receive visual, auditory, and tactile stimuli that were electronically coordinated with the brain-wave recording equipment. In the split second that any stimulus was administered, it was automatically noted on the subject's EEG record at a point opposite the brain waves that were picked up simultaneously. By making contour maps of different planes of the brain in various subjects, Rémond and his collaborators were learning what normal and abnormal EEG contours looked like. With this knowledge they hoped the new method of EEG display would become an important clinical tool for diagnosing malfunctions of the nervous system. The French scientist also saw possibilities for his method in research on the brain's most basic of all functions, learning. He felt that EEG contours made at frequent intervals during the learning process—for example, the learning of a language —might offer comparisons that could help investigators determine why one person learns better than another.

While scientists like Walter and Rémond were analyzing EEG's drawn from the scalp, a basic technique was developed for determining the origin of brain waves in three dimensions that took into account potentials arising inside the organ as well as on the surface. In 1935, medical literature carried two instances of EEG's made from electrodes placed directly upon the exposed cerebral surface in human patients undergoing brain surgery. The technique, "electrocorticography," was slow in developing, and investigators were limited in both the number of subjects and the locations of exposed cortical areas, which were determined by the medical requirements of a surgeon. However, the technique brought the scientist closer to the brain, where natural potentials were more powerful, not having to pass through the skull and scalp. Furthermore, the experimenter could see exactly where on the organ his electrodes were picking up the EEG.

However, he was still confined to a two-dimensional plane. To reach into the third dimension his electrodes would have to be inserted into the depths of the brain, which animal experiments had revealed was possible without inflicting serious damage. By the 1950's long slender depth electrodes were being successfully implanted into human brains for clinical purposes. At first it was done only during brain surgery, but then methods were developed for implanting electrodes via small holes drilled through the skull. It was even found they could be fixed in place and safely left in the brain for long periods of time. While the implantation was always for diagnostic purposes, the electrodes were valuable to researchers.

In the mid-1960's some of the most advanced work with implanted electrodes was conducted at the University of California Medical Center by Paul H. Crandall and his associates for diagnostic purposes. Each depth electrode consisted of two stainless steel wires of only 0.01 millimeter diameter. They were held parallel a few millimeters apart by a center strut. The wires, except for the very forward tips, which projected barely beyond the strut, were insulated with epoxy. When Crandall and his associates were ready to implant such an electrode, they determined exactly where the parallel wires should go in the brain by consulting special anatomical charts of the organ. They then drilled a small hole in the patient's skull at a carefully selected site that had been locally anesthetized. The opening was fitted with a stainless steel receptacle that screwed into the bone to receive and hold the electrode. A precision-built "stereotactic" frame located around the patient's head guided the electrode as a small, hydraulically driven device pushed it ever so slowly through the receptacle and on into the depths of the brain. Electrical impulses continually sent down the electrode during insertion were measured on an instrument that enabled Crandall to determine the moment-by-moment resistance of the nerve tissue between the two points of the electrode tip as it slowly moved inward. This helped the surgeon decide exactly where in the various strata of the brain the tip was located at any given moment. Recent research had found that different strata are characterized by different electrical resistances to such impulses.

Many such electrodes could be thus implanted in a patient's head to help locate the source of problems that surgery might alleviate. The electrodes could be left in place for weeks or months to conduct ongoing tests. A patient was hardly bothered either by the insertion of the many electrodes or by their continued presence in the brain, which suffers no pain. At a seminar on epilepsy in 1966, Crandall asked one of his female patients to appear before visitors from all over the world to demonstrate the use of the implanted electrodes. The lady, wearing a large white bonnet of bandages covering the outer stems of several electrodes, arrived in the room with a nurse after having just been across the street on a brief shopping tour. With such depth electrodes, precisely placed and available for tests over an extended period of time, investigators of brain waves were given a tremendous advantage in determining what happens to various EEG potentials from hour to hour and day to day.

Through all the years of progress in identifying, recording, and analyzing brain waves, electroencephalographers continued generally on the course set by Berger as he tried to find psychological meaning in the endless stream of spontaneous waves coming from people's heads. The continuing research involved subjects at various age levels, in different states of consciousness, subjected to many stimuli, and suffering mental or neurological disabilities.

Some of the most interesting records were drawn from children at various age levels, for their EEG's seemed to offer an inkling to what happens in the maturing brain. A pioneer in this area was Donald B. Lindsley, now at the University of California. Working with his own family, Lindsley found that he could even record the EEG of a child during the seventh fetal month, and he was surprised that the electrical activity could be recorded from the mother's abdominal wall. In a classic community study of 132 children Lindsley repeatedly recorded individual EEG's as he followed the youngsters through several years of development. Another classic EEG study made between 1935 and 1943 by Charles E. Henry of Western Reserve University School of Medicine involved 890 children between the ages of three months and nineteen years.

Essentially the studies of children revealed the development of the alpha rhythm with age. The investigators found that brain waves begin at the age of three or four months as very slow oscillations (delta) and gradually increase from three or four cycles per second to five or six at age twelve months. Subsequently the frequencies increase to ten cycles per second by the end of life's first decade, whereupon the change ceases, although the youngster continues to mature. EEG studies of monkeys revealed similar alpha-wave development starting at fifteen to twenty days of age and continuing at a rate comparable to human change adjusted for differences in life span and rate of maturation.

In the early days of electroencephalography investigators largely neglected older people, except for psychiatric patients, who could hardly offer an EEG portrait of the normal aging brain. One of the earliest studies of normal subjects was made in 1954 by Walter D. Obrist of the Duke University Center of Aging, when he recorded the brain waves of retired men in a fraternal home. He found the alpha-wave frequency significantly, but not dramatically, lower in the later years, with more waves of seven to nine cycles per second than of ten to twelve. The Duke scientist and others compared the EEG's of mentally healthy older subjects and persons having signs of senility, with memory loss, disorientation, less emotional control, and poorer judgment. Records of the less healthy individuals indicated a widespread slowing of waves all over the brain. In the more healthy subjects the slowing was generally localized in the brain's temporal lobes (above the ears), and even then, to the left side. The scientists surmised that the slowing might reflect decreased blood circulation to the brain, probably because of the arteriosclerosis present to some degree in large numbers of older people. This idea was supported by the fact that other investigators had already associated abnormally slow waves with disturbances in cerebral blood circulation caused by congestive heart failure and cerebral thrombosis. Furthermore, medical scientists had found a significant correlation between abnormally slow waves in elderly patients and subsequent post-mortem tests revealing arteriosclerotic brain disease. Obrist noted with interest that the localized slowing, predominantly over the left temporal lobe, occurred on the side of the brain most often subject to vascular problems like stroke. Such experiments naturally raised the question of whether or not reduced blood circulation to the brain might be responsible for the troublesome, but not necessarily serious, memory failures that many people experience as they approach the later years.

Sleep, as Berger's work revealed, was another obvious area of brain function that called for continuing research by electroencephalographers. The early, classic studies of sleep were conducted by Frederic A. Gibbs and his wife at Harvard, but their efforts were only the beginning of an attack on the mysteries of sleep that involved thousands of miles of EEG records drawn from subjects of all ages. By the 1960's some two dozen sleep laboratories were scattered around the United States. One was at Duke University Medical Center, where a 1969 news release told of volunteers spending their nights in soundproof, climate-controlled sleep rooms while electroencephalographs recorded their brain waves. "Sleeping conditions simulate the home atmosphere as closely as possible," said the release. "After getting into their pajamas, volunteers practice such nightly rituals as reading or listening to music. An all-night sleep record consists of fifteen hundred pages and weighs several pounds. These records are examined and evaluated by a computer model that was developed at Duke for surveying sleep records in terms of patterns, shifts, and the difference between normal and abnormal sleep, as well as other pertinent data regarding sleep."

From the EEG records of thousands of volunteers there came a stage-by-stage picture of how a person falls asleep and sleeps. As he grows drowsy, stops moving, and closes his eyes, the comparatively rapid, irregular waves of his EEG synchronize into the regular beat of the alpha rhythm. With their first appearance the alpha waves have a relatively high amplitude, but it gradually decreases with approaching sleep. During this diminishing phase of the alpha waves the person experiences the pleasant, dreamlike state where thoughts come in pieces. In the first stage of actual sleep, the alpha waves are completely replaced by low-amplitude, fast, irregular waves. Meanwhile the subject's respiration evens out and the heartbeat slows down. The person is then barely asleep, and he can be easily awakened. He remains in this state for only a few minutes before slipping into the second sleep stage, which is revealed by the electroencephalograph pens quickly tracing fast potential changes that cause sharp "spindles" to project up from the surrounding waves. This sleep is still comparatively light sleep, and the subject is easily awakened. In the third sleep stage the spindles are replaced by delta waves with high amplitudes and oscillations as slow as one per second. At this time the brain is apparently being closed down for the night. The person is not so easily awakened. His muscles relax, blood pressure drops, temperature declines, heartbeat continues to slow, and breathing becomes all the more even. The fourth and final stage is the deepest sleep of all, and the individual is oblivious to many of the stimuli that would awaken him in the earlier stages. The EEG record reveals that the brain's electrical activity has settled into a continuous train of slow, high-amplitude waves. In this stage one might expect that the brain would fail to receive various stimuli, as when awake, but the EEG indicates that such signals still have an impact on the organ's electrical activity. However, the incoming messages are obviously kept from becoming part of the psychic stream that we call consciousness.

As the EEG phenomenon of sleep was defined and studied in animals and humans between the mid-1930's and the 50's, it was eventually realized that a night's sleep was much more than stage one, two, three, four, from beginning to end. Actually there is a shifting back and forth among the stages, so the sleeper does not simply settle down into the slow-wave, fourth stage and remain there until he awakens. In 1957 two University of Chicago scientists, William Dement and Nathaniel Kleitman, published a fascinating report about the eye movements of people asleep. From this work came recognition of a new sleep stage so different that investigators hesitated to define it as sleep. They named it "paradoxical sleep," although it is more commonly called REM (rapid eye movements) sleep. The first period of REM sleep may occur more than an hour after the typical subject enters stage one. The observer may recognize the onset of the REM stage when the EEG tracings indicate that the sleeper is slipping from the slow waves of stage four back to the spindles of stage two, and then to the erratic oscillations of stage one. The investigator watches the electroencephalograph channels connected with two electrodes attached near the subject's eyes so as to pick up and record electrical potentials created when the eyes move. Suddenly the machine indicates the eyes are shifting around as if the person were looking about the room. The subject is now restive, and his breathing, heart rate, and blood pressure become irregular. In fact, there are many observable signs that the sleeper is experiencing fright. He still can't be awakened easily, but his reactions indicate that certain meaningful stimuli get through to him. Dement and Kleitman decided that this phase of sleep coincided with a period of vivid dreaming, and it became the subject of considerable research in subsequent years.

In another area of EEG investigation, psychiatrists and others made extensive efforts between the 1940's and 60's to find connections between abnormal EEG tracings and abnormal behavior. The research, however, was beset with problems that evolved mainly from the difficulty of determining the normal EEG. Brain waves, like the human beings producing them, appear with many individual variations. For example, epileptiform discharges recorded by an EEG are a pretty good indicator of cerebral trouble, but the same potentials can also appear in people who do not have significant problems. This can happen in the case of an epileptic's relatives. Working with these variations in mind, electroencephalographers turned out miles and miles of records trying to associate abnormal individuals with abnormal EEG's.

In general, behavioral disorders were correlated with an excessive amount of slow-wave activity in both the delta and theta frequency ranges. The abnormal discharge appeared either continuously or intermittently, and either generally or focally (confined to one area of the head). Disorders were also associated with epileptiform discharges that appeared as sharp spikes and complexes of spikes and waves in the EEG records. And the abnormal behavior could be associated with changes in the EEG's responsiveness to various stimuli induced by light, sound, or drugs.

In 1952, for example, Denis Hill, professor of psychiatry at Middlesex Hospital, London, made an extensive EEG study of persons with aggressive psychopathic behavior, and he found considerable EEG abnormality, indicating that the brain had suffered maturational problems. An excess of theta waves appeared on both sides of the head, especially from the temporal and central regions of the brain. Alpha waves varied from the normal. And an abnormal amount of slow-wave discharges appeared from the posterior of the brain's temporal region.

In the early days of studying brain waves, it was felt that the EEG's of criminals might identify abnormal brain functions, and that such records might even be correlated with types of criminal offenses, but experiments did not substantiate this idea. Some early studies of young delinquents and prison populations indicated that their behavior might be evident in their EEG's, but continued work in this area made it less and less likely that electroencephalographers could draw such connections. It appeared that the brain-wave machine's usefulness in this area might be limited mainly to criminals who were aggressive psychopaths, including murderers. Investigations of this class of criminal revealed abnormal EEG's (comparable to the Hill study above) in seventy percent and higher of the cases.

In passing, it is interesting to note that one of the most famous EEG's associated with crime was made in 1964 on Jack L. Ruby, the accused killer of Lee Harvey Oswald, alleged assassin of President John F. Kennedy. The records were analyzed by the veteran Harvard scientist Frederic A. Gibbs, who decided they showed "seizure disorders of the psychomotor variant type." The disorder was once called "hystero-epilepsy." A victim often becomes suddenly unreasonable, and he may have a tantrum or perform some irrational act which may be triggered by a circumstance unconnected with him. Afterwards he frequently can't remember what he did during the attack. The EEG associated with hystero-epilepsy shows high-voltage slow waves located focally in the anterior of the brain's temporal region. Ruby's lawyers were interested in the diagnosis because their defense was based on the defendant having been insane when Oswald was shot.

On a less dramatic level of psychiatric disturbances—personality disorders deemed psychoneurotic—early investigators sought connections between problems and EEG tracings, but again the results were not as definitive as had undoubtedly been hoped for. Here they were dealing with such difficulties as anxiety neurosis, reactive depression, hysterical disorders, obsessive-compulsive disturbances, and mixtures of these problems. In general the electroencephalographers found that the majority of psychoneurotic patients had normal EEG's. However, it was discovered that when large groups of their records were compared with large groups from normal subjects, significant EEG abnormalities showed up just outside the normal range of brain waves. The psychoneurotics had an abnormal amount of theta rhythms between four and seven cycles per second and of beta rhythms over thirteen cycles.

Beginning with Berger in 1931 schizophrenics were tested for EEG abnormalities, but at first he and others felt that the unusual disorder was not evident in brain waves. However, this conclusion was changed as the investigations continued, and eventually it was recognized that EEG's from various groups of schizophrenic patients revealed from twenty to sixty percent abnormalities. The disease, which causes victims to withdraw from reality to a world of fantasy, was associated with an excessive amount of theta activity, particularly in patients who suffered catatonic rather than paranoid states of schizophrenia.

Over the years following Berger's discovery of the EEG in man, investigators applied their electrodes to the heads of people and animals as they tried to correlate brain waves with almost every situation of life. This was illustrated in 1968 when Thomas C. Barnes of the Philadelphia State Hospital published a book entitled *Synopsis of Electroencephalography,* which presents hundreds of short reports of EEG recordings from Berger's time on. Here are some samples:

▪ Aspirin, according to a 1965 report, causes excessive slow waves.

▪ Two cups of coffee stimulate the EEG, said a report in 1963.

▪ A number of studies have indicated that large percentages of patients suffering headaches show abnormal EEG's.

▪ In many recordings over a number of years LSD affected the EEG, and when the drug was administered to a cat the effects lasted up to three weeks.

▪ Marijuana produces "slightly fast waves" in man, said a 1958 study.

▪ An orgasm at the end of coitus, said a 1954 study, is recorded as a "convulsive EEG."

▪ The EEG of Albert Einstein contained nothing unusual.

▪ A 1964 test of an opossum playing dead produced an EEG indicating the animal was most alert.

▪ In the late 1960's a football player's brain waves were monitored by radio telemetering equipment during a game, and it revealed that his alpha waves increased from 9.2 per second to 12.5 after a touchdown.

▪ And a 1960 investigation indicated that yoga and Zen meditation increased alpha waves.

After all the EEG tests, what has been proved? Some authorities would answer, "Very little!" The value of the EEG has almost always been subject to question. In 1944 Edgar Adrian, writing in the journal *Nature*, described the state of the science in this way: ". . . the most that can be said is that if we had to appoint someone to a responsible post and had an unlimited field of candidates, it would be safer to exclude the five percent whose electroencephalogram showed the most unusual feature."

Twenty years later another example of how the EEG remains under question was found in the English medical journal *Lancet*, where W. B. Matthews, consultant neurologist to the Derbyshire Royal Infirmary, expressed serious disappointment in what could be learned from brain waves.

He listed seven questions commonly asked of the EEG and proceeded to show how the answers at best are of limited value. "It must be accepted," he concluded, "that the direct clinical applications, while definite enough, are far more restricted than was at first hoped; at the same time, the technique is still a valuable experimental method."

But what has restricted the science? It has undoubtedly been the inability to answer the most basic question of all: What is a brain wave? In 1949 W. Grey Walter stated the problem vividly: "Even now [after more than a decade of work], we can probably understand less than one per cent of the total information contained in a record. . . . We are rather in the position of a visitor from Mars who is deaf and dumb and has no conception of the nature of sound, but is trying to build up a knowledge of languages by looking at the grooves in a gramophone record."

In the early years of the science, investigators generally felt that the electrical waves picked off the head were a rhythmical summation of the firing of underlying neurons, with each producing its rapid, all-or-none spike and the whole adding up to the relatively slow waves of the EEG. This view undoubtedly reflected all the work that had so recently gone into the study of peripheral nerve activity, where the potentials measured from the surface of a nerve trunk were summations of the electrical activity of the axons within. But in the 1930's and 40's some investigators were not completely ready to accept this proposal. One was George H. Bishop of Washington University, St. Louis, whose intensive studies of the problem led him to alter his views several times in the 40's and 50's. Some of the skeptics questioned the idea that the sharp, fast electrical activity of single neurons get together to make the slow, smooth waves of the EEG. They wondered if perhaps these mysterious, spontaneous potentials might not come from some other electrical facet of the nerve cell. Perhaps the waves were the result of changing potentials along the cell membranes, which, as seen in an earlier chapter, were then under intensive investigation by cell physiologists.

A test of the idea became possible with the development and improvement of ultra-fine microelectrodes capable of getting at single cells or very small groups of them. They offered hope of comparing the activity of individual brain cells with simultaneously recorded EEG potentials to see if they were directly related. One of the earliest investigations of significance was conducted at the Harvard Medical School by Alexander Forbes and two colleagues, B. Renshaw and B. R. Morison. Working on the exposed brains of cats and rabbits, they inserted fine electrodes below the cortical surface to pick up and compare the electrical activity from as few cells as possible with electrical waves recorded simultaneously from the brain's surface. The scientists reported that: "A sharp distinction may be drawn between the axon-like spikes and the slow waves. Although we do not know what the slow waves signify in terms of the activity of neurons, no evidence has yet appeared to indicate that the latter are the summation products of numbers of axon-like spikes or other rapid components. No intermediate forms are seen. Though they have 10 to 100 times the duration of the spikes, the slow waves have contours which are smooth. . . . When the two types of activity occur together in the same record they show no interdependence; neither seems affected by the other even when, as occasionally happens, they are superimposed. One type of activity may occur without the other."

Such assertions, however, needed much more work and improved methods before being definitively pinned down; scientists, therefore, were left to continue wondering about the nature of brain waves. In June 1948, when Herbert H. Jasper gave the presidential address to the American Electroencephalographic Society at Atlantic City, he was still asking: "What is the functional significance of these slow, rhythmic, potential waves derived from neuron aggregates throughout the nervous system?" And he was still questioning the theory that brain waves were a product of the explosive all-or-none electrical activity of the brain's neurons in their active states. There was no satisfactory reply, he admitted.

But four years later Jasper and two other scientists at McGill University and the Montreal Neurological Institute were finally able to reply with the backing of substantial scientific results. Jasper, Choh-luh Li, and Hugh McLennan made a renewed attack on the problem, using the new, infinitesimally slender micropipette electrodes capable of getting at the electrical activity of single cells. The subjects were cats with their brains exposed. In a given experiment a micropipette was first applied to the surface of a cat's cortex close to where larger electrodes were already picking up brain waves of eight to ten cycles per second from a relatively wide area. When the investigator was sure that his micropipette was also receiving the same waves, he inserted the tip into the depths of the cortex and moved it about with the help of a device called a micromanipulator. The probing continued until an oscilloscope indicated that the experimenter was picking up electrical activity from a single neuron.

"These results," reported Li, McLennan, and Jasper, "would seem to prove that the brain waves commonly used by the electroencephalographer as an index of cortical activity may, under certain circumstances, bear little relationship to the active discharge of individual cortical cells, at least of the type from which records can be obtained with microelectrodes. Certainly there is no support for the supposition that the slow waves result from envelopes of spike discharge."

The three scientists hypothesized that brain waves might flow from membrane potentials in the cortical cells. The potentials, they proposed, might be rising and falling synchronously, providing the valleys and summits of brain waves. While such oscillating potentials would make a cell more or less excitable, they would not necessarily cause it to fire by forcing it over the critical threshold potential. Thus brain waves, arising from millions and millions of cells, could very well occur without the underlying neurons reacting with all-or-none discharges.

This view, which was not confined to the Canadian workers, caused scientists to reconsider the neuron as a functional unit. The axon, the neuron's action end, had dominated investigations when brain waves were discovered, so it was naturally assumed that they were the product of axonal activity. But this assumption suffered from some serious contradictions. Berger's alpha waves were on the one hand accepted as signs of cerebral inaction, but on the other hand they were said to be products of neurons in action. When scientists thought about this obvious conflict, it made them consider other parts of the neuron as possible sources of EEG potentials, and this turn away from "axonology" led to a new examination of neuronal functions that could be the foundations of brain waves.

By the mid-1950's attention was focused on dendrites for an explanation of the EEG's slow, spontaneous waves. Here the electrical characteristics were not the all-or-none potentials of cell bodies and axons, but a moment-by-moment summation of inhibitory and excitatory post-synaptic potentials. Moreover, it was realized that dendritic potentials, compared to those on a cell's body and axon, were sizable because they arise from a surface area that is larger in total than any other on the neuron. And finally it was evident that dendritic potentials were not the spike-like discharges so closely identified with cells in action, but more evenly graded electrical changes comparable to the EEG. Many eminent neuroscientists decided that dendrites could very well be the originating sites for brain waves. For example, in 1954 Ichiji Tasaki and two associates wrote: "We propose . . . a hypothesis that brain waves such as Berger [alpha] rhythms are the summations of rhythmical dendritic potentials. . . ." Support for their idea came from the physiologists' work upon the brains of cats with microelectrodes, which revealed that the electrical characteristics of various parts of a brain cell are not all alike. This kind of investigation eventually led to the conclusion that EEG potentials probably originate along the dendrites of the brain's pyramidal cells. These neurons have what are called "apical dendrites," which extend upward toward the cortical surface, as well as toward the electrodes with which the electroencephalographer picks up brain waves.

But from where does the rhythm of the EEG come? What makes millions of dendrites work in time with one another to produce the large summated potentials that Berger originally detected from the human head? The answer remains unknown, although some possible explanations have been proposed. In the 1930's it was thought that the rhythms might reflect changing rates of cell metabolism. Thirty years later scientists were looking for a pacemaker that timed brain waves. Some thought that if such a mechanism exists it might be found in the part of the brain called the thalamus, and this theory was being explored in the 1960's.

Despite all the theories, the complicated amplifiers and recorders, the computers, depth probes, endless miles of records, and millions of words about the EEG in books and journals, the electroencephalographer has forever faced the bothersome fact that he is working with something he really doesn't understand. This was clearly illustrated in 1959 when the journal *Psychological Review* published a paper by John L. Kennedy entitled, "A Possible Artifact in Electroencephalography." The paper did not question that the brain produces electricity "in a great variety of patterns," but it impressed upon the reader that the interpretation of brain waves remains a very risky pursuit because it deals with a subject not fully understood. It is still somewhat like trying to translate a foreign-language radio broadcast from a place we have yet to discover and a people we have yet to meet.

Kennedy made the point by recording alpha waves with EEG electrodes applied to an ultra-simple model of the human skull and brain. It consisted of a ceramic vessel, comparable to the skull, filled with a gelatin mass of the size and consistency of the brain. The only other feature was a mechanical plunger that could be moved back and forth to pulse the gelatin mass in the same way as the living brain is pulsed by blood vessels. When the plunger was in action, Kennedy could record electrical potentials from the ceramic vessel, and like alpha waves they oscillated at about ten cycles per second. A number of factors could vary the frequency, but the most important was the "tightness" of the gel within the model skull. As the gel warmed up and became more liquid, for example, the frequency of the electrical waves dropped to six to eight per second. Local frequency differences could be caused by local changes in the consistency of the gelatin mass. For instance, a gum eraser imbedded into the surface of the gelatin brain could be located through the ceramic skull by locating "slow waves" coming from around the eraser. Varying the rate and direction of the mechanical pulser also could produce a variety of frequencies and wave forms comparable to those taken from the human skull under different circumstances.

The Kennedy paper went on to point out that earlier work indicated: "Possibly 5 per cent of a group of normal subjects will have very poor alpha rhythm, even on repeated testing and a few show no alpha or anterior temporal rhythm at all. They seem to be perfectly normal people, but no brain waves!" Kennedy described an adult male subject who was one of these rare individuals with no alpha waves. The man had received a hole in his skull over the left ear during an auto accident. It was roughly circular and about an inch in diameter. The skin covering the hole was visibly in motion with the normal pulsing of the brain. Kennedy decided to see if brain waves might not appear if the hole were filled and normal intracranial pressure restored. A flat plastic plate was fashioned to fit over the skin above the hole, and a head band was made to press in upon the plate until the pulsing motion ceased. With the plate in place, normal alpha rhythms appeared when the subject closed his eyes. Removing the pressure on the plate removed the alpha waves.

Kennedy's paper is a bad bump in the long flow of EEG literature, a warning of what can happen when modern, high-powered amplifiers are applied to the electrical potentials of the human head. In 1966 the paper was included in a University of California collection of key papers on brain physiology and psychology. The editors' introduction said: "While Kennedy's paper should not be taken as a serious blow to the validity of electroencephalography it does emphasize the extreme care needed when we try to interpret something we do not understand."

13

ELECTRICAL MAPS OF THE
NERVOUS SYSTEM

In 1934 the *Yale Journal of Biology and Medicine* carried a remarkable report from two Yale scientists who had succeeded in electrically stimulating the brain of a monkey as the animal moved around a cage unrestricted by any wires connected to its head. The experiment was one of the earliest attempts to stimulate the brain remotely. The scientists, E. Leon Chaffee and Richard U. Light, had surgically imbedded a small, compact coil of wire into a circular opening in each of several monkeys' heads and then connected the coil to an electrode implanted in a carefully selected site of the brain. An animal so prepared was placed in a small cage mounted inside three large circular coils of wire set in three different planes to make a sphere-like enclosure. When electrical current was passed through the large external coils, the resulting magnetic fields induced current into the coil in the monkey's skull and stimulated the creature's brain through the implanted electrode. In effect, the arrangement became a transformer with the large, external coils acting as the primary winding and the small coil in the monkey's head acting as the secondary winding.

In one monkey, with the electrode placed in the motor cortex, excitation of the coils made the animal's right arm swing vigorously in and out from its body. In another with the electrode placed at a different point along the motor cortex, the electrical excitation produced a "series of chewing and tongue-wagging motions," followed shortly by an extension of the right hand with flexion at the wrist. In a third experiment, the electrode was inserted in a monkey's hypothalamus, a part of the brain that integrates the body's various autonomic functions. When the coils were activated for ten minutes, the stimulation at first appeared to make the animal restless, but then it settled down and yawned several times. When the stimulation stopped, the monkey fell into a deep sleep.

As Chaffee and Light were reporting on their monkey experiments at Yale, Frederic A. Gibbs and his wife were involved at Harvard with experiments that eventually used four hundred cats. With each animal anesthetized the Harvard scientists drilled a burr hole in the skull and inserted a fine needle electrode into the brain. It was held in place by a metal plug fitted into the bone. Hundreds of different sites on the cats' skulls were tested to determine the "convulsion threshold" for various parts of the animal's brain. In the course of the work, the Gibbses encountered a surprising phenomenon. In three of their four hundred subjects, the brain stimuli made the animals purr, as do all happy and contented cats. "This reaction was so striking," said the Harvard couple, "and the region from which it was obtained so definitely localized that we considered it worthy of a special report."

The Yale and Harvard work included but two of the more fascinating experiments in a long line of investigations dating back to 1870 and the development of ESB (electrical stimulation of the brain) by Gustav Fritsch and Eduard Hitzig. By the 1930's ESB had become a primary tool for mapping the nervous system of animals and man. By stimulating hundreds of points on the brain or in the depths of the organ and then observing the subject's reactions, investigators painstakingly constructed a picture of how the nervous system directs messages outward from the brain, and of how subsystems are functionally related within the brain. The grand mapping job with ESB complemented the sensory mapping techniques using evoked potentials, but it had many more ramifications, since ESB began revealing neural bridges between physiological and psychological phenomena in the brain.

In the beginning, as we have already seen, ESB rapidly proved of great value when employed by pioneer researchers like David Ferrier, Victor Horsley, and Charles E. Beevor. Subsequently the technique was used with remarkable success by Sherrington, who experimented between 1901 and 1917 with a series of collaborators on the exposed brains of anthropoids, including chimpanzees, gorillas, and orangutans.

Their results revealed that points on the motor cortex of higher mammals control movements, not on a one-to-one basis, but through an ultra-complex relationship. As Sherrington and his co-workers systematically stimulated point after point of the animals' brains, they recognized that in the same species no two cortical surfaces are exactly matched. For instance, the stimulation point that might obtain a certain movement in one animal could fail to produce it in another. Or in the same animal a point on the left cerebral hemisphere prompting a specific contralateral movement would not necessarily match the point on the right hemisphere eliciting the same contralateral movement.

The experimenters also recognized that even when a point of stimulation was identified as corresponding with a specific bodily movement, it still could not be depended upon to produce the same results under all circumstances. A researcher, for example, might explore until his electrode touched the single point on the brain that would cause one of the animal's fingers to flex, but once that spot was located, the stimulating electrode could be moved away from it, one little step at a time, and the finger would continue to flex, even as the stimulation reached cortical locations where previously no such movement was obtainable. In other words, the sensitivity of one small point on the brain seemed to trail the electrode as it moved away.

It became clear to Sherrington and his co-workers that the cortex of higher animals, like the ape, is a far more sophisticated affair than that of lower animals, like the dog. On the higher nervous scale specific movements obtained from particular cortical points were more "fractional" than on the lower nervous scales. For instance, stimulation of a point on the cortex of a dog might cause the jaws to open symmetrically, but stimulation of a comparable point on the ape's brain might actuate only one side of the jaw, causing an asymmetrical opening of the mouth. This greater fractionalization of brain functions in the higher animal provides it with more refined controls of movements. Thus the ape of our example is capable of a wide variety of facial expressions denied the dog.

In conjunction with this ESB research Sherrington further revealed the brain's amazing capabilities with some fascinating ablation studies in which cerebral tissue was cut out in order to see what effect it would have on the experimental animals. In this research he and his co-workers used ESB to identify cortical areas corresponding to specific movements, and then with the animals anesthetized, the scientists surgically removed the electrically delineated portions of the cortex. When an animal, with its scalp put back in place, regained consciousness, its reactions offered some interesting clues as to the functions of the surgically damaged brain areas.

"A point which impressed us repeatedly," wrote Sherrington, "was the seeming entire ignorance on the part of the animal on its awakening from an ablation experiment, of any disability precluding its performance of its willed acts as usual. Surprise at the failure of the limb to execute what it intended seemed the animal's mental attitude, and not merely for the first few minutes, but for many hours. It was often many hours before repeated and various failures to execute ordinary acts contributory to climbing, feeding, etc., seemed to impress gradually upon the animal that the limb was no longer to be relied upon for its usual services. . . . The surprise seemed to argue unfulfilled expectation, and defect in the motor execution rather than in the mental execution of the act, raising the question whether the function of part of the cortex ablated in such cases be not indeed infra-mental."

But as time went on, the limb function damaged by ablation of the brain returned slowly until the animal was using it normally. "Improvement in the willed actions of the limb," said Sherrington, "set in very early, and progressed until the limb was finally used with much success for many purposes even of the finer kind. Thus after destruction of the greater part of the arm areas of both hemispheres the two hands were freely and successfully used for breaking open a banana and bringing the exposed pulp of the fruit to the mouth. And again, after considerable destruction of one leg area the foot was successfully used for holding on the bars when climbing about the cage."

What had happened in the brain in order for the damaged functions to be restored? The surgically excised areas did not grow back because, once destroyed, nervous tissue does not regenerate. Was recrudescence the answer, with adjoining areas of the brain taking over the lost functions? To answer such questions the scientists re-opened the skulls of their experimental animals and, by applying their electrodes, found that recrudescence was not the explanation. For instance, in an animal where ablation had temporarily removed a hand function, the investigators' electrodes revealed that the cerebral workings had not, as suspected, been transferred to an adjacent area of the brain corresponding with the elbow and shoulder. Stimulation affected the elbow and the shoulder in the normal manner, but not the restored hand movements. Furthermore, cerebral ablation of the elbow and shoulder areas destroyed those functions, but failed to affect the renewed hand functions. Exploration of other nearby cortical areas gave the same results. The English scientists, keeping strictly to the evidence of their experimentation, did not allow themselves to reach any conclusions as to how the brain had regained its damaged functions, but at the time others surmised that the work was taken over by subcortical areas of the organ.

While this line of research was proceeding under Sherrington, a Swiss ophthalmologist, Walter Rudolf Hess, arrived at an important personal decision that led to his becoming one of the century's most important neurological scientists, and a major contributor to the development of brain mapping with ESB. In 1912, at age thirty-one and with a family to support, Hess dropped a lucrative practice to devote his life to basic research in physiology. He became a teaching assistant and took up the studies required by his new career. A dozen years later the Swiss scientist was perfecting a technique of brain exploration that offered an entirely new approach to the study of the nervous system. It provided electrical brain mappers, whose explorations had been largely confined to the cortical surface, with a unique approach to investigations of the depths of the organ. Hess applied his new method to study a part of the brain that communicates directly with the spinal cord, namely the brainstem, which underlies the two great cerebral hemispheres. He became particularly interested in the brainstem's upper section, the diencephalon. In this region his electrodes encountered one of the most important and fascinating parts of the central nervous system, the hypothalamus, the highest integrative center for autonomic and somatic functions, and he found it particularly important to the nature of his inquiry. Hess not only made major contributions toward mapping the anatomical details of the brain in relation to function, but he also, as we shall see, opened up important questions about the relationships between psychological phenomena and brain physiology.

His method depended upon the implantation of extremely fine electrodes deep into the heads of cats while the animals were under anesthesia. The electrodes, consisting of slender wires electrically insulated except for their very tips, were guided with precision through holes in the cats' skulls toward selected points in the diencephalon. When the anesthesia wore off, the cats resumed a relatively normal existence, unaware that their brains had been connected up with the little wires projecting from their heads. Hess then used the implanted electrodes for two purposes. He first employed them to stimulate the deep areas of the brain with tiny electric currents while he observed the behavioral effects upon the cats. When these results were a matter of record, the Swiss scientist sent a comparatively large current into the animals' heads to destroy small areas of brain tissue immediately around the electrodes' tips. He then studied the cats' behavior to determine what functions had been affected by the electrical damage to the neurons. With both these tests completed, the cats were killed and their brains were sliced in thin, serial sections so that Hess could microscopically verify the precise locations of his electrode tips, and determine exactly what neurons were destroyed by electrocution. These experimental steps allowed Hess to make functional maps associated with the detailed anatomical structures of the brainstem.

But his careful exploration was not a simple, easy investigation. As Hess probed the depths of his cats' brains, he soon found that complex interrelationships between minute areas of the brain required a meticulous, point-by-point analysis if his exploration was to offer meaningful results. This required the use of untold numbers of cats. The painstaking, time-consuming work challenged all of the former ophthalmologist's skills for dealing patiently with small precision instruments over long periods of time. Volumes of data were produced by the study, and to be of value they had to be organized in graphic fashion. The exhaustive project became exceedingly expensive, and Hess had to seek special financing. It was obtained from various Swiss foundations and the Rockefeller Foundation of New York.

His wire electrodes precisely implanted in the heads of hundreds of cats led Hess to the control centers for some of life's most basic, spontaneous functions, such as respiration and blood circulation. But the great revelation of his work was that these control areas could not be characterized as isolated centers, each corresponding with some specific function. To the contrary, each function could only be understood if viewed as an integral part of a complicated interrelationship that acts not as separate functions but as a unity of functions. Thus when a wire in a cat's head stimulated one tiny area of the brain that would seem to relate specifically to some internal organ, it could very well set off a whole combination of functions involving both a series of internal organs and the creature's reactions to its external environment. For example, the gentle stimulation of what might seem like a minute, isolated control center for some basic autonomic function could simultaneously prompt the cat to assume a nasty frame of mind with all the attendant feline ferociousness.

"Even a formerly good-natured cat turns bad-tempered," Hess wrote; "it starts to spit and, when approached, launches a well-aimed attack. As the pupils simultaneously dilate widely and the hair bristles, a picture develops such as is shown by the cat if a dog attacks it while it cannot escape."

As the Swiss scientist selected different sites to implant his electrodes in the brain's deeper regions, the responses varied widely, from complete, friendly submission to rage with the urge to fight or flee. Stimulation of one certain part of the brain caused an animal to curl up and go to sleep. It could then be awakened by a gentle nudge or a loud sound, as any cat can be aroused from a normal sleep. Tiny currents introduced into another part of the brain would cause the cat to evacuate its bowels or bladder after assuming the characteristic posture for such acts. And when still other areas were stimulated, the cat's respiration and blood circulation were influenced by the stimuli.

As Hess sorted out these responses in relation to the areas of the brain under stimulation, it became evident that in the small region called the hypothalamus he had recognized an important management center for coordinating some of the most complex functions of the central nervous system. Here he had located the integrative center for two main divisions of the autonomic nervous system, the sympathetic and parasympathetic systems, which were discussed in an earlier chapter.

The sympathetic nerves are those associated with the transmitter substance noradrenaline. The parasympathetic nerves liberate acetylcholine. The two systems are antagonistic. The sympathetic fibers accelerate activity; for instance, speeding up the heartbeat and dilating the pupils of the eyes. The parasympathetic fibers decelerate activity, slowing down the heartbeat and contracting the pupils. When an animal or human exhibits flight or fight, rage or fear, his sympathetic system is activated. When he settles down and feels secure, the parasympathetic system is at work. These various reactions are basic to carnivorous animals, who, in stalking and hunting their food, must be prepared to offer a wide gamut of behavioral responses in daily life. The hypothalamus, as indicated by Hess's work, is the coordination center of the two systems. It allows a creature to use both in a balanced fashion according to its needs. When fear is the order of the moment, the heart has to be speeded up, the eyelids retracted, the pupils dilated, the hair on the back raised, the breath speeded up, certain chemicals secreted, and so on. The hypothalamus gives the directions. When the opposite behavior is required, the brain center also manages the necessary functions to bring the parasympathetic system into action. Thus the two systems are balanced and integrated by the deep region of the brain that Hess so painstakingly studied with his wires.

He also recognized that in its location at the top of the brainstem and tied so closely to the main hemispheres, the hypothalamus connects the autonomic system with the cerebral cortex. The center, therefore, does not work completely on its own. Directives, in a sense, come down from the cortex above. Hess felt that the recognition of these relationships between automatic nervous processes directed toward the inside of the animal and psychological processes directed toward the outside meant that "a bridge is thrown over a gap . . . which lies between the purely somatically oriented physiology and psychophysiology."

"It completes and broadens the insight into psychosomatic relationships," said Hess, "in the way they had been demonstrated by the great Russian physiologist Pavlov, who approached them from another side."

While Hess's implanted wires brought new physiological understandings of complex brain functions, they disturbed some psychologists' long-held views of the brain and emotions. The tiny amounts of electricity introduced into the brains of Hess's cats apparently affected the animals' emotions as well as stimulating motor activity. But were emotions really influenced by the stimuli? The answer is yes—it was subsequently proven so—but back in the 1930's, Hess's results were so alien to current psychological and physiological thought that they were not easily accepted. In fact, the variety of emotions stirred by electrical stimulation of the cats' brains were labeled by critics as "sham rage," which implied that Hess had not really touched upon emotions with his implanted wires but, instead, had simply triggered the physical manifestations of emotions without producing their true psychological manifestations. Emotions, thought the believers in sham rage, arose from some obscure activities in the brain as a whole. Certainly they couldn't be created with a tiny amount of electricity artificially introduced into a small segment of the brain. Hess, who rejected the term, was correct in doing so. To some scientists the Swiss physiologist's success in altering his cats' emotions was one of the most significant events in the history of the neurological sciences.

In 1965 a well-known physiologist at the Yale University School of Medicine, José M. R. Delgado, said: "Although these findings [Hess's] did not produce a significant impact on philosophical thinking, in retrospect they may be considered as important as the nineteenth-century demonstration that the contraction of a frog muscle did not depend on circulating spirits and could be controlled by physical instrumentation."

Hess's major work was published in 1932, but for many years it attracted comparatively little scientific attention. In 1949, however, he was awarded the Nobel Prize for Physiology or Medicine, and soon his implanted-electrodes techniques were playing a major role in brain research. This research will be discussed shortly, but first ESB as applied to human brains should be examined further.

As told in an earlier chapter, one of the first published cases of electrical stimulation of the human brain came from an Ohio physician, Roberts Bartholow, who carried out an unusual experiment on an Irish woman. This experiment was followed by isolated instances of ESB on humans. A particularly notable case was reported in 1892 in the journal *Brain* by William B. Ransom, physician to the General Hospital, Nottingham, England. It was the first published case of ESB producing sensations in a part of the body. Ransom described his patient in a note as follows: "T.F., a young man of 19, came into hospital . . . complaining of fits." Each fit began with a tingling sensation in the left thumb that then spread up the arm to the shoulder and face. When treatment with bromides failed to relieve the young man, he was brought to the operating room, and two bone discs were trephined from his skull exposing an area of the brain about two inches long and an inch wide. This relieved pressure from a cystic accumulation of liquid that had depressed the brain surface. When the depressed area was stimulated with a gentle electric current, the contralateral thumb and fingers flexed. Increasing the current caused contractions to spread up the arm to the shoulder and face, all of which was followed by an epileptic fit. The bone disc was left out of the hole, the scalp was allowed to heal across the opening, and the patient recovered relatively free of fits. Subsequently he agreed to serve as a subject for ESB experiments that Ransom conducted by inserting slender metal electrodes down to the cortical surface through the scalp and the underlying hole in the skull. This was when the English doctor found that his gentle stimuli caused the young man to experience sensations in his hand. A very weak current also caused the subject to see a blue or white light, mostly in the left eye, a phenomenon that had also occurred at the onset of a fit.

One of the most renowned pioneers in the use of ESB on human beings was an American, Harvey Cushing, the first person to devote his career entirely to brain surgery and the founder of modern basic neurosurgical techniques. He was educated at Yale and Harvard medical schools, and in Europe, where he worked as a pupil under Sherrington. In the Englishman's laboratory, he assisted in the stimulation of the brains of higher apes. Back in America in 1903 Cushing applied electrodes to a human patient's brain and produced convincing evidence that the results in apes were also applicable to humans. At the same time he revealed that stimulation of the sensory regions of the brain could provide the conscious patient with sensations he could describe.

Cushing's classic experiment occurred at Johns Hopkins Hospital when he was treating "a sturdy and intelligent boy 15 years of age . . . suffering from 'convulsive attacks originating in right hand and right side of face.' " While the young man was on the operating table, the surgeon applied a "mild faradic current" to a part of the brain called the precentral strip. In his report, Cushing listed the motor responses in the order in which they were caused by the stimulation—as follows:

"(1) An opposing movement of thumb and fingers from points opposite to the unmistakable genu [part of cortex where stimulation occurred].

"(2) Somewhat higher up, extension of the index finger.

"(3) Still higher flexion of the fingers, which carried over to flexion of the wrist.

"(4) At the upper margin of the exposed field, flexion of the elbow.

"(5) Below the evident middle genu the movements, which required a somewhat stronger current, consisted of contraction of the side of the face.

"(6) Movements of palate and fauces, a curious choking sensation being occasioned whenever they were obtained; and

"(7) From the very lowest exposed part of the strip, movements of the tongue occurred, and the patient experienced a sensation of movement in the lower jaw, though this was not certified by the observers."

Cushing went on to explain that the same electrical stimulation applied to another nearby area of the cortex "led to a sensation in the hand, arm and little finger—chiefly in the little finger. . . ." Stimulation lower down on this same area of the cortex "occasioned a sensation of warmth in the arm, but this was rather vague and indescribable."

The surgeon commented that his results raised many questions, such as how did the subject interpret electrical stimulation of a supposedly sensory field in the brain as sensory. ". . . these and many other questions that arise," said Cushing, "are matters rather for the psychologist."

When Cushing's work with ESB is mentioned, a German, Otfrid Foerster, is likely to receive a share of credit for the pioneering work on humans, but the person who most seriously put ESB to work as a surgeon's tool was Wilder Penfield. He was born in Spokane, and educated at Princeton, Oxford, and the Johns Hopkins Medical School. As a Rhodes Scholar, he worked with Sherrington. "In his laboratory at Oxford," said Penfield, "to search for the hidden truths of neurology became a habit of mind, a coloring of all one's thoughts." In 1928 the American surgeon joined McGill University in Montreal, and six years later he became director of the newly established Montreal Neurological Institute. For years Penfield and his co-workers at the institute made medical history with hundreds of patients who were subjected to ESB, as both part of their treatment and a systematic program for mapping the human cortex.

Penfield was mainly interested in treating focal epilepsy through excision of abnormal areas of the brain. As he began his surgery in Montreal, his efforts were confined to comparatively narrow regions of the brain, especially when destructive lesions appeared in the dominant (in most cases the left) hemisphere. Here, usually, are the brain's speech areas, and without knowing their exact limits the surgeon dared not use his knife except in relatively narrow regions of the cortex.

"The most precious and indispensable portion of the adult's cortex," said Penfield, "is the major speech area. It might be worthwhile to forfeit other areas and so lose other functions in order to gain a cure, but never speech. Thus, the need of a method to map the exact territory devoted to speech was urgent."

That method was ESB, and the Montreal surgeon used it extensively to learn where the abnormal tissue was located and whether or not he could remove it without destroying crucial functions, especially speech. Simultaneously he produced the most comprehensive maps of the human cortex ever made with ESB. They augmented and supported other maps from other methods, such as those developed by men like Paul Broca and John Hughlings Jackson, who localized cortical functions by associating their loss with disease-damaged areas of the cortex, and those developed by a number of famous histologists who made extensive cytoarchitectural studies (investigations of cellular structure) of the human cortex.

In a typical brain operation Penfield's patient rested on his side upon the operating table with his head and shoulders under a lean-to-like tent. The surgeon worked to the rear, out of view of the patient, the dome of whose skull projected through a hole in the tent wall where the doctor could operate upon it. A small piece of the skull, locally anesthetized with Novocaine, was cut out and opened up like a trapdoor exposing the brain. Meanwhile, the patient, remaining conscious and alert, could only see one of Penfield's assistants, who sat in front of the tent where he could communicate with both the patient and surgeon. A stenographer recorded all the pertinent remarks made during the procedure, and a photographer within view of the skull opening made a visual record of the proceedings.

With the brain exposed, Penfield worked quickly and carefully to stimulate the cortex while the assistant, following the surgeon's instructions, performed specified tasks and reported upon the patient's reactions. The patient, in one instance, might be shown a series of objects or cards with pictures and asked to describe what he saw. Or he might be instructed to count aloud, or recite from a printed page, or he might be asked to write on a pad of paper. Meanwhile, Penfield would move his electrodes from point to point on the cortex to see if the stimuli influenced what the patient was doing, or to see if he was caused to move or experience certain sensations. When the stimulus prompted a reaction of interest, the surgeon dropped a tiny numbered ticket on the stimulated point as he dictated a note to identify the number with what happened. In the course of an operation, many such tickets might be dropped on the brain, and they would be recorded by the photographer. The pictures and stenographic record provided a visual-verbal account of the surgery, including what was said among the three principals: Penfield, the assistant, and the patient.

From hundreds of operations Penfield and his co-workers compiled volumes of data from which they assembled a composite picture of what functions relate to what areas of the human cortex. They localized the body's many sensory and motor functions to the postcentral and precentral gyri, two convoluted ridges enclosing the brain's central fissure, the "Fissure of Rolando." Thousands of stimulations of these gyri in hundreds of patients told the surgeon-scientist that different sensory and motor functions are, according to their importance, allotted different-sized portions of the cortical surface. The sensory area of the cortex corresponding to the hand, for example, is much larger than that corresponding to the foot. These differences were graphically illustrated by two drawings prepared for Penfield by an artist. One was called the "sensory homunculus," the other, the "motor homunculus," and they soon became familiar to every student of the brain. Each drawing shows the distorted body of a little man stretched around the curved surface of a section of one cerebral hemisphere. The bodily parts of the figurine are distributed opposite the cortical areas to which they relate functionally, and the sizes of the parts are distorted to illustrate the proportion of cortex devoted to each function. By far the largest parts of the motor homunculus are the lips and hands, indicating that their functions require the largest single shares of the motor cortex. In the sensory homunculus the tongue and hands are largest. In both drawings the toes are comparatively small, for relatively little of the cortex is devoted to their movements and senses.

By far the most interesting results from Penfield's electrodes came when they stimulated areas of the cortex relating to speech, hearing, vision, and memory. Here the surgeon's gentle electric currents appeared to influence the brain's most sophisticated functions, and the results seemed to offer insights into the organ's deepest secrets.

When an electrode touched the major speech area of the cortex (there are three such areas, one major and two minor, in the left hemisphere of most human brains), the patient either vocalized or lost his ability to speak. One of the first cases of vocalization occurred in 1935, when an electrode touched a certain point on the precentral gyrus, and the patient, a man, uttered a well-sustained vowel cry that continued until the electrode was removed. The surprised patient remarked that something had forced him to speak. When the electrode was held on the same spot for a long time, the vocalization went on and on, execept for brief interruptions as the patient caught his breath. He was asked to stop making the sound, but he couldn't do anything about it as long as the electrode continued stimulating the cortex. Exploration of the nearby cortical region with the electrodes revealed that two discrete areas, each about two millimeters in diameter, prompted vowel cries when stimulated, and their pitch varied somewhat according to which area was involved.

The arrest of speech was associated with stimulations applied to the small cortical regions corresponding to throat movements. The electrodes either blocked the patient's speech completely or slowed it down. When speech was electrically blocked by the surgeon, the patient could recognize a familiar object like a pencil and think of its purpose, but he couldn't name the object when instructed to do so. Removal of the electrode, however, removed the block, and the word flowed freely out across the tip of the patient's tongue.

With this kind of electrical exploration, Penfield and his associates found they could determine the precise limits of the three speech areas. "And we could remove less useful cortex right up to it," said the Montreal surgeon, "without fear of losing the precious jewel of the brain, speech function. We mapped out the cortical area thus in hundreds of cases and acquired precise scientific information to take the place of anatomical conjecture."

In cases where Penfield's electrodes could explore the occipital lobes at the rear of the brain they produced some fascinating effects on the patient's vision. One of the early cases involved an eighteen-year-old boy who suffered epileptic seizures that began with his seeing "a round, bright-colored object rotating in front of his left eye." When the rear left quarter of the boy's skull was opened, and the occipital lobe was stimulated, the patient reported a number of visual phenomena. As one point was stimulated, he saw two wheels, mostly red and blue, on the left of his visual field. At other points, the electrodes produced impressions of a ball of light, tiny moving lights in color, flashing lights, a long white mark in the right eye, and a red spot in the left eye.

Over the years Penfield's electrodes exploring the occipital lobes of patients obtained many different visual displays: "flickering lights, dancing lights, colors, bright lights, star wheels, blue, green and red colored discs, fawn and blue lights, colored balls whirling, radiating gray spots becoming pink and blue, a long white mark, et cetera." The stimuli, however, never seemed able to assemble a complete picture for the patient, but only the raw material for one. "These visual phenomena," wrote Penfield and a colleague, Theodore Rasmussen, "suggest that, from a functional point of view, there is represented in the occipital cortex no more than elements that go to make up the final image that reaches consciousness during normal vision. The occipital cortex is obviously involved in the complicated elaboration of visual pictures that eventually present themselves at some higher level of nervous integration. But stimulation here is incapable of conjuring up such a picture."

Penfield prompted auditory responses when he electrically stimulated a small area of the brain's temporal lobes, which are located low on either side of the head. The electrical currents prompted many patients to hear simple sounds, but in other cases the stimuli had no effect at all. Sometimes the subject under stimulation indicated "a sense of deafness."

Other times he said the tones of the operating room sounds were changed by the stimulation.

From patient to patient, where auditory responses were obtained, the artificially produced sounds differed considerably. The following descriptions came from a number of patients, as recorded in the surgical team's notes: "ringing sound like doorbell," "low pitched sound 'like a motor,'" "sound like under water, like having a bathing cap on," "continuous clicking like crickets at night," "rushing sound like a bird flying," "'. . . like a house with doors shutting,'" "'I hear boom boom or something,'" and "'key of your voice changed.'"

As with the fragmentary character of visual responses to stimulation, the auditory results could not be characterized as fully developed sounds. "The sounds heard," wrote Penfield and Rasmussen, "are elementary tones which may be high-pitched or low, continuous or interrupted, but always devoid of complicated or changing qualities. The effect upon hearing may be an apparent decrease or increase in volume or change in the tone of the sounds heard."

Quite early in his work at Montreal Penfield happened upon what is undoubtedly the most fascinating aspect of his career. He was exploring a relatively large area of the temporal cortex to which neurologists had been unable to attribute any functions. "One day I stumbled on a clue," said the surgeon. "I applied the electrode to the right temporal cortex (nondominant). The patient, a woman of middle age, exclaimed suddenly, 'I seem to be the way I was when I was giving birth to my baby girl.' I did not recognize this as a clue. I could not help feeling that the suddenness of her exclamation was strange, and so I made a note of it."

Several years later the surgeon was operating upon a fourteen-year-old girl who suffered from epileptic seizures wherein she became frightened, screamed, and sought protection by grabbing onto anyone nearby. The fright usually arose from a vision in which the girl saw herself in a terrifying situation that had occurred when she was seven years old. On a lovely day she had been following her brothers in the high grass of a meadow when a man had suddenly come up from behind and said: "How would you like to get into this bag with the snakes?" She had screamed and run home with her brothers to tell their mother. Subsequently the terrifying event had repeated itself in nightmares, and eventually it had become part of the epileptic attacks. As they occurred, the girl remained conscious of her present environment, however; it seemed that another mind, drawing upon the past, was presenting the picture of herself walking in the meadow with her brothers. In 1938 she became a neurosurgical patient in Montreal, and Penfield was stimulating part of her temporal lobe when suddenly the girl cried out: "Oh, I can see something come at me!" As the electrode was moved to another point on the temporal lobe, the patient was instructed to hold onto a bar above her head over the operating table. A moment later she described her experiential response to this stimulation. "I held onto the bar and the bar seemed to be walking away from me. I saw someone coming toward me, as though he were going to hit me." The stimulus was then applied to another point, and the girl cried out that she heard a number of people shouting. "They are yelling at me for doing something wrong," she said, "everybody is yelling." Asked to identify the voices, the young patient said it was her mother and brothers. Stimulation of another point led her to say, "I imagine I hear a lot of people shouting at me." The surgeon repeated the same stimulus three times without warning, and again the girl heard the people shouting. Touching still another point caused her to yell: "Oh, there it goes; everybody is yelling!" And as the electrode was held in place for a brief interval, the patient said, "Something dreadful is going to happen." Finally the electrode was moved a bit, and she cried out, "There they go, yelling at me; stop them!"

The surgeon decided that an abnormal part of the temporal

cortex, which had developed in infancy during administration of an anesthetic, should be excised. The ESB tests indicated that the area to be removed was responsible for the epileptic seizures and their hallucinatory consequences. The malfunctioning part of the brain was apparently causing abnormal electric discharges that, like the surgeon's electrodes, stimulated the frightening vision. When the operation was over and the girl had recovered, she was free from the seizures and the accompanying hallucinations. However, she could still remember the man in the meadow, and the fear associated with him.

In subsequent cases involving the temporal cortex, Penfield's electrodes produced a variety of hallucinations and perceptual illusions. When the stimulus was applied at a certain point on the brain of a young French Canadian woman, she heard "funny things," and as the electrodes were moved slightly, she heard music, a familiar air, she said. After the surgery the same woman recalled that while on the operating table she had seen people with snow on their clothing enter the operating room, and she had wondered why they had been allowed to enter. As the right temporal lobe of another woman was being stimulated, she exclaimed: "Oh, a familiar memory—an office somewhere. I could see the desks. I was there and someone was calling to me—a man leaning on a desk with a pencil in his hand." When the right temporal lobe was stimulated in a young man who had come from South Africa for surgery, he said: "Yes, Doctor! Yes, Doctor! Now I hear people laughing—my friends—in South Africa." In a 1954 case a woman under stimulation suddenly felt as though she were at home in her kitchen. From outside she could hear the voice of her young son, Frank, against a familiar background of neighborhood noises. Ten days after the surgery, the woman denied that the illusion on the operating table was only a memory. "Oh, no," she said, "it seemed more real than that. Of course, I have heard Frankie like that many, many times—thousands of times." Brain stimulation of another woman caused the patient to hear a Christmas song that had deeply moved her several Christmas eves past at a church back home in Holland. Another patient heard an orchestra playing, and, in addition to recognizing her presence on the operating table, she sensed being present in a theater during the orchestral performance.

Penfield was fascinated by the way an ESB experience unfolded, as if it were a short film whose showing was controlled by the surgeon's electrodes. Time in the ESB sequence was real time. This was verified by asking certain patients to tap or hum along in time with the music they were hearing under stimulation. Furthermore, a memory film always moved forward, never backwards. It could be stopped by removing the stimulus, and often it could be replayed from the beginning by reapplying the electrode at exactly the same spot. Memory films played only one at a time, with all others kept back by some inhibitory mechanism. Thus—if this analogy applies—the brain would seem to be a repository of untold numbers of film clips, each with sound and pictures of something from an individual's past. The brain's electrical activity somehow draws one film at a time from the library and plays it through, unless interrupted by a break in the electrical activity that keeps the show going.

Penfield was also very interested in his patients' conception of their experiences on the operating table under ESB. Although the stimuli appeared to move people to the past and to other places, no one was fooled by the phenomenon. Regardless of the artificially induced feelings and apparitions, patients remained acutely aware of their presence on the operating table with a neurosurgeon electrically stimulating their brains. But they also recognized a peculiar doubling of awareness, which they could think about and discuss as a strange paradox. Moreover, patients realized that the electrically prompted experiences from the past were not simply the product of ordinary memory. They were more like dreams, and some were described as flashbacks upon the patients' lives.

From all the ESB work on hundreds of patients, Penfield and his associates drew some interesting conclusions about the functional development of the human brain. From birth, they decided, parts of the cortex are committed to the fixed jobs of taking care of the brain's sensory and motor functions, but other areas are uncommitted in the earliest years of life. The temporal lobes, one on each side of the brain, are "uncommitted cortex" reserved for speech and perception. "It will make possible the memory and use of words," said Penfield, "as well as the memory and interpretation of experience." As a child piles up experiences and learning, he commits more and more of the uncommitted cortex with functional connections that will serve for life. Development of the major speech center, said Penfield, is the prime example. It occupies the posterior half of the uncommitted cortex of the left hemisphere. If the area is damaged in a youngster's early years, the affected speech center is likely to re-establish itself in another part of the uncommitted cortex. When damage occurs prior to three or four years of age, the speech function may even migrate from the left to the right side of the brain in the search for a new, healthy region of the cortex. Meanwhile the child suffers a temporary loss of speech or disability. But as an individual matures, the growing commitment of the cortex makes such changes less and less possible. Soon after life's first decade much of the previously blank slate is taken up with the business of perception, and damage to the speech cortex is a much more serious matter, for the function has less free territory into which it may move. And severe damage to the brain's speech mechanism at age twenty or over can very likely inflict permanent speech disability or loss upon a person.

Penfield's experiences with ESB in the operating room led him to some provocative ideas about the teaching of languages. He felt that teachers should recognize the matter of the brain's changing plasticity as a crucial factor determining when the mother tongue and other languages can be most effectively taught. "The brain of the child is plastic," said Penfield. "The brain of the adult, however effective it may be in other directions, is usually inferior to that of the child as far as language is concerned." In life's first decade, Penfield explained, the uncommitted cortex makes its general functional connections. At the time the process may be easily directed toward forming neural connections that can most readily enable an individual to learn languages, his own and others. In this period, said Penfield, a youngster can, with comparative ease, develop facilities for learning other languages directly, as opposed to word-by-word translation. This is accomplished, the surgeon concluded, by development of "a remarkable switch mechanism that enables him to turn from one language to another without confusion, without translation, without a mother tongue accent." With this facility well developed in a child, the surgeon believed, the person was cerebrally prepared to learn new languages in later life by the direct method.

Penfield held that his conclusions were borne out in homes and in countries where young children are naturally exposed day by day to more than one language. Not only do such children grow up multilingual, he pointed out, but as adults they display a natural facility for learning additional tongues. Penfield recommended that language teaching, which had traditionally been reserved for the later years of school, begin early in education, simply by exposing the youngest pupils to more than one tongue in their daily educational routines. He referred to such a program as the "mother's method." "The mother," he said, "does her teaching when the child's brain is ready for it. In three or four years she may give the child only a few hundred words, but he gets the set, acquires the units, creates the functional connections of the speech cortex. . . . If a nation is to be bilingual or trilingual or multilingual, the schools should adopt the mother's direct method for the first stage of foreign-language teaching."

In stimulating the brains of hundreds of patients of various ages, Penfield came to think of the organ's development as passing through four cerebral seasons. "Man's mind," he said, "has its own peculiar calendar. There is a time to plant, a time to wait on increase, a time for the harvest of knowledge, and, at last, a time for wisdom."

The ESB techniques developed by the Montreal surgeon had the dual benefit of providing basic procedures that are now routine in brain operations and of conducting a systematic exploration of the human cortex. But the exploratory efforts were naturally limited. The subject was always a neurosurgical patient whose malfunction confined the experimenter to the relatively small area of the brain under treatment. The experimenter was also limited to the time of an operation and other confinements of an operating room. Finally, the circumstance allowing investigation of the human brain—a diseased condition—meant that the results might not be duplicated in a healthy brain. At best, the scientific exploration had to be a by-product of the experimenter's primary concern: treating a neurological disease.

ESB investigations of healthy brains were, and still are, confined to animals in the manner of Hess and his experiments on cats. In the post-World War II years, when Hess received the Nobel Prize, important advances with ESB appeared at a relatively rapid rate. The techniques employed were an outgrowth of Hess's methods enhanced by the wealth of technical improvements that came from the war, especially in electronics.

One of the most remarkable discoveries was reported in 1949 from Northwestern University by two physiologists, one an American, Horace W. Magoun, and the other an Italian, Giuseppe Moruzzi. They were exploring a web of neural tissue in cats that runs longitudinally through the brainstem, which lies at the base of the organ and on top of the spinal column. During investigation of this tissue, called the "reticular formation," Magoun and Moruzzi made a discovery that provided a new understanding of the brain's transitions from sleep to wakefulness or from states of relaxation and drowsiness to alertness and attention.

The nature of the reticular formation had been indicated in 1935 by a European physiologist, Frédéric Bremer, when he found that transection of a cat's brainstem above the reticular formation resulted in the animal remaining in a deep sleep from which it could not be awakened. With this surgical preparation, called *cerveau isolé*, the cat's EEG and the appearance of its eyes confirmed that it was sound asleep. When a transection of the stem was performed below the reticular formation, in a preparation called *encéphale isolé*, Bremer found that the cat could remain awake, and the EEG and eye signs were those of a state of wakefulness. Bremer concluded, without a full understanding of what was happening, that wakefulness was dependent on the inflow of impulses to the brain from the brainstem, and when this inflow was cut off sleep resulted.

Magoun and Moruzzi worked with cats under a sleep-inducing anesthesia, or a surgical preparation patterned on Bremer's *encéphale isolé*. The two scientists then implanted electrodes in the animals' reticular formations and applied minute electric currents. They found that introduction of a small, gentle current would awaken a sleeping cat as peacefully as a child's voice calling a drowsing kitty to a saucer of milk. During their ESB experiments Magoun and Moruzzi recorded their cats' EEG's and observed what happened when the animals were awakened by electrical stimulation of the brainstem. When a cat was asleep, the electroencephalograph traced slow, high-voltage, synchronized waves associated with sleep, but stimulation of the reticular formation changed the tracings to the fast, low-voltage electrical activity that is characteristic of arousal from sleep.

The discovery made at Northwestern was of basic importance to understanding the central nervous system. Probing the brainstem with their electrodes, Magoun and Moruzzi had encountered the main part of a general alarm system for the brain. They named it the "reticular activating system" (RAS). Previously authorities had felt that the brain's arousal was controlled by the amount of inflowing sensory impulses, but the Northwestern scientists showed that the RAS alerts the brain for action. Anatomical studies that had been made of the reticular formation supported this conclusion. They revealed that nerve fiber tracts passing through the brainstem have many branches leading off into this formation. The Northwestern ESB studies indicated that sensory signals moving along these tracts activate the system via the branchings. The RAS in turn alerts the cortex to make it ready to deal with the incoming sensory messages. When, for example, a drowsy automobile driver suddenly finds his car headed for the ditch, he snaps to a state of alertness and swerves back onto the road. In the process visual signals trigger the RAS, and it alerts the cortex, which then deals with the mental exercises necessary for getting the car headed back down the road.

In the years following this basic discovery at Northwestern, Magoun, Moruzzi, and other scientists learned a good deal more about the RAS, and, as has so frequently happened in the study of brain physiology, the system turned out to be far more complicated and sophisticated than the original discovery might have indicated.

It became apparent, for example, that the RAS is trainable. It may learn to alert the cortex of one individual under certain conditions while neglecting to do so in another under the same circumstances. The city dweller's RAS, for example, learns to leave his brain asleep with the worst imaginable roar of traffic coming through the bedroom window every night, but the same person, on a visit to the country, is kept miserably awake at dawn on a quiet Sunday morning by the peeping of a baby robin. Another example is the young mother who is aroused by the cries of her baby while the father slumbers on in the same room.

Continued investigation indicated that the RAS goes to

work not only when triggered by afferent sensory signals, but also when signaled by the cortex itself. In other words, the cortical activity of a thought may operate the alarm system. Thus the brain alerts itself for action. This was demonstrated experimentally by ESB applied to a certain point on a monkey's cortex, causing the animal to suddenly perk up, as if to say, "What was that?" The stimulation didn't frighten the monkey, but simply alerted it.

Further studies indicated that the reticular formation exerts controls over motor signals from the brain involving movements in the body. Electrical stimuli applied to the RAS revealed that the system, according to where it is stimulated, can either enhance or inhibit both voluntary and reflex activities. This fact was demonstrated by an unusual experiment using an anesthetized monkey with a pen attached to a toe so as to trace movements of the animal's leg upon a rotating drum as repeated taps on the knee caused the limb to kick reflexively. Meanwhile an investigator stimulated various areas of the RAS and observed the effect on the knee jerks. In one area of the brainstem, the electrodes caused the jerks to become larger, but as the eletrodes were applied lower down on the reticular formation, the stimuli reduced the reflexive action.

One of the scientists involved in these experiments, John D. French of the University of California, Los Angeles, once referred to the RAS as an "integrating machine" for the nervous system. "It awakens the brain to consciousness and keeps it alert," he said; "it directs the traffic of messages in the nervous system; it monitors the myriads of stimuli that beat upon our senses, accepting what we need to perceive and rejecting what is irrelevant; it tempers and refines our muscular activity and bodily movements. We can go even further and say that it contributes in an important way to the highest mental process—the focusing of attention, introspection and doubtless all forms of reasoning."

While the discovery of the RAS was a most important

accomplishment of the post-World War II period, it was but one of several that came from probing the brains of cats, rats, and monkeys with stimulating electrodes. Among the most outstanding contributors was a professor of psychology at the University of Michigan, James Olds, whose subjects were rats.

In the 1950's Olds was conducting some tests with implanted electrodes through which stimuli were received over a wire leading away from the animal's head, like a leash. In each case a rat was placed in a box with corners labeled A, B, C, and D. As the animal moved around the box, the experimenter would deliver an electric current to the brain whenever the rat headed toward corner A. In a series of animals serving in a test that involved stimulation of the reticular system, the results with one particular animal were remarkably different. The stimuli associated with corner A seemed to develop in the animal a liking for that area of the box. Soon an application of the stimulus, regardless of where the animal was standing in the box, caused the rat to go to corner A. The following day the creature's good feeling for the corner seemed to have been reinforced. For some reason, it was in love with corner A.

On the third day Olds and his associates tried a variation of the test on the same rat. By careful application of their stimuli, they tried to draw the rat away from corner A and attract it to corner B. Whenever it made a move in that direction they gave its brain a tiny shock. Soon it had more or less forgotten A and was favoring B. The experimenters then found they could direct the rat with the wired-up brain to almost any point in the box by giving it repeated stimuli whenever it moved toward the selected spot.

Subsequently this same rat, now an unusual character in Olds's laboratory, was made to perform on a T-shaped platform. As it moved down the leg of the T and turned toward one of the arms, its brain was shocked if it turned right, but not if it turned left. On repeated trips down the T the animal always turned right. The experimenters then reversed the procedure and soon had their subject repeatedly turning left.

Finally, they conducted a test on the T, the results of which seemed most surprising of all. They withheld food from the animal for twenty-four hours and then brought the hungry rat back to the T, where mash had been placed at the extremity of each arm. The animal would walk down the leg of the T and turn onto either arm to head for some food, but halfway out on the arm a brain shock was delivered by the experimenter and there the rat stopped, satisfied, as if it had already eaten.

What was going on? It was discovered that there was a difference between this rat and the others in the experiment. When the electrode was implanted in its brain, it had been aimed, as in other cases, at the reticular system, but it had missed and ended up in a nerve pathway from a part of the organ called the rhinencephalon. Olds and his co-workers had accidentally hit upon a new center of the brain. At first they thought it was a kind of curiosity center, one that made the animal go back to a place for continued exploration. But as the tests continued, the scientists realized that their electrode had accidentally located a "pleasure center," an area that rewards a creature when electrically activated. In other words, it wasn't a matter of the rat falling in love with a particular corner of the box; it was a case of its liking what happened in its brain when it moved toward that area. In the experiment with the food on the T it obviously liked the brain stimulus better than the mash, even though it was famished.

This contention was substantiated when Olds stimulated the same area of the brain in other rats while they performed in a special box patterned after one that had been developed earlier by the famous Harvard psychologist B. F. Skinner. The Skinner box contained a lever that, when pressed by an animal's paw, would reward the animal with a food pellet ejected through an opening. Experiments employing the equipment without pellets revealed that in a given period an animal would press the lever by chance a certain number of times, but with the pellet-rewards the number of actions was increased by purposeful pressing ten to twenty times. The actual number, in fact, could be varied by supplying different kinds of pellets, so that the results became a measure of how much the animal valued the reward.

Olds's modified Skinner box contained a paw lever that actuated a switch connected so as to turn on stimuli that were then transmitted through a leash-like wire leading to an electrode implanted in a pleasure center of the brain. Thus the rat could stimulate its own brain by pressing the lever with a paw. The first subject proved, beyond a doubt, that the stimulus was truly rewarding to the animal. After a few minutes in which the rat learned about the lever, it pressed it repeatedly, about once every five seconds. It continued the self-stimulation for a half hour, and then the electrical source was turned off. The animal gave a few more tries, realized the good feeling was gone, and stopped pressing the lever.

With this technique Olds and his associates began a systematic study of rat brains to map out the pleasure centers more carefully. When their electrode tips touched upon the classical sensory and motor regions of an animal's brain, the rate of lever pressings would remain extremely low—ten to twenty-five times an hour—indicating that the actions resulted from chance. But as electrodes were implanted closer to reward areas, the number of presses would increase—and tremendously so when the most powerful centers were encountered. The highest numbers of presses resulted from stimulation of areas of the hypothalamus and certain points in the midbrain in areas that Hess and others had associated with the control of such processes as digestion, excretion, and sex. An animal with an electrode in these pleasure centers might stimulate itself as many as five thousand times an hour.

When the tiny stimuli reached the most productive pleasure areas in a hungry rat, the urge for electrical self-stimulation overrode its desire to partake of a tasty meal placed beside it in the box. Some of Olds's rats loved the self-stimulation so much that they tirelessly pressed the paw lever more than two thousand times per hour for twenty-four consecutive hours.

By the 1960's Olds had mapped rewarding areas over a large region in the depths of the brain extending through the midline. The response to stimulation measured by bar presses per hour varied considerably from point to point within the region, indicating that the electrical stimulus produced varying degrees of pleasure according to where it was applied. The powerful drive to obtain the electrical stimulation of a high-response pleasure center in the brain was illustrated in several ways. Rats on a runway, for example, would run much faster to receive an electric shock to the brain than they would to receive food. In some tests, rats were trained to suffer shocks in crossing an electric grid in order to receive either food or brain stimuli. When the shocks were increased, it was shown that the rats would suffer greater punishment to receive the stimulation than they would for food—even when they had been deprived of the latter for twenty-four hours.

Olds's fabulous techniques of self-stimulation gave neurology and psychology an important tool for studying behavior. Not only did he bring scientists closer to understanding some of the basic drives mediating behavior, but also, through his ingenious techniques, he provided a way of quantifying the processes.

Throughout this period of the 1950's and 60's, many other investigators, in laboratories from Michigan to Texas to Germany, were probing the brains of rats, cats, monkeys, and other animals to study the fascinating regions of cerebral tissue involved with the control of various psychological and physiological phenomena. An outstanding example of the work occurred at the Yale University School of Medicine, where Neal E. Miller and several collaborators used ESB to study a number of drives in animals.

While Olds investigated the pleasure centers of rat brains, the Yale workers stimulated areas of cat brains that produced "pain-fear-like reactions," grouped under the single, descriptive title of "alarm reactions." These responses, which the cats disliked, were elicited when the scientists' electrodes reached a number of specific points in the midbrain and diencephalon.

In one experiment the researchers employed a box with a grid floor that could deliver an unpleasant shock to a cat's paws. At one end of the box a paddle wheel projecting up through the grid would turn off the shock if rotated by a cat's paw. An animal soon learned to seek relief from the discomfort of the grid by turning the paddle wheel. Miller and his co-workers then arranged for the paddle-wheel switch to interrupt electrical stimulation reaching an alarm center in the cat's brain via an implanted electrode. Now, without the grid shock in operation, the animal still flipped the paddle wheel to seek relief from the unpleasant reaction caused by the brain stimuli. In fact, a new cat that had never suffered paw shocks would still learn to use the paddle wheel, solely on the basis of seeking a remedy for the unpleasant responses forced by the brain stimuli.

This series of experiments with the alarm reaction revealed that it could be conditioned in a cat. Immediately prior to stimulation, the investigators sounded a tone that did not in itself influence the cat, but after a number of such trials, they found that the tone minus the stimuli could elicit the same alarm reaction produced by the brain stimulation. The Yale scientists also used their stimuli in conditioning a cat to experience an adverse reaction to a compartment that previously had no effect upon the animal. Once conditioned the cat found the compartment so unpleasant that it tried to escape. Finally, the Yale workers discovered that they could teach a hungry cat to avoid food for some time if an alarm point was stimulated as it approached a tempting meal.

Continued animal experiments by Miller and his associates led to the study of points in the brain where stimulation caused such reactions as rage, flight, hunger, and sexual behavior. The investigations involving sex were conducted on rats with implanted electrodes aimed at sites near the hypothalamus. In a number of the sites the stimuli caused male rats to ejaculate. In some cases the ejaculations could only be elicited by repetitive bursts of stimulation that Miller described as ". . . a pattern suggestive of the series of normal copulations required before ejaculation in the rat." In no instance did the stimuli produce such sexual behavior as mounting, which is possible when large doses of the male hormone, testosterone, are administered to rats.

As the brains of cats and rats were being electrified at Yale, a European team at the Max Planck Institute for the Physiology of Behavior worked for several years with tiny electrodes studying the brains of chickens. Erich von Holst and Ursula von Saint Paul proved that their fine, inserted wires could electrically prompt the birds to go through nearly their entire behavioral repertory, most of which was well known from studies already made at the institute.

Through their investigations, the two scientists compared the strengths of various drives by activating them concurrently and observing what behavior emerged at given moments under given circumstances. This research allowed the scientists to measure the inner dynamics of drives, which is impossible to do solely through visual observation. Simply to look at a hen eating, cackling, standing, or sitting tells nothing about the combination of drives causing a particular action. But when the scientists' multiple electrodes were known to be simultaneously activating multiple drives the investigators were presented with a clearer picture of what the bird was most likely to do in responding to the various forces.

In other laboratories around the world ESB brain mapping was also applied to the autonomic functions of the central nervous system that depend on certain small areas of the brain for the control of visceral activity. Many studies revealed that electric stimuli applied to selected points in the brain could influence such functions as heart rate, blood pressure, respiration, gastric secretion, and vasomotility. A great deal of work was done studying the autonomic reactions of the pupil of the eye, especially in cats, dogs, and monkeys. From a number of control points in the brain the investigators found that with stimulating equipment wired to cerebral electrodes they could dilate and constrict an animal's pupils by the twisting of dials on their electronic equipment. In experiments at Yale, ESB permitted a scientist to vary the pupils of a monkey's eyes to any desired diameter by the turn of dials, as precisely as one adjusts the diaphragm aperture behind the lens of a camera.

In most of the experiments discussed thus far, animals with implanted electrodes were stimulated through flexible wires leading to their heads. These, however, imposed serious limitations to various behavioral studies. For example, the wires made it difficult to observe the effects of ESB on the social relationships in a colony of animals. The solution was in remote stimulation, which, as the opening of this chapter described, was tried with serious technical handicaps at Yale in 1934. Effective remote stimulation was eventually provided by World War II developments in electronic miniaturization and the postwar invention of the transistor. They made possible tiny radio sets that could be carried freely by moving animals to receive stimuli from transmitters located some distance away.

Remote radio stimulation first succeeded around 1950 when several experimenters used small crystal receiving sets attached to animals. For example, three scientists at the Yale University School of Medicine built a receiver using a germanium diode rectifier sealed in a pure polyethylene envelope small enough for implantation under a membrane on a monkey's head. A stimulating electrode projecting from the envelope entered the animal's brain through a small hole in the skull. Electrical stimuli were received by the device from a nearby transmitter. But diode rectifiers, without amplification by the relatively large, heat-producing vacuum tubes of the day, were incapable of receiving anything but powerful signals transmitted from only a few feet away. However, the transistor soon became the basis of tiny radios sensitive enough to utilize comparatively feeble signals transmitted over fairly long distances.

A transistorized receiver was built at the UCLA School of Medicine in 1953 by two neuroscientists, Marcel Verzeano and John D. French, with two technical assistants. Its size prevented implantation under an animal's skin, but it was still an extremely small device. The receiver, sealed in plastic, measured only 1⅛ × ½ × 2 inches. Along with its hearing-aid battery the equipment was easily carried on a cat's collar, from where it was connected to an electrode implanted in the brain. Stimuli could be transmitted effectively up to eighty feet, which allowed the experimenter to remain out of sight and out of earshot of an animal so as not to influence the results. This kind of miniaturized equipment, which continued to shrink as the electronic arts developed, became valuable in many ESB experiments designed to map animal brains in relation to behavior. For example, some of the chicken experiments conducted at the Max Planck Institute employed tiny, twenty-five-gram radio receivers carried by the birds for remote control tests.

Some of the most publicized work with remote stimulation was conducted at Yale in the 1950's and 60's by the Spanish-born physiologist José Delgado. In an experiment at Yale with a colony of six cats, one animal was subjected to remote radio stimulation of the roof area of the midbrain (near the top of the brainstem), which caused it to prowl in search of trouble among other animals known to be its subordinates.

Despite the stimulated hostility, it still avoided one cat that in past encounters had proved to be its superior.

"It was evident," explained Delgado, "that brain stimulation had created a state of increased aggressiveness, but it was also clear that the cat directed its hostility intelligently, choosing the enemy and the moment of attack, changing tactics and adapting its motions to the motor reaction of the attacked animal . . . brain stimulation seemed to determine the affective state of hostility, but the behavioral performance seemed dependent on the individuality of the stimulated animal, including its learned skills and previous experiences."

In Delgado's cat experiment, the intensity of the stimuli was relatively high, and the brain was activated for only short periods of time. In another case, stimulation at reduced intensity was applied for extended periods to one of six cats chosen for its friendliness, one that liked to be held and petted. A radio-stimulated electrode activating part of the brain's amygdala (a nugget-like mass of gray matter in the temporal lobe) was turned on for two hours, and the otherwise friendly cat withdrew to a corner where it occasionally uttered sullen growls. If another animal approached, it was greeted with hisses and similar threats of attack. When the experimenter tried to pet the radio-stimulated cat, spats and hisses warned him to keep back. But when the stimulus was turned off, the cat returned to its normal friendly behavior.

Delgado's experiments with radio-controlled monkeys were all the more provocative because of the influences exerted by brain stimulation upon their autocratic societies, in which groups are dominated by boss monkeys. In a number of experiments the Yale scientist stimulated certain areas of a boss monkey's brain and, in effect, heightened his aggressiveness to make him more autocratic than ever. Such a monkey— who normally takes more territory in a cage than his fellow inmates, feeds first, and is generally avoided—stepped up his boss tactics against the most submissive of his subjects. He chased them around and bit them, showing particular aggressiveness toward male monkeys that threatened his authority. His favorite female partner, however, was not subjected to his added hostility.

"These results," explained Delgado, "confirmed the finding in cat colonies that aggressiveness induced by cerebral stimulations was not blind and automatic, but selective and intelligently directed."

The more humorous of ESB experiments were found in Delgado's electrical taming of rhesus monkeys, described by the scientist as "destructive and dangerous creatures which do not hesitate to bite anything within reach, including [wire] leads, instrumentation, and occasionally the experimenter's hands." Stimulation in the caudate nucleus* of a rhesus monkey strapped in a chair and making angry faces at the researcher suddenly curbed its aggressiveness enough for Delgado to dare insert a finger into the monkey's mouth. By switching the stimulus off and on, the animal could be switched back and forth from a bad monkey to a good monkey.

Once able to electrically tame a rhesus monkey, the scientist did so via radio to a boss caged with his subjects. When the stimuli were transmitted, the boss's autocracy rapidly crumbled. The subjects quickly recognized that their top monkey had somehow lost his punch, and they began roaming the cage much more freely. Indeed, they occasionally crowded him without fear of the usual reprisal it would bring. After an hour of intermittent stimulation, the chief had lost his traditional claim to his extra-large territory, and there was a marked reduction in the percentage of time that he was on his feet aggressively tending his bossy chores. However, twelve minutes after the radio transmission had been turned off he had re-established himself as head of the realm.

---

* The central nervous system has many nuclei, small masses of gray matter, or groups of nerve cells, named to indicate their anatomical locations; many are found deep in the brain and are associated with emotional and motivational behavior.

In one of these experiments, control of the stimuli was given to the monkeys themselves. Their cage was fitted out with a lever, and when it was pressed, stimulation was radioed to the boss monkey's brain. In a remarkably short time the subordinate animals found that the lever turned off the boss's rough tactics, and they used it to cut him down to size.

One of Delgado's experiments brought him popular fame, including a front-page story in *The New York Times*, the kind of publicity some of his contemporaries felt should be avoided by scientists. The Yale investigator, who was born in Ronda, Spain, returned to his homeland, where he wired up the brain of a brave bull with a small radio receiver attached to the animal. The bull was released in a ring where Delgado, in the role of a toreador, stood with a cape in one hand and a small, self-contained radio transmitter in the other. The radioed bull charged the scientist-toreador, but as he arrived within a few feet of Delgado, the Yale physiologist pressed a transmitter button sending a tiny stimulus to the caudate nucleus of the bull's brain. The beast—suddenly transformed into a Ferdinand—stopped, turned, and trotted away passively.

Some of the most provocative of Delgado's results came from experiments where a single stimulus produced an entire sequence of events that were repeatable upon subsequent stimulation of the same point in the brain. This pattern was shown in an aggressive female monkey named Ludi, the boss in a colony of four other monkeys, two male, two female. When a stimulus was applied to a point of her brain's red nucleus (in the midbrain), the monkey went through a complex sequence of responses that interrupted whatever she was doing and ended with resumption of that activity. The sequential acts began with a change in facial expression, followed by her turning her head to the right, standing up, rotating to the right, walking upright, touching the walls of the cage or grasping a swing, climbing a pole, descending, uttering a low tone, threatening subordinate monkeys, and finally, changing her aggressive attitude to a peaceful one and approaching members of the colony in a friendly manner. Whenever the red nucleus was stimulated, Ludi repeated the sequence. Even on subsequent days, stimulation caused consistent repetition of the step-by-step performance.

In another female monkey, radio stimulation of the nucleus medialis dorsali evoked a comparable sequence, also repeatable again and again. In the last act of the sequence, the monkey returned to the starting point, bent over on all fours and raised her tail, whereupon the male monkey mounted her. In a series of stimulations lasting over ninety minutes, the sequence was repeated eighty-one times, each ending with the boss monkey mounting the female subject.

By the 1970's the technology of ESB had become highly sophisticated. Delgado was using "stimoceivers," extremely small solid-state radio receivers that could be well hidden under the skin to receive stimuli and relay them through fine wires to the brain. The Yale scientist received another measure of popular publicity—again including the front page of *The New York Times*—when he and co-workers were reported as having established "direct two-way radio communication between an animal's brain and a computer." The subject was a chimpanzee named Paddy, whose head was equipped with a small two-way radio and a great many steel electrodes leading into the depths of his brain. The tiny radio transmitter sent EEG signals from the animal's amygdala to a nearby computer programmed to recognize spindle patterns in the brain waves. When they appeared, the computer radioed stimuli back to Paddy's minute receiver and the signals were led by electrodes to the animal's reticular formation. This chimp-to-computer-to-chimp feedback resulted in a lowering of the EEG spindling until the computer no longer responded and stopped radioing stimuli. After several days of give-and-take between brain and computer, spontaneous spindling almost disappeared. Meanwhile Paddy became less aggressive, not so excitable, and comparatively uninterested in food. When the computerized system was shut off, the personality changes lasted for about two weeks, but then Paddy slowly returned to his normal self, the EEG spindling also reappearing.

"We are now talking to the brain without the participation of the senses," said Delgado. "This is pure and direct communication—I call it 'nonsensory communication.'" He foresaw such a system at work on humans, serving as a kind of "brain pacemaker" to deal with cerebral dysfunctions that a computer could recognize from the EEG and take steps to alleviate. The steps might include an automatic injection of a chemical triggered by radio, or stimuli radioed to the appropriate region of the brain. The "brain pacemaker" might, for example, prevent epileptic fits.

As Hess, Olds, Delgado, and other scientists were artificially electrifying the brains of animals, with fascinating results for a quarter of a century, they were restrained in human experimentation related to deep regions of the brain until the increasing therapeutic use of implanted electrodes —described in the previous chapter—provided an entirely new dimension for human brain research by ESB. Patients with implanted electrodes were not confined to an operating table and the relatively short time of most surgical procedures. Once electrodes were set in well-defined cerebral regions, they might remain there for weeks or months. The subject, in a short time, was free of the disturbing trauma that accompanies any surgical procedure. With these advantages, a number of ESB investigators produced a variety of results by deep stimulation of the human brain during the 1950's and 60's.

In a seven-year period Robert G. Heath and Walter A. Mickle at the Tulane University School of Medicine, New Orleans, implanted electrodes in the brains of fifty-two patients at cortical and subcortical levels. Most of the patients were chronic schizophrenics. In all of them with subcortical electrodes, various deep cerebral structures were tested with ESB for behavioral responses. Heath's and Mickle's results were summarized in five parts.

When they stimulated a middle region of the brain, patients experienced a general sense of good feeling. They appeared more alert and spoke more rapidly. Some asked for more stimulation. Patients with intractable pain experienced immediate relief.

Stimulation of a part of the hypothalamus produced an opposite reaction. The patients became uncomfortable and anxious, and they complained that their hearts were speeding up and that their skin was flushing. They rejected the idea of more such stimulation.

When certain regions of the diencephalon and mesencephalon were stimulated, the patients had painful experiences. They developed tension and rage and complained of diplopia (double vision of a single object).

Stimulation of the caudate nucleus often made the patients appear drowsy, although they had no subjective complaints about the feeling.

An "emergency reaction of either rage or fear" came from stimuli in the amygdala and certain parts of the hippocampus (an elongated ridge of gray matter behind the brain's temporal lobe), and no subject wanted to repeat the experience. On one occasion the patient reported what seemed to be an illusion.

In this same period other interesting studies were being conducted with humans at the Gauster Mental Hospital, Oslo, Norway, by Carl W. Sem-Jacobsen and Arne Torkildsen. In experiments comparable to Olds's work with animals, the Norwegian workers gave their human subjects a button for stimulating their own brains at will. When they stimulated cerebral pleasure areas, patients usually responded with high rates of button pressings. With electrodes that acted upon the strongest pleasure areas of the brain, some patients actually stimulated themselves into convulsions, and then, as the current was shut off by the investigator, they lay smiling and happy.

In one case a patient amused himself by interrupting his own speech. He would press the ESB button while talking or counting, and it would stop him, no matter how hard he tried to continue. He attempted a kind of running start by counting fast with the idea that inertia might help him continue beyond the moment of stimulation, but it never worked. The whole experience frequently left him laughing at himself.

Sem-Jacobsen and Torkildsen tried to map out what had been previously labeled the "positive" and "negative" systems in the brain. The positive systems produce good feelings, while the negative produce anxiety, fright, horror, and depression. The positive systems were easily tested in human subjects, because people enjoyed the stimulation, and it could be repeated. Stimulation of the negative systems, however, was unwelcome, and repetition was avoided. Still, the scientists were able to make enough comparisons of the two systems to draw some interesting conclusions. The areas of the brain prompting each kind of response were often only one half to one centimeter apart, and areas with similar strengths of response appeared to be adjacent to one another. A mild negative area, for example, would be located right next to a mild positive area.

"It seems as if the positive and the negative regions," the Norwegian scientists wrote, "are parts of two complete different systems, closely located as one entity, like the inhibitory and excitatory innervation systems."

All the scientists investigating human subjects with implanted electrodes had difficulties in drawing valid scientific conclusions from their results. A tiny stimulus in the depths of a human brain acts at the source of thousands of cerebral forces responsible for wide ranges of behavior. The investigator has the difficult job of ascertaining objectively what is or is not the product of his stimulation. What should he think when stimulation of a female brain elicits a desire from the patient to marry the scientist? Delgado reported that it happened twice to him. One patient, a thirty-six-year-old woman under temporal lobe stimulation, talked about the scientist's nationality, background, and friends. "Spaniards are very attractive," she said. "I would like to marry a Spaniard."

At the University of Pittsburgh School of Medicine, a professor of psychology, H. E. King, interviewed patients before a sound movie camera as their brains were stimulated. In one film a young woman is being interviewed while her amygdala is occasionally stimulated. During a short sequence when the stimulus was off, she described her general frame of mind before coming to the hospital: "Like I can't be a part of anything," she said, pensively. "Like I don't belong and everything is a dream or something." Then the tiny stimulus was turned on, and the woman's expression suddenly showed tension.

"How do you feel now?" the interviewer asked.

"I feel like I want to get up from this chair!" she exclaimed in a high voice. "Please don't let me!"

Her expression changed to that of a person pleading for something, and she said: "Don't do this to me. I don't want to be mean."

"Feel like you want to hit me?" the interviewer asked.

"Yeah, I just want to hit something," she said, angrily. "I want to get something and just tear it up. Take it so I won't." She handed a scarf to the interviewer. He returned a sheaf of paper, and the patient tore it into shreds. "I don't like to feel like this," she said. The strength of the stimulus was reduced slightly and this relieved the patient's anxiety. When it was increased again, the extremely hostile feelings returned.

After the current was turned off, the subject couldn't describe her feelings under stimulation. They were not painful, she said, but she didn't like the sensations, whatever they were. Then she decided that somehow they made her feel better by reducing her worry.

Through such limited observations of behavior in response

to stimuli, commendable progress was made in mapping the unbelievably intricate systems behind the control of life and thought. Meanwhile, the ESB experiments naturally stirred up concern that scientists were leading us to mass thought control—an excellent subject for speculation by an imaginative writer.

Esquire magazine, for example, carried a commentary on Delgado's work, entitled: "Someone to Watch Over You (For Less than 2¢ a Day)." The author envisioned an "electroligarchy" run by a few boss people whose untapped, non-stimulated brains run the computers that control all other brains in a three-layer society below. The top layer, the "Electrons," would enjoy only a few carefully implanted electrodes to maintain happiness and creativity. Second in line would be the "Positrons," with cerebral wiring that would preserve them as white collar workers. And on the bottom the "Neutrons," each with many electrodes in his brain, would be completely robotized so they could serve in such jobs as ditch digging and love every moment of it.

Science fiction? Yes, but not completely so. In the mid-1960's neurological control systems were a serious enough matter for federal officials at Bethesda, Maryland, to consider a twelve-year plan for developing the mechanisms. The National Institute of Neurological Diseases and Blindness (the word Blindness is now changed to Stroke) hoped to establish a laboratory to study the possibilities. Three areas of research would be involved:

First, the study of nervous system controls over the things immediately around us. On a relatively simple level, this research might lead to artificial limbs controlled by the nervous system. Federal money was granted for this, and in 1968 a neurologically controlled mechanical arm, developed with a $100,000 grant, was demonstrated at the Massachusetts General Hospital in Boston. The "Boston arm" was controlled by nerve impulses picked up from muscle in the stump of an amputated arm. An amputee could flex the artificial arm simply by thinking about it. The developers were with the Harvard Medical School and Massachusetts Institute of Technology.

Second, the proposed research program would study control of the central nervous system from external sources comparable to what we have seen in reviewing ESB techniques.

Third, the research would consider the cybernetics of information processing as related to the first two considerations.

As of this writing, the full-fledged program has not been started.

All this aside, the mass wiring of brains in large numbers of people is not likely to happen, not soon, anyway. Forgetting the ethical considerations, which would be a serious deterrent to mass brain wiring, insertion of electrodes in millions of heads would be an extremely formidable undertaking, even if the subjects held still for it. At best, the brain wirers could only impose one or a few behavioral traits at the most on masses of people—a difficult goal, since anatomical and physiological differences, as many as there are humans, would force the electrode implanters to work from detailed and careful studies of each and every subject's brain. Would it be worth all the trouble? It might be better to concentrate on more effective public speaking, an ancient method for mass brain control.

"Scientific discoveries and technology," Delgado once told an audience at the American Museum of Natural History, "cannot be shelved because of real or imaginary dangers, and it may certainly be predicted that the evolution of physical control of the brain and the acquisition of knowledge derived from it will continue at an accelerated pace, pointing hopefully toward the development of a more intelligent and peaceful mind of the species without loss of individual identity, and toward the exploitation of the most suitable kind of feedback mechanism: the human brain studying the human brain."

14

THE SEARCH FOR THE ENGRAM

At age sixteen or seventeen, Karl S. Lashley, who became one of America's great psychologists, was at the University of West Virginia, where he had intended to major in Latin or English until a chance encounter with a neurologist turned his interests to the biological sciences. Soon after, the young Lashley happened upon a set of microscope slides displaying a frog's brain prepared with the Golgi stain. He was fascinated and naïvely proposed to an instructor that he, Lashley, should work out all the connections in the tiny brain. "Then we should know how the frog works," the young man said. In later years he often joked about spending all of his life trying to figure out how the frog works.

Actually, Lashley devoted a large share of his career to a more difficult pursuit. He spent some three decades trying to locate where memories are stored by the brain. Most of his subjects were rats.

For centuries men assumed that when a memory lodged in the brain, some change occurred within the head. The early Greek philosophers thought of the mind as a tablet inscribed by experience. In the seventeenth century, René Descartes attempted to explain memory with this proposal about the pineal gland, which he thought was the seat of the soul: "When the mind wills to recall something, this volition causes the little gland, by inclining successively to different sides, to impel the animal spirits toward different parts of the brain, until they come upon that part where traces are left of the thing which it wishes to remember; for these traces are nothing else than the circumstance that the pores of the brain through which the spirits have already taken their course on presentation of the object, have thereby acquired a greater facility than the rest to be opened again the same way by the spirits which come to them; so that these spirits coming upon the pores enter therein more readily than into the others."

In 1904 a French scientist, Richard Semon, named Descartes' memory "traces." Whatever it might be, a trace was called an "engram." Some time later Lashley began his thirty-year "search for the engram" in rats and monkeys, and in a few chimpanzees. In most of the experiments the animals were trained to varying degrees, from making simple associations to solving comparatively difficult problems. Rats, for example, were trained to react in different ways to various lights, and monkeys were taught to open and enter latch boxes. Once trained, the animals were anesthetized and their skulls opened so that carefully selected parts of their cerebral cortexes could be surgically removed. After a postoperative recovery period, the subjects were observed and tested to see what effect, if any, the excision of brain tissue had on the learning. With another but similar method the scientist performed the surgery prior to the training as he tried to discover what the damaged brain would fail to learn. In either instance the animals were finally killed and their brains analyzed to see exactly what parts had been destroyed. Lashley, who began the work at the Institute of Juvenile Research in Chicago, systematically searched thousands of animal brains in hopes of locating the engram.

In 1950 Lashley summarized his efforts in a paper entitled "In Search of the Engram," and there he said: "This series of experiments has yielded a good bit of information about what and where the memory trace is not. It has discovered nothing directly of the real nature of the engram. I sometimes feel, in reviewing the evidence on the localization of the memory trace, that the necessary conclusion is that learning just is not possible. It is difficult to conceive of a mechanism which can satisfy the conditions set for it. Nevertheless, in spite of such evidence against it, learning does sometimes occur."

Lashley concluded that the engram was not stored at a specific point in the brain, for memories seemed to settle over wide areas of the cortex. This was indicated by the way the removal of brain tissue caused animals to forget what they had been taught. The amount of forgetting was related to the brain tissue removed. If about half the cortex of a trained animal was removed, it forgot about fifty percent of the experimental learning. If seventy-five percent of the tissue was removed, about twenty-five percent of the learning remained. Lashley could only conclude that memory was a diffuse process involving the entire cortex and not a discrete event in one definable location of the vastly intricate brain. He could not explain why.

The search for the engram is certainly the most challenging of all the explorations of the nervous system. Memory, difficult and baffling even to contemplate as a physical function, is central to everything human. An understanding of how it works would have an incalculable impact on all human life. Men have forever tried to comprehend the nature of memory, and they inevitably come back to the notion expressed by Descartes and followed by Lashley: that intellectual exercise leaves residual changes in the brain. The idea has been stretched to the absurd by quacks, frequently rejected for the utter lack of evidence, and overridden by other theories, but it survives and is still central to the search for the engram in modern times.

It received substantial attention around 1800 in the principles of phrenology, an empirical system of psychology promoted by a Viennese physician, Franz Joseph Gall. As discussed in Chapter 3, Gall tried to develop a functional map of the brain's surface. He also correctly pointed out that the white matter of the brain serves as connecting material for the active gray matter. While he was credited with such sound observations, Gall with his followers, especially J. K. Spurzheim, was not so well remembered for phrenology. According to its principles, the mental powers of man could be listed as a number of independent faculties, each having a definite place on the surface of the brain. These various surface regions, the phrenologists proposed, differed in size from person to person according to how large a part the corresponding mental faculties played in an individual's character. Gall's followers went on to make the dubious claim that variations in the cerebral surface could be detected in the physical structure of the skull. They proposed, therefore, that a trained observer could analyze a person's character and disposition by studying the shape of his head. The foundations of this cult rested on the phrenologist's assumption that physical growth of the brain's various regions corresponded to the growth of the related mental faculties. Spurzheim talked in terms of the brain increasing with exercise. "This may certainly happen in the brain as in the muscles," he wrote in 1815; "nay, it seems more than probable, because the blood is carried in greater abundance to the parts which are excited, and nutrition is performed by the blood."

As phrenology became the practice of quacks, a good descriptive word was lost to the science of the brain, and the memory of Gall was tainted for his part in the spurious affair. However, the downfall of phrenology by no means ended the idea that mental capacity might be physically revealed in the brain. For example, Charles Darwin decided that the organ was enlarged by mental exercise, like muscle with physical exercise. In 1874 he wrote that the domesticated rabbit's brain was "considerably reduced in bulk" compared to the same organ in the wild rabbit or hare, which had been forced for generations to use its intellect, instincts, senses, and voluntary movements much more than his homebound cousin. Many medical men believed the same to be true of the human brain, as evident in the common practice of the 1800's of measuring and weighing the brains of great men to see if differences could be attributed to their intellectual attainment. As microscopes and other tools improved, scientists continued studying the brains of the famous and infamous. As revealed earlier, Lenin's death in 1924 was followed by an intensive study of his brain in a former industrialist's mansion adapted for a laboratory. Russian scientists, especially trained for the investigation, devoted two and a half years to serially sectioning the Soviet leader's brain for detailed investigation. An early report compared an abnormal growth of pyramidal cells found in the association cortex (part of the cerebral cortex not responsible for primary motor or sensory functions) with the hypertrophy of muscle resulting from continuous physical exercise.

But this kind of research offered no sound conclusions, and for a period of time in this century, the idea that mental activities produced residual changes in the brain was pretty much abandoned in favor of theories that explained learning and memory strictly in terms of the brain's electrical activity. They proposed that storage of information depended upon the ongoing electrical activity in some kind of neural circuitry. Lashley, who expressed one of these theories, talked about "complex patterns of reverberatory circuits." He proposed: "Recall involves the synergetic action or some sort of resonance among a large number of neurons. The learning process must consist of the attunement of the elements of a complex system in such a way that a particular combination or pattern of cells responds more readily than before the experience. The particular mechanism by which this is brought about remains unknown."

Such theories were strenuously tested in several ways in

the decade and a half following World War II. All the experimenters felt that if memory was somehow imposed upon the continuing electrical activity of the cerebral neurons, one might disrupt memory by disrupting the electrical activity.

Several scientists tried to do so by "scrambling" the brain's electrical activity with electro-convulsive shocks. One of the earliest shock experiments was conducted on thirty albino rats by Carl P. Duncan of Brown University. They were trained three times a day for fifteen days to run down the leg of a T maze and turn left to obtain a reward of a small portion of wet mash. On the sixteenth day, the animal's habit was reversed by repeatedly luring it to the right arm of the T for a relatively large reward of mash. When the rat's left-turn habit had been overridden by a right-turn habit, twenty of them were administered brief, eighty-volt convulsive shocks with two electrodes, one applied to each ear. The other ten (control) rats did not receive the shocks. Subsequent tests revealed that fourteen of the twenty shocked animals had reverted to the left-turn habit—as if the memory of the right turn had been knocked out of their heads. Eight of the ten control rats continued the right-turn habit.

"It is argued," Duncan wrote, "that one of the effects of shock may be to cause an amnesia or a disorganization for recent habits, thereby allowing older incompatible habits to regain dominance."

Other researchers with variations on Duncan's experiments arrived at essentially the same conclusion. The shock treatment disrupted recent memories, but once information had time to settle into the brain, electrical interference had no effect on the memory.

Other scientists literally tried to freeze memories out of rat brains by cooling them so much that the process interfered with the natural electrical activity. In one study conducted by R. K. Andrus and three co-workers in London, rats were cooled down to between zero and plus one degree Centigrade so that the electrical activity of the brain was arrested

90 to 120 minutes. When they were "reanimated" with normal temperatures, the animals were tested to see if they retained some simple maze habits learned earlier. They showed no serious loss of memory. ". . . our results," the researchers reported, "are difficult to explain if long-term memory is dependent upon the continuous activity of the brain."

These and other techniques that interfered with the brain's continuing electrical activity failed to disrupt long-term memories, although they clearly indicated that immediately after a learning experience the related memories are vulnerable to attack. The results undermined the reverberatory-circuit theories, and the search for the engram turned back to the idea that residual changes in brain tissue might still be found to explain the storage and retrieval of information. In the post-World War II years some illuminating studies were conducted on the brains of animals and humans. One series was somewhat reminiscent of Lashley's surgical approach to memory. This was the "split-brain" research made famous by Roger W. Sperry and his colleagues at the University of Chicago and the California Institute of Technology (Cal. Tech.). Their investigations, conducted with animals and humans, are not ordinarily identified strictly as investigations of memory, but the results had a good deal to say about the place of the engram in the brain.

Sperry, Hixon Professor of Psychobiology at Cal. Tech., worked on various aspects of the nervous system for more than three decades, but he is undoubtedly most renowned for his split-brain experiments that have, in his words, "enabled us to pinpoint various centers of specific brain activity, . . . suggested new concepts and new lines of thought and . . . opened up a wealth of new possibilities for investigating the mysteries of the mind."

The mammalian brain is a double brain, as almost any picture of the organ reveals. It has two hemispheres, each associated with the opposite side of the body, each with a set of motor and sensory systems for that side. However, the anatomical connections between the two hemispheres are not obvious in an ordinary picture. In the deepest regions of the brain, the hemispheres are joined by a common brainstem, which connects with the spinal cord. Above that, there are several connections, bundles of nerve fibers called commissures. The most prominent, the "great cerebral commissure," or "corpus callosum," has millions of fibers connecting the two halves of the cerebral cortex. These bridges between the hemispheres, it would seem clear, tie the brain together so it can function as a unit. In the split-brain experiments, started in the early 1950's, Sperry and his colleagues severed the hemispheric links, first in cats and then in monkeys and chimpanzees. The cuts, made while the animals were anesthetized, severed all the fibrous connections between hemispheres, down to and including the upper parts of the brainstem. When the animals returned to consciousness, the scientists observed them to see the effects of the split brain.

At first it seemed that nothing had happened. The split-brain animal functioned normally. In fact, some standard tests indicated that it even learned as well as the animal with an intact brain. Sperry concluded that the differences imposed by the split brain would have to be revealed by special tests, and these were designed and administered beginning in 1951 by Ronald E. Myer, a doctoral candidate in Sperry's laboratory.

In this work, Myer severed both the corpus callosum and the optic chiasm, a fibrous structure that feeds nerve signals from each eye to both cerebral hemispheres. The surgery broke the main communication lines between the two halves and ensured that messages from each eye would feed only to its corresponding side of the brain. This provided a way of visually training one side of the brain at a time. The one-sided learning could be accomplished and tested in the following way: an animal, wearing a patch over one eye, was taught to solve a simple problem. The patch was then shifted

VISUAL FIELDS
(LEFT)   (RIGHT)

LEFT
HEMISPHERE

RIGHT
HEMISPHERE

OPTIC
CHIASM

CORPUS
CALLOSUM

Diagram to show paths of visual input to both hemispheres of human brain. Information presented to one visual field goes only to opposite hemisphere: left visual field to right hemisphere and vice versa. In a normal brain incoming information limited to one hemisphere is communicated to other hemisphere via corpus callosum. In split-brain operation the corpus callosum is severed (between arrows), thereby interrupting communication from one side to the other. Experimenter can then give information to only one hemisphere, by presenting it to opposite visual field.

to the other eye, and the animal was presented with the same problem, but now it couldn't solve it. The test revealed that only one hemisphere had benefited from the learning. If the opposite half of the brain were to learn how to solve the problem, it had to be trained independently. A normal animal had no such difficulty when learning was presented in such a way that it was channeled over visual pathways to only one side of the brain. It was evident that the intact organ had internal means of transferring learning from one side to the other. Clearly, the split-brain animal was a creature whose single brain had been divided into two relatively independent brains.

Comparable experiments with different training problems were conducted on other animals, and the results were the same. Sperry and his colleagues even used the eye-patch technique on a split-brain animal to train each of the two hemispheres with one of two ways to solve a single problem. Offering a normal animal double solutions is a frustrating experience for the creature, but it was not so for the animal with two brains, one trained for each solution. The possibility for conflict had been removed in splitting the brain.

"In short," Sperry wrote, "it appears from the accumulated evidence that learning in one hemisphere is usually inaccessible to the other hemisphere if the commissures between the hemispheres are missing. This means that the corpus callosum has the important function of allowing the two hemispheres to share learning and memory."

He proposed that in the learning process, engrams are either established (1) in both sides of the two-sided mammalian brain, or (2) in only one side, although in that case the learning is available to the opposite hemisphere upon call. In either case, Sperry said, the corpus callosum is the bridge that allows both hemispheres to use the same memory.

The Cal. Tech. scientist and his colleagues found they could determine whether engrams were set down in only one or in both hemispheres. They simply trained a normal brain, severed the corpus callosum, and then tested the hemispheres independently for the learning. This was done in cats and monkeys, and even in humans who underwent split-brain surgery, which will be discussed below. The double-engram system, that simultaneously provides both halves of the brain with the same learning, was found more often in cats than humans. The single-engram system, directly involving only a single hemisphere, was more often the rule for the human brains. Monkey brains had more of a mixture of the two memory systems than either those of cats or humans. The single-engram system was especially evident in human memories related to language, which is normally consigned to the dominant (left) hemisphere of the brain.

When split-brain experiments on animals indicated that severing the corpus callosum did not seriously affect mental faculties, neurosurgeons were encouraged to perform such surgery on human patients to confine epileptic seizures to one hemisphere in cases where the dysfunction was expected to migrate to the opposite hemisphere. The operations were even more successful than anticipated. They not only confined the seizures to one side of the brain, but also reduced the original, unilateral attack, as if the intact commissure between hemispheres had something to do with organizing the seizures.

In 1961, split-brain surgery was performed on a forty-eight-old war veteran at the White Memorial Hospital in Los Angeles by two surgeons of the California College of Medicine, Joseph E. Bogen and Philip J. Vogel. They had agreed to work with Michael S. Gazzaniga from Sperry's laboratory in testing the patient after the surgery. The neurosurgeons severed several commissures of the man's brain, including the corpus callosum. The operation succeeded, and the veteran became the first of ten such cases operated upon by Bogen and Vogel and tested by Gazzaniga.

When these split-brain patients recovered from the surgery, they seemed surprisingly normal, with their same general temperament, personality, and intelligence. One patient was a thirty-year-old housewife with two children. Upon recovery, she returned home and led a normal, active life, with no complaints. However, the close observer of these patients could see that each favored the right side, which is controlled by the opposite and dominant hemisphere of the brain. The person seemed relatively unaware of his left side for some time after the operation. If an object were passed to his left hand, he seemed unaware of it, or if he bumped into something with his left side, he didn't seem to notice.

Some specially designed tests clarified what was happening beneath the split-brain patient's outwardly normal facade. When one of the subjects was asked to watch a horizontal line of lights, each of which flashed briefly in sequence from one end of the line to the other, the patient seemed to see only the flashes appearing in his right visual field sending signals back to the left side of the brain—or at least that is what he said. Flashes that signaled only the right hemisphere via the opposite (left) visual field were apparently not seen, according to the patient. Then Gazzaniga and his colleagues discovered that the apparent blindness of the right hemisphere was evident only when a patient was asked to report verbally on seeing the lights. When instructed to point at the light flashes, the subject indicated that he saw all the lights regardless of the hemisphere involved. This test by gesture revealed that the right side of the brain was registering the vision as well as the left, but it simply couldn't say so with words because the speech faculty was limited to the left hemisphere. The right, when split from the left, was, in effect, mute.

The muteness of the right hemisphere was demonstrated in a number of ways. A picture, a familiar object, or a simple sentence visually presented only to the left hemisphere was easily described or read off, either orally or in writing. But the same display entering only the right hemisphere produced no such response. A common object, like scissors, passed to the patient when his hands were hidden from his view by a small screen was easily described when it was held by the right hand (dependent on left hemisphere); but if first passed to the left hand, the individual could only guess what he was holding.

While tests requiring verbal responses made the right hemisphere appear feeble-minded, tests requiring non-verbal responses revealed it had a high level of intelligence. For example, the patient might be shown a cigarette so the image was in the visual field of the right hemisphere. Meanwhile, that hemisphere's hand (the left) could feel around behind a screen and pick out an ashtray from among several other objects unrelated to the cigarette. This kind of test revealed that learning had been laid down in the right hemisphere, but the mechanisms for expressing it were missing and the speech equipment of the left hemisphere could not be used because of the split in the brain.

"This [muteness of the right hemisphere] is illustrated in many ways," Sperry explained in a paper presented at the Vatican in 1965. "For example: the subject may be blind-folded and some familiar object like a pencil, a cigarette, a comb or a coin placed in the left hand. Under these conditions the mute hemisphere connected to the left hand feeling the object perceives and appears to know quite well what the object is. Though it cannot express this knowledge in speech or in writing, it can manipulate the object correctly, it can demonstrate how the object is supposed to be used, and it can remember the object and go and retrieve it with the same hand from among an array of other objects either by touch or sight. While all this is going on, the other hemi-sphere meanwhile has no conception of what the object is and, if asked, says so. . . ."

One would assume that separating the mute and the speech hemisphere would be a devastating handicap to the split-brain patient, but it isn't. The lost communication is com-pensated for by the fact that most situations influence both sides of the split brain. Even if only by inference, the left can usually learn what the right learns. Sounds entering both ears, or tactile sensations coming through both hands might, for example, tip off the left hemisphere of things seeming to involve only its opposite half.

This was demonstrated by the blindfolded patient. ". . . let the right hand cross over and touch the test object in the left hand," Sperry said, "or let the object itself touch the face or head as in demonstrating the use of a comb, a cigarette or glasses; or let the object make some giveaway sound, like the jingle of a key case, then immediately the speech hemisphere also comes across with the correct answer."

The split-brain surgery and subsequent tests helped confirm some important ideas about the brain that had been current for nearly a century. In 1874 Carl Wernicke of the University of Breslau published a classic, seventy-two page paper entitled "The Symptom Complex of Aphasia," and it became a major influence on the anatomical study of aphasia (loss of power to use or comprehend speech). From this and other work that followed, it was decided that if the brain's right hemisphere were to perform with language, it depended upon the communication of verbal information across the corpus callosum.

Support for this idea came from the study of brain dysfunctions, one of which was described as "pure alexia without agraphia" (the inability to read without the inability to write). In 1892 a French doctor, J. J. Déjérine, made a post-mortem study of a patient with pure alexia without agraphia. The patient had developed a defect in his right visual field (which is related to the left hemisphere), and it completely robbed him of the ability to read. However, he could still copy down the very words that he could not understand. Furthermore, he could write something spontaneously, but then he could not read it. In the post-mortem examination, Déjérine found that the left visual cortex and the posterior of the corpus callosum had been destroyed. From this finding he came up with an explanation of the perplexing syndrome:

With the left visual cortex destroyed, a viewing of written language only registered in the right visual cortex. However, the right side could not deal with the incoming signals as language, for this required communication with the left hemisphere speech mechanism via the corpus callosum, which had been destroyed. The patient could, therefore, deal with writing only as non-verbal symbols, not as language laden with ideas.

Another dysfunction, "callosal disconnection," was described and confirmed in post-mortem examinations by a group of Wernicke's students, who found that the victims' corpus callosums had been destroyed by lesions. These patients, whose brains had been split by disease, had many of the symptoms seen in later years in the split-brain surgical cases.

The split-brain experiments on humans proved that our so-called single brain is literally two brains, each with immense capabilities of its own. Indeed, there were indications that one hemisphere is in some ways more efficient than the normal, two-part brain. Gazzaniga and a colleague, E. D. Young, found that split-brain monkeys can handle twice as much information as a normal monkey. They also determined that a split-brain person can simultaneously employ both halves of his brain to complete two tasks in the time it takes the average individual to complete one.

The scientists were often asked, perhaps facetiously, how the two brains of a split-brain individual got along with one another. Does the person with a will of his own recover from split-brain surgery with two wills of his own and find they don't agree? In the veteran who became the first such patient, a conflict of the two half-brains seemed to be a problem. He might be drawing on his pants with one hand and the other hand would try to pull them off. The patient's wife became aware of the conflict; as her husband's left hand beckoned her to come near, the right might indicate she should stay away. However, the differences never became serious, for there always seemed to be enough unifying forces acting upon both sides of the brain to keep them pretty much in harmony.

But why do we have two brains in one cranium? The split-brain scientists could not say—except that the explanation might lie in some grand quirk of evolution. Sperry, in the 1964 James Arthur Lecture on the Evolution of the Human Brain at the American Museum of Natural History, said: ". . . the brain-bisection studies leave us with a strong suspicion that evolution may have saddled us all with a great deal of unnecessary duplication, both in structure and in the function of the higher brain centers.

"Space in the intracranial region is tight, and one wonders if the premium item could not have been utilized for better things than the kind of right-left duplication that now prevails. Evolution, of course, has made notable errors in the past, and one suspects that in the elaboration of the higher brain centers evolutionary progress is more encumbered than aided by the bilateralized scheme which, of course, is deeply entrenched in the mechanisms of development and also in the basic wiring plan of the lower nerve centers." Sperry added that he felt the human head could probably do very well with a "single unified set of brain controls."

"With the existing cerebral system," he said, "most memories have to be laid down twice—one engram for the left hemisphere and another engram copy for the right hemisphere. The amount of information stored in memory in a mammalian brain is a remarkable thing in itself; to have to double it all for the second hemisphere would seem in many ways a bit wasteful. It is doubtful that all this redundancy has had any direct survival value. . . ."

Human survival as a whole person with only half a brain is proven possible by the history of an operation called a "hemispherectomy." With this surgery, reported in medical literature for many years, one side of the brain is removed to save an individual from fatal problems such as a brain tumor. Hemispherectomies have been performed hundreds of times on children, who have not only survived but have also recovered the functions that resided in the excised half of the brain. Even removal of the left hemisphere has been followed by the right half, ordinarily the mute side, taking over the speech functions. This kind of transfer, which was said to be possible up to age fifteen, was attributed to the "functional plasticity" of the young brain, an advantage supposedly lost in adulthood.

In 1966, however, two authors in *Science* magazine, Aaron Smith and C. W. Burland of Omaha, Nebraska, presented "the first reported case of an adult . . . who is continuing to improve in many functions more than seven months after removal of the entire left cerebral hemisphere because of glioma [brain tumor]." Immediately after the surgery, the forty-seven-year-old male patient suffered paralysis of the right side of the body, blindness in the right visual field, and severe aphasia, but in time the functions began to return partially. Ten weeks after the operation, a nurse happened to ask the patient, "Did you have a B.M. today?" and surprisingly he replied, "What does B.M. mean?" Until he died, two years and four days after the operation, the patient's communication of thoughts and ideas improved slowly, and he was able in various degrees of proficiency to speak, write, perform arithmetic problems, carry out abstract mental tasks, sing, and discriminate between colors. The general success of hemispherectomies was added evidence that man might survive without the duplication in his double brain.

Sperry suggested that the dominance of one of our cerebral hemispheres may be "definite evidence of a belated tendency in evolution to try to circumvent some of the duplication difficulties." As other scientists had already noted, the phenomenon apparently exists only at the very top of the evolutionary scale, in the human brain. Man is the only mammal, as far as we know, having a brain with one side devoted to a single class of learning.

In 1968 two neuroscientists of the Boston University School of Medicine, Norman Geschwind and Walter Levitsky, reported on some revealing studies concerning cerebral dominance. They questioned a widely held assumption that there were no significant differences between the two halves of one brain. Geschwind and Levitsky proved this false by carefully measuring and comparing the two hemispheres in a hundred adult human brains made available for post-mortem studies. "We demonstrated that . . . differences exist and are indeed readily visible to the naked eye," Geschwind wrote in a 1970 report. "The area that lies behind the primary auditory cortex in the upper surface of the temporal lobe is larger on the left side in 65 percent of brains, and larger on the right in only 11 percent. This region on the left side is, on the average, nearly a centimeter longer than its fellow on the opposite side—that is, larger by one-third than the corresponding area on the right. . . . This region which is larger in the left hemisphere is, in fact, a portion of Wernicke's area, whose major importance for speech was first shown nearly 100 years ago. It is reasonable to assume that there are other anatomical asymmetries in the hemisphere of the human brain, reflecting other aspects of dominance." The Geshwind-Levitsky findings were confirmed by other investigations.

The discovery of these physical differences in functional areas of the human cortex could hardly surprise anyone who had read the reports of some fascinating work on rat brains in progress for many years at Berkeley, California. At least, it wouldn't surprise anyone who had dared think that the rat-brain results might apply to human brains—something that scientists are reluctant to do, although they sometimes can't keep themselves from the temptation.

In 1953 two psychologists, David Krech and Mark R. Rosenzweig, joined a biochemist, Edward L. Bennett, to study the relationships between intelligent animal behavior and brain chemistry. Around 1960 these scientists, working at the University of California, Berkeley, were surprised to find that experience modified not only the chemistry of their animals' brains but also the anatomy. With this information, the chemist and two psychologists asked an anatomist, Marian C. Diamond, to join the research team. Their work had major significance for the long and baffling attempts to discover whether learning causes changes in the brain detectable by physical means.

In the general design of their experiments, the Berkeley scientists claimed to have followed the second half of a proposal made by the phrenologist J. K. Spurzheim in 1815, when he asked if the brain might not increase with exercise. "In order . . . to be able to answer this question positively, he wrote, "we ought to observe the same person when exercised and when not exercised; or at least observe many persons who are, and many others who are not, exercised during all periods of life." Bennett, Diamond, Krech, and Rosenzweig used rats (over ten thousand) instead of people, and they compared many that were mentally exercised with many that were not.

The scientists worked with large colonies of rats that were enough alike so that the main variable between animals would be the different experiences to which each would be subject in the laboratory. The tests were actually run on "littermate pairs" always chosen from the same family. They were taken at weaning (about twenty-five days) and separated so that each baby rat would experience a vastly different life from its sibling during the next eighty days. One was placed in an "impoverished environment," which meant solitary confinement in a small, quiet, dimly lighted cage. Although it enjoyed all the food and water it desired, the impoverished rat received none of the stimulation that comes from social life. Meanwhile the sibling rat grew up in an "enriched environment." It lived among ten or a dozen other rats with plenty of space and light and lots of fun with "toys," like ladders, wheels, boxes, and platforms. And every day a laboratory worker gave small groups of these lucky rats a chance to explore a special area with barriers rearranged in different patterns each day.

"Rat pups are as playful and as amusing to watch as kittens in these situations," Rosenzweig explained. "After about 30 days in this permissive free play environment, some formal training is given in a series of mazes. In the home cage they have food and water ad lib. Thus these animals are stimulated by their cagemates, by their complex environment and by trials in several apparatuses."

On the eightieth day of their disparate lives the littermate pairs, now young adults, were removed from their respective cages and killed. The two brains in each instance were removed, divided into several samples, and analyzed. Finally, the data was compared to see if cerebral differences had developed between the impoverished rat and the enriched rat.

This fate came to innumerable pairs of rats from the 1950's up into the 1960's. While the general design of the experiments remained the same, some variations were introduced to study more specific effects of experience on rat brains. At first the Berkeley researchers confined their analysis to brain chemistry, but then they made an accidential discovery that led to a broader study. As part of measuring chemical activity per unit of brain tissue, they routinely weighed the samples, but after a few years they recognized that small weight differences could be associated with the different experiences. This led to the group's inclusion of the anatomist, and in continuing analyses, they considered structural changes caused by experience.

By the mid-1960's the California scientists listed five major differences between impoverished and enriched rat brains.

First, the typical rat with the permissive background had a bigger cortex than its severely restricted sibling. The cortex enriched by experience was some four percent heavier than the impoverished cortex. In addition, the depth of the enriched cortex had increased some six percent. The increases were not part of an over-all rise in body weight, for the active rat came to the end of its days weighing about seven percent less than its confined littermate. Even the total brain weight reflected this difference; it weighed slightly less in the enriched animal. So it was only the cortex, the highest level of the brain, that was apparently influenced by experience.

Someone who questioned the results suggested that the difference in cortical weight might reflect an increase in the organ's motor regions because of all the physical exercise in the enriched experience. The Berkeley group checked on this by confining both littermates of a pair in impoverished cages, with the exception that one cage was equipped with a wheel upon which the inmate could exercise at will. Comparisons of both rats' brains showed no significant difference in cortical weight. "It proved to us that the increase in weight was not just the athletic program," Krech once stated. "The coach will never take the place of the professor."

Some more enlightening evidence was found when the researchers weighed specific regions of the enriched cortex and found differences between them. The brain's occipital region (which contains the visual area) showed the greatest weight change (some six percent), while the somesthetic area (area of cortex receiving sensory signals from skin) had the least increase (two percent). Most fascinating of all was the way the scientists could modify the weight of certain areas of cortex by modifying an animal's experience. For example, rats raised in the dark ended up with less visual cortex. If rats were kept in the dark, but in a relatively complex cage with "toys," their somesthetic areas were heavier than in rats living in the same complex cages with light.

The second difference between the impoverished and enriched brains was in enzymatic activity. Chemical studies of the cortex indicated over-all increases of both cholinesterase and a closely related enzyme, acetylcholinesterase, both of which speed up the hydrolysis of the nerve transmitter substance acetylcholine. A close analysis, however, showed that only the cholinesterase increased in relation to the greater weight of enriched cortex, while acetylcholinesterase decreased per unit weight. This data was difficult to explain until a third difference between the two brains was found through histological observations.

This third difference was an increase in the glial cells of the enriched brains—which supported a growing belief that the glia is more than just packing material for neurons. In noting the increase in glia, the microscopists also found fewer neurons per unit weight of enriched brain tissue, apparently because they were pushed farther apart by the larger numbers of glial cells. This evidence explained the per-unit-of-tissue increase in cholinesterase, which is associated chiefly with glial cells, and the decrease in acetylcholinesterase, associated mainly with neurons.

The fourth difference was that the enriched neurons were enlarged. Histological studies showed that their nuclei had increased in size compared to those in the same cells in the sibling rat.

Finally, the experimenters recognized that the capillaries of the enriched cortex had increased in diameter. This appeared to be a physiological response to the need for a larger blood supply to the more active brain.

If the five differences were indicative of mental development, the impoverished animals were obviously losers. But was the loss permanent? To answer this question, the Berkeley group treated rats to impoverished environment for 105 days and then switched them to the enriched environment for 50 days of the good life. Analysis of their brains showed that the tissue had become endowed with the cerebral features of the enriched rats of the original tests.

How did all this sacrifice of rats to science explain memory? It didn't, although it was an indirect, but important, contribution toward an understanding. The work set into place one part of the grand puzzle of the mind and made the total solution a little more possible. Bennett, Diamond, Krech, and Rosenzweig put it in the following way:

"We wish to make clear that finding these changes in the

brain consequent upon experience does not prove that they have anything to do with storage of memory. The demonstration of such changes merely helps to establish the fact that the brain is responsive to environmental pressure—a fact demanded by physiological theories of learning and memory."

About three years before the Berkeley studies started, two psychologists at the University of Chicago, J. J. Katz and Ward C. Halstead, proposed that the engram might exist as a molecular change in the nerve cell, and they pointed to protein as possibly playing the central role in memory. The theory, however, was ahead of its time, and most of a decade went by before the idea was seriously explored. Meanwhile scientists were making some highly relevant discoveries about the nucleic acids, DNA (deoxyribonucleic acid) and RNA (ribonucleic acid). In 1957, F. H. C. Crick, a physicist turned molecular biologist at the University of Cambridge, wrote: "If proteins are the principal stuff of life, the nucleic acids are its blueprint—the molecules on which the Secret of Life, if we may speak of such a thing, is written." Crick won the 1962 Nobel Prize in Physiology or Medicine with James D. Watson and Maurice H. F. Wilkins for discovery of the molecular structure of DNA, which had previously been identified as the material of genes (biological units containing heredity information).

It had been learned that most DNA resides in the nucleus of cells and most RNA is found outside the nucleus, in the cytoplasm. It had also been concluded that the complicated DNA molecule manages the physiological processes of a cell by directing the manufacturing of the closely related RNA molecule, which in turn directs the synthesis of protein, "the principal stuff of life." And it had been demonstrated that DNA contains the "genetic code" with an organism's "ancestral memories." In other words, it provides the memory that reminds an embryo what it shall grow up to be—an elephant, a Canadian goose, or a blue-eyed brunette. RNA, geneticists decided, has the day-to-day job of carrying out the directions of the genetic code.

Around 1960, Holger Hydén, the director of the Institute of Histology at the University of Göteborg, Sweden, theorized that RNA might also be the "memory molecule," serving the memory processes within an organism's lifetime. He felt that in RNA the long search for the engram might come to a successful finish. RNA might be, in Descartes' words, "that part where traces are left of the thing which [the brain] wishes to remember." The traces might be found as changes in the chemical code of the RNA molecule, decided Hydén, and he and his associates did some remarkable experiments that tested and strengthened the theory.

First, Hydén analyzed RNA from individual nerve cells that he removed from small mammals, usually rats and rabbits. The removal of cells, a tremendous accomplishment in itself, was done "freehand." Hydén used a stereomicroscope with a magnification of eighty to a hundred diameters trained on nerve tissue from which he virtually unwrapped one minuscule nerve cell from the surrounding glia. He did it with an ultra-fine steel thread, a tenth the diameter of a human hair, which he gingerly wielded as a scapel. Once the cell was free, he measured its RNA by some complicated "micromicro" techniques developed by a colleague, Jan-Erik Edström. The unimaginable difficulty of this work is graphically reflected in the fact that one cell offered only 45 to 1,550 micromicrograms of RNA (a micromicrogram is one million-millionth of a gram). With these infinitesimally small quantities, the scientists learned a great deal about RNA as related to the nervous system.

The most striking result showed that in terms of RNA content nerve cells rank among the highest of all cells in the body. Hydén decided that the largest neurons of the nervous system were the body's "most highly specialized cells for producing RNA and protein."

Using Edström's "micromicro" capabilities, the Swedish

investigator and another colleague, E. Egyházi, designed experiments to learn if "the neurons may be linked with the capacity of the central nervous system to store information." In one well-known experiment, white rats, whose diet had been held to a minimum, were placed in a cage that had food on a small shelf affixed to the wall about thirty inches above the floor. To get at the food, a rat had to learn to walk a fine tightwire slanting upward from the floor to the shelf. It wasn't easy. The average rat took four days to master the stunt. Once it made the tightwire grade, an animal would carry a piece of food back down the wire so it could dine on the floor. While one group of animals was being trained on the tightwire, a control group from the same litter was kept in single cages with food, water, and room in which to roam. Finally, both the trained and untrained rats were killed, and nerve cells of their vestibular nuclei (a part of the brain that would be stimulated by learning to walk the wire) were analyzed. The results showed significant increases of RNA in tightwire rats compared to the control animals. Nerve cells from the trained rats had 751 micromicrograms of RNA per cell compared to 683 in the untrained rat. While these quantitative results suggested that learning was related to RNA, exactly how remained a mystery.

Hydén's interest in the RNA of nerve cells led him to many experimental situations, including tests on barracuda that he caught by trawling every morning during "a pleasant stay at a laboratory in the Caribbean." In a less exotic situation, the Swedish scientist analyzed nerve cells from the spinal cords of human victims of traffic accidents, and he learned that RNA increases from ages three to forty, remains at that level until age sixty, and then drops off rapidly.

Although Hydén's experiments did not prove that the memory trace is in the RNA molecule, he proposed a complicated three-step theory that supported this idea. The theory, later altered in light of new information, remained neither proven nor disproven, but it was the catalyst for a great deal of work by many scientists on the biochemistry of memory.

One unusual but often cited discovery about RNA and memory came from an incidental observation by Frank Morrell at the Stanford University School of Medicine, Palo Alto, California. He was studying a phenomenon found in epilepsy where a lesion on one brain hemisphere repeats itself in a "mirror focus" on the opposite side. Morrell found he could artificially produce a mirror focus in an animal. In one hemisphere he applied a certain chemical or a freezing technique that produced an epileptogenic lesion, complete with characteristically abnormal brain waves. Any time from a few days to three weeks a similar lesion would then appear at a comparable location on the opposite half of the brain, even though the area had not been exposed or damaged in any way. Development of the mirror focus could be prevented, Morrell learned, by severing the animal's corpus callosum. This observation led to the conclusion that information, even though pathological, passes from one hemisphere to the other. He also found that a mirror focus, once established, continues its electrical abnormality even when the original lesion on the opposite hemisphere has been surgically removed.

These findings made the Stanford scientist suspect that the mirror-focus cells continued their abnormal activity because of structural or biochemical alterations, not because of continuing electrical directions received across the corpus callosum from the original lesion. In effect, the cells were remembering to behave as they did. To check this assumption, Morrell devised and conducted a complicated experiment on such a focus, and it supported his contention that the mirror focus remained intact essentially because of memory.

During this work Morrell made the above-mentioned "incidental observation." A certain kind of stain applied to tissue of a mirror focus indicated it was high in RNA. Formal tests comparing focus tissue with nearby normal tissue definitely showed the former to have a higher concentration of RNA. Morrell's discovery was another piece of evidence that this nucleic acid might be the memory molecule.

Meanwhile other scientists decided the role of RNA in memory might be tested with drugs that inhibit or enhance the synthesis of the nucleic acid. The drug 8-azaguanine was one of two known to interfere with RNA synthesis. In 1961 it was used on rat brains by Wesley Dingman and Michael B. Sporn, then working at the University of Rochester, New York. Dingman and Sporn injected rats with 8-azaguanine radioactively labeled so the scientists could be sure it was incorporated into the brain RNA during a two-part experiment. First, the researchers found that the 8-azaguanine did not affect the learning of rats that had been trained to swim through a maze made in a water tank. However, for the second part of the experiment injections were made before training, and ability to learn the water maze was reduced. The results led Dingman and Sporn to postulate "that memory traces in the nervous system are produced by the formation of altered RNA molecules." In the 1960's magnesium pemoline, which enhances RNA synthesis, was used in several experiments on animals and even humans to see if it might improve memory, but the results were generally negative.

Still another type of attack was made on the puzzle of RNA and memory. If the quantity of RNA had something to do with memory, the experimenters decided they might improve memory by increasing RNA in the subjects' bodies. This was tried on aged patients at McGill University in Montreal by D. Ewen Cameron and several co-workers, who extracted RNA from yeast and administered it intravenously or orally. All of the early results from a battery of memory tests taken by the elderly subjects were called "favorable," and fifty percent were listed as "good." The best responses to the RNA came from people suffering from poor memories and confusion. Later experiments with better methods had poorer results, but they still indicated memory improvements in patients at different levels of senility. However, the McGill scientists were not certain whether the good results proved that RNA had uplifted the human memory mechanisms or that some extraneous factor had stimulated the process.

The same kind of mixed results came from comparable animal experiments with yeast RNA. Then the very idea of producing a better memory from RNA injections into the brain via the body received a serious setback when H. Eist and Ulysses S. Seal of the Veterans Administration Hospital, Minneapolis, found that radioactively labeled RNA could not pass from the body to the brain because it would be blocked by what is called the "blood-brain barrier."

All the research on RNA and memory was provocative but inconclusive. Certainly the nucleic acid remained as a candidate for the role, but it began to look as if RNA in the drama of memory really had a subordinate role or co-role, for protein was receiving attention in many laboratories. In fact, some researchers were turning back from RNA to the Katz-Halstead protein theory formulated around 1950 at the University of Chicago. Scientific journals began receiving papers about investigations of protein as the memory molecule.

The best-known protein experiments, conducted at the University of Pennsylvania by Josefa B. Flexner, Louis B. Flexner, and Eliot Stellar, employed the antibiotic puromycin, which interferes with protein synthesis. They worked with mice trained on a Y maze so they would walk out one arm to avoid an electric shock delivered to trespassers on the other arm. Twenty-four hours after training was over, the mice were injected with puromycin so that it entered directly into certain areas of the brain. Memory of the Y-maze experience disappeared completely. If the mice were injected anywhere from eleven to forty-three days after training, the "long-term memory" was also erased, but this time the puromycin had to be injected into more areas of the brain to do the job. In continuing work, puromycin was used in various other experiments that tried to shed light on the relationship between memory and protein. For example, the Flexner group found that they could make a rat's memory impregnable by "overtraining." Originally the experimenters considered a rat trained if he could travel the Y maze correctly nine out of ten times. By repeating the number of such successful trials some sixty times, they apparently drilled memory of the experience so thoroughly into the rat's mind that the antibiotic could not dislodge it.

Two Massachusetts scientists at the McLean Hospital in Belmont and at the Harvard Medical School also reported on puromycin experiments with rats. Samuel H. Barondes and Harry D. Cohen, using the Y maze for a learning experience, tested mice that had received brain injections five hours before training. The animals learned the Y maze and, according to tests, still retained the memory fifteen minutes later, but in the ensuing two and three quarter hours the learning faded progressively to a low level. A similar experiment with like results was conducted on goldfish by Bernard W. Agranoff and co-workers at the University of Michigan. "This indicated to us," Agranoff stated, "that puromycin didn't block the short-term memory demonstrated during learning, but did interfere with the consolidation of long-term memory."

In 1967 the two Flexners, writing in *Science* with Richard B. Roberts of the Carnegie Institution of Washington, explained the memory process involving RNA and protein as follows: "We assume that the initial learning experience triggers synthesis of one or more species of mRNA [a type of nucleic acid, messenger RNA]. This mRNA alters the synthetic rate of one or more proteins which are essential for the expression of memory. These proteins are thought to modify the characteristics of synapses concerned in a learning process so that the passage of impulses between nerve cells is facilitated."

At the University of Pennsylvania the Flexners and Stellar

also wrote what seemed like a summary befitting most of the research on the biochemical basis of memory: "The initial purpose of these investigations was to determine the molecular basis of the 'memory trace.' This goal still remains distant, although there are some indications that protein synthesizing systems are involved. This objective, though of enormous interest, is to be regarded only as a necessary first step. Whether new proteins or some other molecules cause the changes in synapses thought to underlie memory, this knowledge of itself will contribute only a beginning to our understanding of the events which account for the functioning of the brain."

As one might imagine, controversy marked this search for the engram on the molecular level. The extremely difficult methods, the elusive evidence, and the great chance for subjective judgments provided fuel for heated discussion and criticism. However, the controversy that swirled around the work that we have just reviewed was a summer breeze compared to the gales whipping another line of research in progress at the same time. The investigative route was very different, but it sought the same goal just discussed—the molecular basis of memory.

The work is said to have begun at the University of Texas in 1953 when two graduate students in psychology, James V. McConnell and Robert Thompson, started looking for a very simple organism with synapses in which to study the changes that learning might bring to the nervous system. Thompson, who became a professor of psychology at Louisiana State University, suggested that the common flatworm, the lowest animal on the phyletic tree, might be a good subject, if it could be trained. Planaria like this had reportedly been trained in simple ways for experiments in Europe and the United States during the 1920's and 30's.

McConnell and Thompson devised a test in which a planarian would go down a plastic trough of water arranged with electrodes so an electric shock could be delivered to the

THE SEARCH FOR THE ENGRAM

animal whenever the experimenter wished. The shock caused a flatworm's body to contract vigorously. The students also suspended lights above the trough for a conditioning stimulus. The training occurred by turning on the lights for two seconds and then transmitting the shock in a third second. With enough trials, a worm would respond to the lights alone, just as if he were being jolted by the missing shock. When the trained animals' behavior was statistically compared to that of untrained animals, McConnell and Thompson decided that it was evidence of "clear-cut classical conditioning in planarians." Their work was published in 1955 in the *Journal of Comparative Physiological Psychology*. McConnell then went to the University of Michigan, where he set up a laboratory to experiment with flatworms.

He once wrote: "To most people, I suppose, the flatworm (planarian) is famous not because it is the lowest animal with a rudimentary brain and a true synaptic type nervous system, but rather because it possesses enormous powers of regeneration. . . . If one cuts this animal in half transversely, the animal does not die; rather the head grows a new tail and the tail grows a new head, and each regenerated piece will eventually become as large as the original organism. Indeed, under the best of conditions, one may cut the animal into as many as 50 pieces and each section will regenerate into an intact, fully functioning organism."

When McConnell and Thompson were in Texas, the latter had suggested an experiment with trained planarians. Cut them in half, he had said, and then test the two regenerated halves of each to see where the memory goes. Thompson and McConnell never got around to the experiment, but in Michigan McConnell and two students attempted it. They improved the original Texas training program so that flatworms responded to the light without shock ninety-two percent of the time. The lab workers then cut each trained worm in half and waited a month for the two pieces to regenerate. The plan of the experiment called for retraining each half up to the ninety-two percent level to see if it took more or less time than the original learning period. The researchers were mildly surprised to find that the head end of each severed worm had retained the ninety-two-percent level of training.

"But what of the tails?" McConnell asked. "They had to regrow an entire new brain and replace most of their vital organs during the month's regeneration. How could one expect a regenerated tail to remember anything at all? The answer is, of course, that one could *not* expect the tails to remember at all—but they did. In fact, many of the tails showed almost perfect retention of the original training. . . . Furthermore, we soon found that if we cut the trained worm in thirds, or even fourths, each regenerated piece would show a significant retention of the memory.

These results were reported in 1959 in the same journal that carried the McConnell-Thompson paper on training planarians. This time, however, critical response was quite different. McConnell, with a scientist's understatement, said the results "were at first considered somewhat unbelievable." The disbelief continued, although McConnell argued that the doubts were dissipated when the experiments were repeated successfully in other laboratories around the world. But valid or not, the experiments still left the simple, obvious question: How could the tail remember?

About this time McConnell became aware of Hydén's idea that RNA might be central to memory, and the Michigan scientist wondered if the nucleic acid might not hold the answer to why the engram seemed to spread through the entire body of the flatworm.

Hardly before he could begin to test the idea, a University of Rochester professor, E. Roy John, and a student of his, William Corning, provided an answer. They used the McConnell-Thompson flatworm training technique. The subjects were then cut in half and allowed to regenerate, but this time the tails were made to regrow in a weak solution of ribonuclease, an enzyme that breaks down RNA. Now when worms were fully regenerated from the tail, they did not remember the original training. This experiment was intended to show that the destroyed RNA was responsible for the missing memory.

At Michigan, McConnell and his students subjected the RNA hypothesis to still another experiment, and again they came up with startling results that some authorities had difficulty believing. They obtained a species of Planaria, *Dugesia dorotocephala,* that cannibalizes when hungry. One group, labeled "victims," was trained in the usual way. Another group of victims was left untrained. Then both groups were fed to untrained cannibals that had been properly starved for the feast. The cannibals ate, and turned out to be trained, at least to a significant degree.

"The results were clear cut," McConnell reported; "the cannibals that had ingested 'trained' victims were, on the very first day of training, significantly superior to the cannibals that had eaten untrained animals."

The work was duplicated in McConnell's laboratory, and during the next few years, the cannibalistic transfer experiments were successfully carried out in ten other university laboratories. McConnell, whose lighter side occasionally transfers to his published papers, said the studies confirmed "our 'Mau Mau' hypothesis," and he warned that "one obviously should not generalize these results to the human level too readily."

With these provocative findings, planarian research spread all over the world. In 1967 a paper presented to a symposium of the American Association for the Advancement of Science reviewed eighty-two different Planaria studies on learning. Sixty-two had reported positive results. The work even gave birth to its own journal, the *Worm Runner's Digest,* described on the masthead as "an Informal International Journal of Comparative Psychology, Published Irregularly by the Planarian Research Group at the University of Michigan."

With McConnell in the editor's chair, the *Digest* was probably history's most informal scientific journal. For example, Volume VIII, Number 1, April 1966, was half filled with serious papers and half with humorous articles, stories, poems, cartoons, skits, and other entertaining features printed upside down from the serious half. The editor's page stated that the masthead reference "published irregularly" meant "damned irregular," and readers were begged to stop asking when the next issue would appear.

Some of the satire in the unusual journal indicated that Planaria experiments were not wholeheartedly accepted by everyone. In fact, deadly serious publications, like the *Journal of Comparative Physiological Psychology,* were carrying works of persistent critics whose arrows flew mainly at the methodology used by the Planaria researchers. For example, the critics did not easily accept the idea that flatworms could be really trained with the basic procedures designed in Texas by McConnell and Thompson and used extensively in subsequent experiments. How can one claim that learning has been transferred from one animal to another, asked the critics, if the learning really can't be proven in the donor animal? They also questioned the validity of the investigators' observations. How could anyone really tell if learning had occurred by training or transfer in such small creatures? The detractors wondered if perhaps the researchers might not be influenced by what they expected to see, as opposed to what was really happening with a planarian.

Despite their scalding in the classic caldron of criticism, the experiments pointed up a valuable tool for approaching the chemical basis of learning. If scientists could literally move a substance from one brain to another and simultaneously transfer memory, they could surely say the memory molecule had been captured. Then it would be a matter of analyzing the substance until the real basis of memory was finally understood. The planarian research offered encouragement and stimulated similar work in higher animals.

In most of these studies, the higher animal was the rat. The first work was done in 1964 by D. J. Albert at McGill University, using a procedure that permitted him to train only one hemisphere of a rat's brain. He then turned around and, in effect, cut out part of the memory by surgically removing tissue from the trained cortex. Finally, he injected a mixture of the excised tissue back into the animal's brain, and now his tests indicated that part of the excised learning had been restored to the rat.

Albert waited until 1966 to publish this work; meanwhile, papers from Czechoslovakia and Denmark told of scientists transferring learning from trained to untrained rats. The Czech research depended upon the transfer of brain homogenates from trained to naïve animals. The Danish workers extracted RNA from the brains of trained rats for injection into untrained animals. But in this same period of time, the first such memory-transfer experiments in the United States became the most famous of all because of the controversy they fired up.

They were conducted at the University of California, Los Angeles, by Allan L. Jacobson and his laboratory associates. The group claimed that not only could they transfer memory, but they could even transfer the ingredients necessary for specific skills. In one experiment, for example, a group of rats was trained to press a foot lever for food when a light flashed. Another group learned to do the same when some clicking sounds were heard. Neither group, however, would react to the other's stimulus. The experimenters then injected RNA extracted from the trained rats into the brains of untrained rats. The extract from the click-oriented donors made click- (but not light-) oriented donees—and the extract from light-trained rats made their recipients respond just to flashes, not to clicks.

These results were important news in the neurosciences, but soon papers began to arrive at journals reporting on comparable RNA-transfer experiments that didn't work. The most notable paper was published in *Science*, August 5,

1966, and it had twenty-three authors, from Berkeley, Yale, McGill, MIT, the Albert Einstein College of Medicine, the Squibb Institute for Medical Research, and Rutgers. Citing two reports of the Jacobson group, one in *Science,* one in the *Worm Runner's Digest,* the scientific squad led by William L. Byrne stated:

"We summarize here our separate attempts to reproduce the results reported. Each of the sets of experiments was independently undertaken in one of our laboratories; the unanimity of our results became apparent only in the course of subsequent informal discussions. We all found that the reported transfer of training due to RNA was not, in our laboratories at least, a demonstrable phenomenon.

"In 18 experiments no clear evidence of a transfer of any of these kinds of training from trained donors to recipients was found. The detailed reports from all our laboratories have been compiled and are available for examination."

At the end of their short paper, the twenty-three tempered their criticism, saying: ". . . we feel that it would be unfortunate if these negative findings were to be taken as a signal for abandoning the pursuit of a result of enormous potential significance. This is especially so in light of several other related but not identical experiments that support the possibility of transfer of learning by injection of brain extracts from trained donors. Failure to reproduce results is not, after all, unusual in the early phase of research when all relevant variables are as yet unspecified."

In *Science* two months later, Byrne and David Samuel, who had been second of the many signers, reported on a successful transfer experiment of their own using brain extract from rats trained to pass bars for rewards.

And that's the way the transfer work proceeded for the remainder of the 1960's—a controversial field troubled by now-we-can-now-we-can't reports. They were once treated satirically in a *Worm Runner's Digest* feature on Dr. W. Labcoat's study showing that rats fed Liederkranz cheese learn a maze faster than rats fed on bacon rind—all of which failed when Professor R. Centrifuge tried the same experiments. Perhaps one or both gentlemen faked their data, mused the *Digest* piece, or one had become a better rat trainer than the other, or: "It could be that the 'cheese' effect works with rats only when they are trained in the dark of the moon; thus, although Prof. Centrifuge replicated the methodology of Dr. Labcoat's experiment exactly, he simply ran his animals at the wrong time of the month."

As the 1970's began, two authors from Yale, Jack R. Cooper and Robert H. Roth, and one from the National Institute of Mental Health, Floyd E. Bloom, wrote: "At the present time one can only state that protein and RNA synthesis may occur along with learning, but the experiment has yet to be designed that explicitly relates these two events. The somewhat chaotic condition of this field is due not only to an inordinate amount of dross that has been presented, but to monistic interpretations of data. Caveat emptor."

Finding the engram, whether in RNA, protein, or another substance, has been anticipated with tremendous excitement, but will the discovery really delineate memory? No, for there will still be much more to learn about the fantastic circuitry, the systems of the brain and how they function in using the memory trace. As the 1970's began, neurophysiologists continued unraveling the complex systems of brain and nerve, and new theories were being added to the many, many ideas on how the brain works.

One of the most important theories came from Karl H. Pribram of Stanford University. In the 1960's he spent countless hours seeking an explanation for something that Lashley had recognized three decades earlier when he found that a rat could remember and perform complex tasks even after major nerve pathways had been severed in the brain and ninety percent of the primary visual cortex had been cut out. Pribram, working with monkeys, used electrical recording equipment to follow changes in their brains caused by training in specific activities. He gathered data from more than 950 monkeys. One of the time-consuming experiments took seven years. Pribram's work forced revisions of earlier concepts of how the brain works when something is learned and remembered. From his studies came a hypothesis that held up well under his tests and satisfied much already known about the brain. It depended on analogy, and, as true far back into the past, the scientist turned to one of the most complicated models available. Pribram, an amateur photographer, decided ". . . the brain may exploit, among other things, the most sophisticated principle of information storage yet known: the principle of the hologram." A hologram is a photograph in which the scene is recorded on a plate in complex patterns that are meaningless in normal light: however, if the plate is illuminated with a laser beam, the image is reconstructed for the viewer. More than that, the viewer can see the entire scene even by looking at a small part of the hologram. Should a corner break off the plate, the viewer would still see the entire scene in the broken piece—just as the brain grasps a fragment and reconstructs the entire image, often instantaneously.

The search for the engram is likely to continue, unsettled, for a long time, but the value of the quest is as clear as it can be for any scientific venture. If man locates and explores the domain of memory, he may solve some of the most difficult, trying problems of all time. Consider the meaning in only two areas of human concern: education and nutrition.

Ages of educators have tried endless theories of learning yet have been unable to explain the physical changes that teaching methods bring to the organ being educated: the brain. In the Croonian Lecture of 1965, J. Z. Young put it this way: ". . . it is certainly a defect that almost all of our knowledge of the process of learning is empirical, consisting at best of rules for memorizing, based on no theory of the physical nature of memory. So long as we remain ignorant of this all our educational theory must remain in this sense primitive." But as memory research continues it becomes conceivable that the educator's capabilities for producing effective learning may be tested and improved, not by time-worn scholastic examinations, but by physical measurements of students' brains. A preview may be seen in the work of Helmer R. Myklebust of Northwestern University, who had indications in the 1960's that new tests of effective learning may be found through computer analysis of the EEG.

What does food have to do with learning? Plenty! appears to be the answer from numerous studies on humans and animals. The work has strongly suggested in recent years that malnutrition during the formative stages of the brain, prenatal and postnatal, may diminish the organ's ability to learn. At Wayne State University, for example, John Churchill found in a study of identical twins that the one born heavier (indicating better nourishment in the womb) grew up with a higher I.Q. In animal studies conducted at Johns Hopkins University, Bacon Chow fed pregnant rats protein-rich diets, and then, during a second pregnancy with the same fathers and mothers, he deprived the females of protein and some calories. The offspring from the second pregnancy were poorer at learning mazes and lever-pressing exercises than the siblings from the first pregnancy. A 1971 paper by two MIT scientists, Richard J. Wurtman and William J. Shoemaker, reported on studies of very young rats showing that chemical transmitters in the brain, noradrenaline and dopamine, were reduced by low-protein diet in the animal's formative days. The results made it appear that the brain's learning capacity may be reduced by malnutrition. These and other animal investigations support what a number of human studies have suggested: that learning can be impaired by malnutrition in life's earliest days and months.

The study of memory as the primary function of the nervous system leads to the center of human existence, where all souls are tossed and turned by memories retained as individuals and modulated by powerful ancestral memories inherent in humanity. When these engrams are found, analyzed, and understood, the explorers of nerve and brain may have finally complied with Cervantes' admonishment: "Make it thy business to know thyself, which is the most difficult lesson in the world."

Bigelow, Henry J. (1850), "Dr. Harlow's Case of Recovery from the Passage of an Iron Bar Through the Head," *Amer. J. Med. Sci.,* 39: 2.

Bishop, G. H. (1958), "The Dendrite: Receptive Pole of the Neurone," *EEG Clin. Neurophysiol.,* Suppl. 10: 12.

Blinkov, Samuel M., and Glezer, Ilija I. (1968), *The Human Brain in Figures and Tables,* New York: Basic Books.

Bodian, David (1952), "Introductory Survey of Neurons," *Cold Spring Harbor Symp.,* 7: 1.

Brazier, Mary A. B. (1957), "The Evolution of Concepts Relating to the Electrical Activity of the Nervous System 1600 to 1800," from the Anglo-American Symposium (1958), *The History and Philosophy of Knowledge of the Brain and Its Functions,* Oxford: Blackwell.

Brazier, Mary A. B. (1961), *A History of the Electrical Activity of the Brain,* New York: Macmillan.

Brazier, Mary A. B. (1962), "The Analysis of Brain Waves," *Sci. Amer.,* 206: 142.

Brazier, Mary A. B. (1964), "The Flectrical Activity of the Nervous System," *Sci. Amer., 146:* 1423.

Brazier, Mary A. B. (1968), *The Electrical Activity of the Nervous System,* 3rd ed., Baltimore: Williams and Wilkins.

Bremer, F. (1958), "Cerebral and Cerebellar Potentials," *Physiol. Rev., 38:* 357.

Brody, Jane E., "Surgery Revises Idea About Brain," *The New York Times,* July 23, 1966, p. 27.

Bülbring, Edith, and Burn, J. H. (1941), "Observations Bearing on Synaptic Transmission By Acetylcholine in the Spinal Cord," *J. Physiol., 100:* 337.

Burns, B. Delisle (1951), "Some Properties of Isolated Cerebral Cortex in the Unanesthetized Cat," *J. Physiol, 112:* 156.

Busse, Ewald W., and Obrist, Walter D. (1963), "Significance of Focal Electroencephalographic Changes in the Elderly," *Postgrad. Med., 34:* 179.

Byrne, William L., and 22 others (1966), "Memory Transfer," *Science, 153:* 658.

Byrne, William L., and Samuel, David (1966), "Behavioral Modification by Injection of Brain Extract Prepared from a Trained Donor" (Abstract), *Science, 154:* 418.

Cannon, Dorothy F. (1949), *Explorer of the Human Brain,* New York: Schuman.

Cannon, W. B. and Bacq, Z. M. (1931), "A Hormone Produced by

Sympathetic Action on Smooth Muscle," *Amer. J. Physiol., 96:* 392.

Chaffee, E. Leon, and Light, Richard U. (1934), "A Method for the Remote Control of Electrical Stimulation of the Nervous System," *Yale J. Biol. Med., 7:* 83.

Chamberlain, T. J.; Rothschild, G. H.; and Gerard, R. W. (1963), "Drugs Affecting RNA and Learning," *Proc. N.A.S., 49:* 918.

Clark, Sam L., and Ward, James W. (1937), "Electrical Stimulation of the Cortex Ceribri of Cats," *Arch. Neurol. Psychiat., 38:* 927.

Cole, Kenneth S. (1968), *Membranes, Ions and Impulses,* Berkeley: U. of Cal. Press.

Cole, Kenneth, "Of All the Nerve," unpublished, undated manuscript provided by author.

Corrodi, Hans, and Jonsson, Gösta (1965), "Fluorescence Methods for the Histochemical Demonstration of Monoamines: 4. Histochemical Differentiation Between Dopamine and Noradrenaline in Models," *J. Histochem. Cytochem., 13:* 484.

Crandall, Paul H.; Walter, Richard D.; and Rand, Robert W. (1963), "Clinical Applications of Studies on Stereotactically Implanted Electrodes in Temporal Lobe Epilepsy," *J. Neurosurgery, 20:* 827.

Crick, F. H. C. (1954), "The Structure of the Hereditary Material," *Sci. Amer., 191:* 54.

Crick, F. H. C. (1957), "Nucleic Acids," *Sci. Amer., 197:* 188.

Crick, F. H. C. (1962), "The Genetic Code," *Sci. Amer., 207:* 67.

Crick, F. H. C. (1966), "The Genetic Code III," *Sci. Amer., 215:* 55.

Cushing, Harvey (1909), "A Note Upon the Faradic Stimulation of the Postcentral Gyrus in Conscious Patients," *Brain, 32:* 44.

Dale, Sir Henry (1937), "Acetylcholine as a Chemical Transmitter of the Effects of Nerve Impulses," *J. Mount Sinai Hosp., 4:* 401.

Dale, Henry H., "Some Recent Extensions of the Chemical Transmission of the Effects of Nerve Impulses," Nobel Lecture, Dec. 12, 1936.

Dale, Sir Henry (1937), "Transmission of Nervous Effects by Acetylcholine," *The Harvey Lectures* 1936–7, Baltimore, p. 229.

Dale, H. H., and Dudley, H. W. (1929), "The Presence of Histamine and Acetylcholine in the Spleen of the Ox and Horse," *J. Physiol., 68:* 97.

Dale, H. H.; Feldberg, W.; and Vogt, M. (1936), "Release of Acetylcholine at Voluntary Motor Nerve Endings," *J. Physiol., 86:* 353.

Dawson, G. D. (1951), "A Summation Technique for Detecting Small Signals in a Large Irregular Background," *J. Physiol., 115:* 2P.

Delgado, José M. R. (1964), "Personality, Education, and Electrical Stimulation of the Brain," from *Innovation and Experiment in Modern Education,* Report of 29th Ed. Conf., pub. by Amer. Council on Ed.

Delgado, José M. R. (1965), "Evolution of Physical Control of the Brain," James Arthur Lecture, New York, Amer. Mus. of Nat. Hist.

Dement, W., and Kleitman, N. (1957), "The Relation of Eye Movements During Sleep to Dream Activity: An Objective Method for the Study of Dreaming," *J. Exptl. Psychol., 53:* 339.

Denny-Brown, D., ed. (1940), *Selected Writings of Sir Charles Sherrington,* New York: Harper.

De Robertis, Eduardo D. P., and Bennett, H. Stanley (1954), "Some Features of the Submicroscopic Morphology of Synapses in Frog and Earthworm," *J. Biophy. Biochem. Cytol., 1:* 47.

De Robertis, Eduardo D. P., and Bennett, H. Stanley (1954), "Submicroscopic Vesicular Components in the Synapse," *Fed. Proc., 13:* 35.

De Robertis, E.; De Iraldi, A. Pellegrino; Rodriguez, Georgina; and Gomez, C. J. (1961), "On the Isolation of Nerve Endings and Synaptic Vesicles," *J. Biophy. Biochem. Cytol., 9:* 229.

Dingman, Wesley, and Sporn, Michael B. (1961), "The Incorporation of 8-Azaguanine Into Rat Brain RNA and Its Effect on Maze-Learning By the Rat: An Inquiry Into the Biochemical Basis of Memory," *J. Psychiat. Res., 1:* 1.

Dingman, Wesley, and Sporn, Michael B., (1964), "Molecular Theories of Memory," *Science, 144:* 26.

Duncan, Carl P. (1948), "Habit Reversal Induced by Electroshock in the Rat," *J. Comp. Physiol. Psychol., 41:* 11.

Eccles, John C. (1957), *The Physiology of Nerve Cells,* Baltimore: Johns Hopkins Press.

Eccles, John C. (1958), "The Physiology of Imagination," *Sci. Amer., 199:* 135.

Eccles, J. C. (1964), "Ionic Mechanisms of Postsynaptic Inhibition," *Science, 145:* 1140.

Eccles, Sir John (1965), "The Synapse," *Sci. Amer., 212:* 56.

Eccles, Sir John (1965), *The Brain and the Unity of Conscious Experience,* Cambridge at the U. Press.

Erlanger, Joseph, "Some Observations on the Responses of Single Nerve Fibers," Nobel Lecture, Dec. 12, 1947.

Evans, C. R., and Robertson, A. D. J. (1966), *Key Papers: Brain Physiology and Psychology*, Berkeley: U. of Calif. Press.

Fernandez-Moran, H. (1954), "The Submicroscopic Structure of Nerve Fibres," *Prog. Biophysics Biophys. Chem., 4:* 112.

Field, John, ed. (1959), *Neurophysiology, Handbook of Physiology*, Vol. I, Sec. 1, Washington, D.C.: American Physiol. Soc.

Field, John, ed. (1960), *Neurophysiology, Handbook of Physiology*, Vol. II, Sec. 1, Washington, D.C.: American Physiol. Soc.

Fisher, Alan E. (1964), "Chemical Stimulation of the Brain," *Sci. Amer., 210:* 60.

Flexner, Louis B.; Flexner, Josefa B.; and Roberts, Richard B. (1967), "Memory in Mice Analyzed with Antibiotics," *Science, 155:* 1377.

Foerster, O. (1936), "The Motor Cortex in Man in the Light of Hughlings Jackson's Doctrines," Brain, 59: 135.

Forbes, Alexander (1953), "Presidential Address, Third Int. Congress of EEG and Clin. Neurophysiol.," *EEG Clin. Neurophysiol.,* Suppl. 4: 3.

Forbes, Alexander, and Thatcher, Catherine (1920): "Amplification of Action Current with Electron Tube," *Amer. J. Physiol.,* 52: 409.

French, J. D. (1957), "The Reticular Formation," *Sci. Amer.,* 196: 54.

French, John D., ed. (1962), *Frontiers in Brain Research*, New York: Columbia U. Press.

Frommer, Gabriel P., and Livingston, Robert B. (1963), "Arousal Effects on Evoked Activity in a 'Nonsensory' System," *Science, 139:* 502.

Fuhrman, Frederick A. (1967), "Tetrodotoxin," *Sci. Amer.,* 217: 60.

Fulton, John F., and Cushing, Harvey (1936), "A Bibliographical Study of the Galvani and the Aldini Writings on Animal Electricity," *Annals Sci., 1:* 239.

Fulton, John F., and Wilson, Leonard G. (1966), *Selected Readings in the History of Physiology*, 2nd ed., Springfield, Ill.: C. C. Thomas.

Furshpan, E. J., and Potter, D. D. (1959), "Transmission at the Giant Motor Synapses of the Crayfish," *J. Physiol., 145:* 289.

Gasser, Herbert S. (1937), "The Control of Excitation in the Nervous System," *The Harvey Lectures*, Mar. 18, 1937, Baltimore.

Gasser, Herbert S., "Mammalian Nerve Fibers," Nobel Lecture, Dec. 12, 1945.

Gasser, H. S., and Newcomer, H. S. (1921), "Physiological Action

Currents in the Phrenic Nerve: An Application of the Thermionic Vacuum Tube to Nerve Physiology," *Amer. J. Physiol.*, 57: 1.

Gasser, H. S., and Erlanger, Joseph (1922), "A Study of the Action Currents of Nerve with the Cathode Ray Oscillograph," *Amer. J. Physiol.*, 62: 496.

Gazzaniga, Michael S. (1967), "The Split Brain in Man," *Sci. Amer.*, 217: 24.

Gazzaniga, M. S.; Boyen, J. E.; and Sperry, R. W. (1965), "Observations on Visual Perception After Disconnexion of the Cerebral Hemispheres in Man," *Brain*, 88: Part II, 221.

Gengerelli, J. A., and Cullen, John W. (1955), "Studies in the Neurophysiology of Learning: II. Effect of Brain Stimulation During Black and White Discrimination of Learning Behavior in the White Rat," *J. Comp. Physiol. Psychol.*, 48: 311.

Gerard, Ralph W. (1953), "What is Memory?", *Sci. Amer.*, 189: 702.

Geschwind, Norman (1970), "The Organization of Language and the Brain," *Science*, 170: 940.

Geschwind, Norman, and Levitsky, Walter (1968), "Human Brain: Left-Right Asymmetries in Temporal Speech Region," *Science*, 161: 186.

"Giant Brain Model Shows How a Thought Is Born," News Release for the Upjohn Company by Farley Manning Associates, New York, June 15, 1964.

Gibbs, E. L., and Gibbs, F. A. (1936), "A Purring Center in the Cat's Brain," *J. Comp. Neurol.*, 64: 209.

Gibbs, F. A.; Davis, H.; Lennox, W. G. (1935), "The Electro-Encephalogram in Epilepsy and in Conditions of Impaired Consciousness," *Arch. Neurol. Psychol.*, 34: 1133.

Glaser, Gilbert H. (1963), *EEG and Behavior*, New York: Basic Books.

Gloor, Pierre (1969), "Hans Berger on the Electroencephalogram of Man," *EEG Clin. Neurophysiol.*, Suppl. 28.

Goff, William R. (1968), "Electrical Signals of the Brain in Sensory Perception," *Yale Scientific Magazine*, 47: 16.

Grass, A. M., and Gibbs, F. A. (1938), "A Fourier Transform of the Electroencephalogram," *J. Neurophysiol.*, 1: 521.

Gray, E. G. (1959), "Axo-Somatic and Axo-Dendritic Synapses of the Cerebral Cortex: An Electron Microscope Study," *J. Anat.*, 93: 420.

Gray, E. G., and Whittaker, V. P. (1959), "The Isolation of Nerve Endings from Brain: An Electron Microscope Study of Cell Fragments Derived by Homogenization and Centrifugation," *J. Anat.*, 96: 79.

Grundfest, Harry (1958), "Electrophysiology and Pharmacology of Dendrites," *EEG Clin. Neurophysiol.*, Suppl. 10: 22.

Grundfest, Harry (1960), "Electric Fishes," *Sci. Amer.*, 203: 115.

Gurowitz, Edward M. (1969), *The Molecular Basis of Memory*, Englewood Cliffs, N.J.: Prentice-Hall.

Hamberger, Carl-Axel, and Hydén, Holger (1945), "Cytochemical Changes in the Cochlear Ganglion Caused by Acoustic Stimulation and Trauma," *ACTA Oto-Laryngologia*, Supp. 61.

Harlow, J. M. (1848), "Passage of an Iron Rod through the Head," *Boston Med. Surg. J.*, 39: 20.

Henry, C. E. (1944), "E.E.G. of Normal Children," *Mon. Soc. Res. Child Dev.*, Natl. Res. Coun.

Hess, W. (1932), "The Autonomic Nervous System," *Lancet*, 222: 1199.

Hess, Walter R. (1967), "Causality, Consciousness and Cerebral Organization," *Science*, 158: 1279.

Hess, Walter Rudolf, "The Central Control of the Activity of Internal Organs," Nobel Lecture, Dec. 12, 1949.

Hill, Denis (1963), *Electroencephalography*, London: Macdonald.

Hillarp, N. A.; Fuxe, Kjell; and Dahlström, Annica (1966), "Demonstration and Mapping of Central Neurons Containing Dopamine, Noradrenaline, and 5-Hydroxytryptamine and Their Reactions to Psychopharmaca," *Pharmacol. Rev.*, 18: 727.

Hoagland, Hudson (1940), "A Simple Method for Recording Electrocortigrams in Animals Without Opening the Skull," *Science*, 92: 537.

Hodgkin, A. L. (1964), "The Ionic Basis of Nervous Conduction," *Science*, 145: 1148.

Hodgkin, A. L. (1964), *The Conduction of the Nervous Impulse*, Springfield, Ill.: C. C. Thomas.

Hoffer, A. (1965), "D-Lysergic Acid Diethylamide (LSD): A Review of Its Present Status," *Clin. Pharmacol. Ther.*, 6: 183.

Hoffer, A., and Osmond, H. (1967), *The Hallucinogens*, New York: Academic Press.

Holmes, Gordon (1954), *The National Hospital Queen Square*, Edinburgh: E. & S. Livingstone.

Holst, Erich von, and Saint Paul, Ursula von (1962), "Electrically Controlled Behavior," *Sci. Amer.*, 206: 50.

Huxley, A. F. (1964), "Excitation and Conduction in Nerve Quantitative Analysis," *Science*, 145: 1154.

Huxley, A. F. (1954), "Electrical Processes in Nerve Conduction," in

Clarke, H. T., ed., *Ion Transport Across Membranes*, New York: Academic Press.

Hydén, Holger (1943), "Protein Metabolism in the Nerve Cell During Growth and Function," *ACTA Physiol. Scand.*, Suppl. XVII.

Hydén, Holger (1961), "Satellite Cells in the Nervous System," *Sci. Amer.*, *205*: 62.

Hydén, Holger, "The Neuron," from Brachet, Jean, and Mirsky, Alfred E., eds. (1960), *The Cell*, Vol. 4, New York: Academic Press.

Hydén, H., and Egyházi, E. (1962), "Nuclear RNA Changes of Nerve Cells During a Learning Experiment in Rats," *Proc. N.A.S.*, *48*: 1366.

Hydén, H., and Egyházi, E. (1963), "Glial RNA Changes During a Learning Experiment in Rats," *Proc. N.A.S.*, *49*: 618.

Hydén, H., and Egyházi, E. (1964), "Changes in RNA Content and Base Composition in Cortical Neurons of Rats in a Learning Experiment Involving Transfer of Handedness," *Proc. N.A.S.*, *52*: 1030.

Illinois Institute of Technology Research Institute (1968), *Technology in Retrospect and Critical Events in Science*, Vol. 1, prepared for Natl. Sci. Foun.

Jasper, Herbert H. (1936), "Localized Analysis of the Function of the Human Brain by the Electro-Encephalogram," *Arch. Neurol. Psychiat.*, *36*: 1131.

Jasper, Herbert H. (1948), "Charting the Sea of Brain Waves," *Science*, *108*: 343.

Jasper, Herbert (1949), "Electrocorticograms in Man," *EEG Clin. Neurophysiol.*, Suppl. 2: 18.

Katz, Bernard (1966), *Nerve, Muscle, and Synapse*, New York: McGraw-Hill.

Katz, Joseph J., and Halstead, Ward C. (1950), "Protein Organization and Mental Function," in "Brain and Behavior" (Symposium), *Comp. Psychol. Mono.*, *20*: 1.

Kennedy, Donald (1963), "Inhibition in Visual Systems," *Sci. Amer.*, *209*: 122.

Kennedy, Donald (1967), "Small Systems of Nerve Cells," *Sci. Amer.*, *216*: 44.

Kennedy, John L. (1959), "A Possible Artifact in Electroencephalography," *Psychol. Rev.*, *66*: 347.

Kimble, Daniel P., ed. (1965), *The Anatomy of Memory*, Vol. 1, Palo Alto, Calif.: Science and Behavior Books.

Kimura, Jun; Gerber, Henry W.; and McCormick, William F. (1968), "The Isoelectric Electroencephalogram," *Arch. Intern. Med., 121:* 511.

Klee, M. R. et al. (1965), "Cross-correlation Analysis of Electroencephalographic Potentials and Slow Membrane Transients," *Science, 147:* 519.

Knott, John R. (1953), "Automatic Frequency Analysis," *EEG Clin. Neurophysiol.,* Suppl. 4: 17.

Koshtoyanti, Kh. S. (1946), *Essays on the History of Physiology in Russia,* Moscow-Leningrad: Pub. House Acad. Sci. USSR.

Krech, D.; Rosenzweig, M. R.; and Bennett, E. L. (1963), "Effects of Complex Environment and Blindness on Rat Brain," *Arch. Neurol., 8:* 403.

Krech, David; Rosenzweig, Mark R.; and Bennett, Edward L. (1966), "Environmental Impoverishment, Social Isolation and Changes in Brain Chemistry and Anatomy," *Psychol. Behav., 1:* 99.

Kristiansen, Kristian, and Courtois, Guy (1949), "Rhythmic Electrical Activity from Isolated Cerebral Cortex," *EEG Clin. Neurophysiol., 1:* 265.

Lashley, K. S. (1929), *Brain Mechanisms and Intelligence,* Chicago: U. of Chicago Press.

Lashley, K. S. (1950), "In Search of the Engram," in *Physiological Mechanisms in Animal Behavior,* New York: Academic Press.

Lemke, Rudolf (1956), "Personal Reminiscences of Hans Berger," *EEG Clin. Neurophysiol., 8:* 708.

Lettvin, J. Y.; Maturna, H. R.; McCulloch, W. S.; and Pitts, W. H. (1959), "What the Frog's Eye Tells the Frog's Brain," *Proc. Inst. Radio Eng., 47:* 1940.

Li, C.; McLennan, H.; and Jasper, H. (1952), "Brain Waves and Unit Discharge in Cerebral Cortex," *Science, 116:* 656.

Liddell, E. G. T. (1960), *The Discovery of Reflexes,* Oxford: Clarendon Press.

Lillie, Ralph S. (1918), "Transmission of Activation in Passive Metals as a Model of the Protoplasmic or Nervous Type of Transmission," *Science, 58:* 51.

Lillie, Ralph S. (1924), "Factors Affecting Transmission and Recovery in the Passive Iron Nerve Model," *J. Gen. Physiol., 7:* 473.

Lindsley, D. B. (1964), "Brain Development and Behavior: Historical Introduction," *Prog. Brain Res., 9:* 1.

Livingston, Robert (1966), "How Man Looks at His Brain," *Oregon Holiday Sci. Lect. Series,* Ore. State U.

Loewi, Otto (1934), "The Humoral Transmission of Nervous Impulse," *The Harvey Lectures*, 1933, Baltimore.

Loewi, Otto, "The Chemical Transmission of Nerve Action," Nobel Lecture, Dec. 12, 1936.

Lucas, Keith (1912), "The Process of Excitation in Nerve and Muscle," Croonian Lecture, *Proc. Roy. Soc., B 85.*

Luce, Gay Gaer (1965), *Current Research on Sleep and Dreams*, P.H.S. Ser. Pub. 1389, U.S. Govt. Print. Off.

Magoun, H. W. (1965), "Neuroscience and Learning," *UCLA Med.*, Aug. 1965, p. 9.

Magoun, H. W. (1963), *The Waking Brain*, Springfield, Ill.: C. C. Thomas.

Magoun, H. W.; Harrison, F.; Brobeck, J. R.; and Ransom, S. W. (1938), "Activation of Heat Loss Mechanisms by Local Heating of the Brain," *J. Neurophysiol., 1:* 101.

Maron, Louise; Rechtschaffen, Allan; and Wolpert, Edward A. (1964), "Sleep Cycle During Napping," *Arch. Gen. Psychiat., 11:* 503.

Marshall, Wade H.; Woolsey, Clinton N.; and Bard, Philip (1937), "Representation of Tactile Sensibility in the Monkey's Cortex as Indicated by Cortical Potentials," *Amer. J. Physiol., 119:* 372.

Masserman, Jules H. (1941), "Is the Hypothalamus a Center of Emotion?", *Psychosomat. Med., 3:* 3.

Matthews, Bryan H. C. (1928), "A New Electrical Recording System," *J. Physiol., 65:* 225.

Matthews, W. B. (1964), "The Use and Abuse of Electroencephalography," *Lancet, 2:* 577.

Mauro, Alexander; Wall, P. D.; Davey, L. M.; and Scher, A. M. (1950), "Central Nervous Stimulation by Implanted High Frequency Receiver," *Fed. Proc., 9:* 86.

McConnell, James V. (1966), "Comparative Physiology: Learning in Invertebrates," *Ann. Rev. Physiol., 28:* 107.

McConnell, James V. (1966), "Worms (and Things)," *Worm Runner's Digest, 3:* 1.

McConnell, J. V., "The Modern Search for the Engram," in Corning, W., and Balban, B., eds. (1967), *The Mind: Biological Approaches to Its Functions*, New York: Interscience Publishers.

"The Medical Case of Jack Ruby," *MD Medical News Magazine, 8* (Mar. 1964): 94.

Mitchell, J. F. (1961), "Acetylcholine Release from Cerebral Cortex During Stimulation," *J. Physiol., 158:* 20P.

Mitchell, J. F. (1963), "The Spontaneous and Evoked Release of Acetylcholine from the Cerebral Cortex," *J. Physiol.*, *165:* 98.

Morrell, Frank (1959), "Experimental Focal Epilepsy in Animals," *A.M.A. Arch. Neurol.*, *1:* 141.

Morrell, Frank (1960), "Secondary Epileptogenic Lesions," *Epilepsia*, *1:* 538.

Morrell, Frank (1961), "Microelectrode Studies in Chronic Epileptic Foci," *Epilepsia*, *2:* 81.

Morrell, Frank (1963), "Information Storage in Nerve Cells," in *Information Storage and Neural Control*, Springfield, Ill.: C. C. Thomas.

Moruzzi, G., and Magoun, H. W. (1949), "Brain Stem and Reticular Formation and Activation of the EEG," *EEG Clin. Neurophysiol.*, *1:* 455.

Mosler, Ursula (1966), "The Annotated Bibliography of Research on Planarians, Part VIII," *The Worm Runner's Digest*, *3:* 48.

Myklebust, Helmer R. (1969), "Learning and Electrocortical Functions," Unpub. Paper from Northwestern U. Info. Office.

Nachmansohn, David (1954), "Metabolism and Function of the Nerve Cell," *The Harvey Lectures*, 1953–4, Baltimore.

Nachmansohn, David (1959), *Chemical and Molecular Basis of Nerve Activity*, New York: Academic Press.

Nathan, Peter (1969), *The Nervous System*, Philadelphia: Lippincott.

Newton, H. F.; Zweiner, R. L.; and Cannon, W. B. (1931), "The Mystery of Emotional Acceleration of the Denervated Heart After Exclusion of Known Humoral Accelerators," *Amer. J. Physiol.*, *96:* 377.

Obrist, Walter D. (1963), "The Electroencephalogram of Healthy Aged Males," from *Human Aging: A Biological and Behavioral Study*, P.H.S. Pub. 986, U.S. Govt. Print. Off.

Obrist, Walter D.; Busse, Ewald W.; Henry, Charles E. (1961), "Relation of Electroencephalogram to Blood Pressure in Elderly Persons," *Neurology*, *11:* 151.

Olds, James (1956), "Pleasure Centers of the Brain," *Sci. Amer. 195:* 105.

Overton, Richard K. (1959), "The Calcium Displacement Hypothesis: A Review," *Psychol. Rep.*, *5:* 721.

Page, Irvine H. (1958), "Serotonin (5-Hydroxytryptamine); The Last Four Years," *Physiol. Rev.*, *38:* 277.

Palay, S. L. (1958), "The Morphology of Synapses in the Central Nervous System," *Exper. Cell Res.*, Supp. 5: 275.

Pearlman, Chester A., Jr.; Sharpless, Seth K.; and Jarvik, Murray E. (1960), "Retrograde Amnesia Produced by Anesthetic and Convulsant Agents," *J. Comp. Physiol. Psychol.*, 54: 109.

Penfield, W. (1947), "Some Observations on the Cerebral Cortex of Man," *Proc. Roy. Soc.*, 134: 329.

Penfield, Wilder (1964), "The Uncommitted Cortex, The Child's Changing Brain," *Atlantic*, 214: 77.

Penfield, Wilder (1937), "The Cerebral Cortex and Consciousness," *The Harvey Lectures*, 1936, Baltimore.

Penfield, W., and Jasper, H. (1954), *Epilepsy and the Functional Anatomy of the Human Brain*, Boston: Little-Brown.

Penfield, Wilder, and Rasmussen, Theodore (1950), *The Cerebral Cortex of Man*, New York: Macmillan.

Penfield, Wilder, and Roberts, Lamar (1966), *Speech and Brain Mechanisms*, New York: Atheneum.

Perlman, David, "The Search for the Memory Molecule," *The New York Times Magazine*, July 7, 1968, p. 8.

Peterson, Lloyd R. (1966), "Short-term Memory," *Sci. Amer.*, 215: 90.

Porter, R.; Adey, W. R.; and Kado, R. T. (1964), "Measurement of Electrical Impedance in the Human Brain," *Neurol.*, 14: 1002.

President's Council on Aging (1964), *On Growing Older*, Washington, D.C.: U.S. Govt. Print. Office.

Pribram, Karl H. (1969), "The Neurophysiology of Remembering," *Sci. Amer.*, 220: 73.

Purpura, D. P. (1959), "Nature of Electrocortical Potentials and Synaptic Organizations in Cerebral and Cerebellar Cortex," *Intern. Rev. Neurobiol.*, 1: 47.

Ramey, Estelle R., and O'Doherty, Desmond S. (1960), *Electrical Studies on the Unanesthetized Brain*, New York: Harper.

Ramón y Cajal, S. (1937), *Recollections of My Life*, trans., Philadelphia: Amer. Philo. Soc.

Ramón y Cajal, S. (1954), *Neuron Theory or Reticular Theory?*, trans., Madrid: Inst. Ramón y Cajal.

Randal, Judith (1966), "Hunger: Does It Cause Brain Damage?" *Think Magazine* (pub. by IBM), 32: No. 6, p. 8.

Ransom, S. W. (1937), "Some Functions of the Hypothalamus," *The Harvey Lectures*, 1936–7, Baltimore.

Ransom, W. (1892), "A Case Illustrating Kinaesthesis," *Brain*, 15: 437

Reinhold, Robert, "Chimp's Brain Signals Itself by Computer," *The New York Times*, Sept. 15, 1970, p. 1.

Rémond, Antoine (1961), "Integrated and Topological Analysis of the EEG," *EEG Clin. Neurophysiol.*, Suppl. 20: 64.

Rémond, A., and Lesèvre, N. (1965), "Distribution Topographique des Potentiels Evoqués Visuels Occipitaux chez l'Homme Normal," *Revue Neurologique, 112:* 317.

Renshaw, B.; Forbes, A.; and Morison, B. R. (1940), "Activity of Isocortex and Hippocampus: Electrical Studies with Microelectrodes," *J. Neurophysiol., 3:* 74.

Roberts, Eugene, and Frankel, Sam (1950), "Gamma-Aminobutyric Acid in Brain: Its Formation from Glutamic Acid," *J. Biol. Chem., 187:* 55.

Robertson, J. David; Bodenheimer, Thomas S.; and Stage, David E. (1963), "The Ultrastructure of Mauthner Cell Synapses and Nodes in Goldfish Brains," *J. Cell Biol., 19:* 159.

Rosenblith, Walter A. (1967), "The Brain," *Internat. Sci. Tech.*, Sept.: 34.

Rosenzweig, Mark R. (1966), "Environmental Complexity, Cerebral Change, and Behavior," *Amer. Psychol., 21:* 321.

Schade, J. P., and Ford, Donald H. (1965), *Basic Neurology*, Amsterdam: Elsevier.

Schaltenbrand, Georges, and Woolsey, Clinton (1964), *Cerebral Localization and Organization*, Madison, Wisc.: U. of Wisc. Press.

Schmeck, Harold M., Jr., "Brain Signals in Test Foretell Action," *The New York Times*, Feb. 13, 1971, p. 1.

Schmitt, Francis O. (1950), "The Structure of the Axon Filaments of the Giant Nerve Fibres of Loligo and Myxicola," *J. Exper. Zool., 113:* 499.

Schmitt, Francis O. (1965), "The Physical Basis of Life and Learning," *Science, 149:* 931.

Schmitt, Francis O., and Melnechuk, Theodore (1966), *Neurosciences Research Symposium Summaries*, Cambridge, Mass.: M.I.T. Press.

Schmitt, Francis O., and Samson, Frederick E., Jr. (1968), "Neuronal Fibrous Proteins," *Neurosci. Res. Program Bull., 6:* 113.

Schmitt, Francis O., and Samson, Frederick E., Jr. (1969), "Brain Cell Microenvironment," *Neurosci. Res. Program Bull., 7:* 277.

Schwartz, Henry G., and Kerr, Alan S. (1940), "Electrical Activity of the Exposed Human Brain," *Arch. Neurol. Psychiat., 43:* 547.

Sechenov, Ivan M. (1965), *Reflexes of the Brain*, Cambridge, Mass.: M.I.T. Press.

Sem-Jacobsen, C. W. (1968), *Depth-Electrographic Stimulation of the Human Brain and Behavior*, Springfield, Ill.: C. C. Thomas.

Sheer, Daniel E. (1961), *Electrical Stimulation of the Brain*, Austin, Texas: U. of Texas Press.

Shenker, Israel, "Drug Brings Parkinson Victims Back Into Life," *The New York Times*, Aug. 26, 1968, p. 35.

Sherrington, C. S. (1906), *The Integrative Action of the Nervous System*, New Haven: Yale U. Press.

Sherrington, C. S. (1928), "Sir David Ferrier, 1843–1928," *Proc. Roy. Soc., 103B:* viii.

Sherrington, Charles Scott, "Inhibition as a Coordinative Factor," Nobel Lecture, Dec. 12, 1932.

Sherrington, C. S. (1935), "Santiago Ramón y Cajal 1852–1934," *Obit. Notices Roy. Soc.,* No. 4: 425.

Shoemaker, William J., and Wurtman, Richard J. (1971), "Perinatal Undernutrition: Accumulation of Catecholamines in Rat Brain," *Science, 171:* 1017.

Sperry, R. W. (1964), "The Great Cerebral Commissure," *Sci. Amer., 210:* 42.

Sperry, Roger W. (1964), "Problems Outstanding in the Evolution of Brain Function," James Arthur Lecture, New York, Amer. Mus. of Nat. Hist.

Sperry, R. W. (1965), "Brain Bisection and Mechanisms of Consciousness," *Pontificiae Academiae Scientiarum Scripta Varia,* 30.

Solomon, Philip (1966), *Psychiatric Drugs*, New York: Grune.

Spurzheim, J. G. (1815), *The Physiognomical System of Drs. Gall and Spurzheim*, London.

Stevens, William, "Amputee's Will Flexes Artificial Arm," *The New York Times*, Sept. 13, 1968, p. 1.

Tasaki, Ichiji (1939), "The Electro-Saltatory Transmission of the Nerve Impulse and the Effect of Narcosis Upon the Nerve Fiber," *Amer. J. Physiol., 127:* 211.

Tasaki, Ichiji (1953), *Nervous Transmission*, Springfield, Ill.: C. C. Thomas.

Tasaki, I.; Polley, E. H.; and Orrego, F. (1954), "Action Potentials from Individual Elements in Cat Geniculate and Striate Cortex," *J. Neurophysiol., 17:* 454.

Tasaki, Ichiji; Singer, Irwin; and Lerman, Lawrence (1967), "Effects of Tetrodotoxin on Excitability of Squid Giant Axons in Sodium-Free Media," *Science, 155:* 95.

Thompson, Robert, and Dean, Waid (1955), "A Further Study on the

Retroactive Effect of ECS," *J. Comp. Physiol, Psychol.*, *48*: 488.

Twarog, Betty M., and Page, Irvine (1953), "Serotonin Content of Some Mammalian Tissues and Urine and a Method for Its Determination," *Amer. J. Physiol.*, *175*: 157.

Udenfriend, Sidney (1950), "Identification of Gamma-Aminobutyric Acid in Brain by the Isotopic Derivative Method," *J. Biol. Chem.*, *187*: 63.

Udenfriend, Sidney, and Martin, A. R. (1970), "Nobel Prize: Three Share 1970 Award for Medical Research," *Science*, *170*: 422.

Van Heyningen, W. E. (1968), "Tetanus," *Sci. Amer.*, *218*: 69.

Verzeano, Marcel, and French, John D. (1953), "Transistor Circuits in Remote Stimulation," *EEG Clin. Neurophysiol.*, *5*: 613.

Vogt, Marthe (1954), "The Concentration of Sympathin in Different Parts of the Central Nervous System Under Normal Conditions and After Administration of Drugs," *J. Physiol.*, *123*: 451.

von Euler, U. S. (1946), "A Specific Sympathomimetic Ergone in Adrenergic Nerve Fibres (Sympathin) and its Relations to Adrenaline and Nor-Adrenaline," *ACTA Physiol. Scand.*, *12*: 73.

Waggoner, Karen (1970), "Psychocivilization or Electroligarchy: Dr. Delgado's Amazing World of ESB," *Yale Alumni Magazine*, *33*: 20.

Walker, A. Earl (1949), "Electrocorticography in Epilepsy," *EEG Clin. Neurophysiol.*, Suppl. 2: 30.

Walker, W. Cameron (1937), "Animal Electricity Before Galvani," *Annals Sci.*, *2*: 84.

Walsh, E. Geoffrey (1964), *Physiology of the Nervous System*, 2nd ed., London: Longmans.

Walter, W. Grey (1936), "The Location of Cerebral Tumours by Electroencephalography," *Lancet*, *2*: 305.

Walter, W. Grey (1949), "Electroencephalography," *Endeavor*, *8*: 194.

Walter, W. Grey (1953), "Toposcopy," *EEG Clin. Neurophysiol.*, Suppl. 4: 7.

Walter, W. Grey (1954), "The Electrical Activity of the Brain," *Sci. Amer.*, *190*: 54.

Walter, W. Grey (1961), "Frequency Analysis," *EEG Clin. Neurophysiol.*, Suppl. 20: 14.

Walter, W. G. (1964), "Depth Recording from the Human Brain," *EEG Clin. Neurophysiol.*, *16*: 68.

Walter, W. Grey (1953), *The Living Brain*, New York: Norton.

Ward, Arthur A. (1958), "Conclusion and Summary, A Symposium on Dendrites," *EEG Clin. Neurophysiol.*, Suppl. 10: 58.

Weiss, Paul, and Hiscoe, Helen B. (1948), "Experiments on the Mechanism of Nerve Growth," *J. Exper. Zool.*, *107*: 315.

Werre, P. F. (1957), *The Relationships Between Electroencephalographic and Psychological Data in Normal Adults*, Leyden: Leyden U. Press.

Wever, Ernest Glen, and Bray, Charles W. (1930), "The Nature of Acoustic Response: The Relation Between Sound Frequency and Frequency of Impulses in the Auditory Nerve," *J. Exper. Psychol.*, *8:* 373.

Whitfield, Vance (1969), "Duke Doctors Say You Dream Every 90 Minutes Each Night," Release Dec. 28, 1969, Office of Info. Serv., Duke University, Durham, N.C.

Whittaker, V. P. (1965), "The Application of Subcellular Fractionation Techniques to the Study of Brain Functions," *Progr. Biophy. Molec. Biol.*, *15:* 41.

Whittaker, V. P.; Michaelson, I. A.; and Kirkland, R. Jeanette A. (1964), "The Separation of Synaptic Vesicles from Nerve Ending Particles ('Synaptosomes')," *Biochem. J.*, *90:* 293.

Whittaker, V. P., and Sheridan, M. N. (1965), "The Morphology and Acetylcholine Content of Isolated Cerebral Cortical Synaptic Vesicles," *J. Neurochem.*, *12:* 363.

Wiener, Norbert (1961), *Cybernetics*, 2nd ed., Cambridge, Mass.: Wiley.

Wiersma, C. A. G. (1959), "Coding and Decoding in the Nervous System," *Engineering and Science* (pub. by Cal. Inst. of Tech.), Oct. 1959, p. 21.

Wiersma, C. A. G., and Yamaguchi, T. (1965), "Interneurons Selecting Information from a Fixed Direction in Space," *Physiologist, 8:* 311.

Wiersma, C. A. G., and Yamaguchi, T. (1965), "Responses of Interneurons in the Optic Nerve of Crayfish," *Fed. Proc., 24:* 275.

Wilkins, Robert H. (1965), *Neurosurgical Classics*, New York: Johnson Reprint Corp.

Wilson, Irwin B., and Nachmansohn, David (1954), "The Generation of Bioelectric Potentials," in Clarke, H. T., ed., *Ion Transport Across Membranes*, Symposium at College of Physicians and Surgeons, Columbia U., New York, 1953.

Wooldridge, Dean E. (1963), *The Machinery of the Brain*, New York: McGraw-Hill.

Woolsey, C. N.; Marshall, W. H.; and Bard, P. (1942), "Representation of Cutaneous Tactile Sensibility in Cerebral Cortex of Monkey as Indicated by Evoked Potentials," *Bull. Johns Hopkins Hosp.*, *70:* 399.

Young, John Z. (1936), "Structures of Nerve Fibres and Synapses in Some Invertebrates," *Cold Spring Harbor Symp. Quant. Biol., 4:* 1.

Young, J. Z. (1964), *A Model of the Brain,* Oxford at the Clarendon Press.

Young, J. Z. (1965), "The Organization of a Memory System," *Proc. Royal Soc.,* B. *163:* 285.

Young, J. Z., "A Unit of Memory," *New Scientist,* Dec. 23, 1965, p. 861.

Young, J. Z., "Life's Balance," Pamphlet that accompanied series of ten lectures on BBC, April 25–June 27, 1965.

INDEX

A NOTE ABOUT THE AUTHOR

Leonard A. Stevens is the author of twelve books and many magazine articles, most of them concerning aspects of science and technology, such as electronic miniaturization, computers in medicine, and water and air pollution. His firsthand research has led him to many parts of the world. To write about volcanos, Mr. Stevens once accompanied a volcanologist of Chicago's Field Museum on an expedition to Central America; for material on the wolverine he joined a winter expedition in Alaska commissioned by the St. Louis Zoo; and one January, to cover the world's windiest weather observatory, he hiked to the summit of Mount Washington, New Hampshire. In two Atlantic crossings Mr. Stevens became thoroughly acquainted with the world's largest ocean liner in order to write *The Elizabeth: Passage of a Queen* (Alfred A. Knopf, 1968).

Mr. Stevens, who is active in politics, has long been interested in the impact of speech on society—which is reflected in two of his books. He is co-author of *Are You Listening?* and author of *The Ill-Spoken Word;* both discuss the effects of our general low regard for oral language.

In the 1960's Mr. Stevens was commissioned by the President's Council on Aging to write *On Growing Older* (U.S. Government Printing Office, 1965). This led to a writing project for the National Institute of Neurological Diseases and Stroke, and to this book.

The author, who lives with his wife and four children in Bridgewater, Connecticut, was born in Lisbon, New Hampshire. He holds B.A. and M.A. degrees from the University of Iowa. During World War II he was a captain with the Air Force on Guam. Before and during the war he studied electronic engineering, which has served him well in science writing, especially about the nervous system.

A NOTE ON THE TYPE

The text of this book is set in Caledonia, a type face designed by W(illiam) A(ddison) Dwiggins for the Mergenthaler Linotype Company in 1939. Dwiggins chose to call his new type face Caledonia, the Roman name for Scotland, because it was inspired by the Scotch types cast about 1833 by Alexander Wilson & Son, Glasgow type founders. However, there is a calligraphic quality about Caledonia that is totally lacking in the Wilson types. Dwiggins referred to an even earlier type face for this "liveliness of action"—one cut around 1790 by William Martin for the printer William Bulmer. Caledonia has more weight than the Martin letters, and the bottom finishing strokes (serifs) of the letters are cut straight across, without brackets, to make sharp angles with the upright stems, thus giving a "modern face" appearance.

W. A. Dwiggins (1880–1956) began an association with the Mergenthaler Linotype Company in 1929 and over the next twenty-seven years designed a number of book types, the most interesting of which are the Metro series, Electra, Caledonia, Eldorado, and Falcon.

This book was composed, printed and bound by the Haddon Craftsmen, Scranton, Pennsylvania. Typography and binding design by Arthur Beckenstein.